Chorionic Villus Sampling

CLINICAL AND BIOCHEMICAL ANALYSIS

A series of monographs and textbooks

EDITOR

Morton K. Schwartz

Chairman, Department of Biochemistry
Memorial Sloan-Kettering Cancer Center
New York, New York

1. Colorimetric and Fluorimetric Analysis of Organic Compounds and Drugs, *M. Pesez and J. Bartos*
2. Normal Values in Clinical Chemistry: Statistical Analysis of Laboratory Data, *Horace F. Martin, Benjamin J. Gudzinowicz, and Herbert Fanger*
3. Continuous Flow Analysis: Theory and Practice, *William B. Furman*
4. Handbook of Enzymatic Methods of Analysis, *George G. Guilbault*
5. Handbook of Radioimmunoassay, *edited by Guy E. Abraham*
6. The Hemoglobinopathies: Techniques of Identification, *Titus H. J. Huisman and J. H. P. Jonxis*
7. Automated Immunoanalysis (in two parts), *edited by Robert F. Ritchie*
8. Computers in the Clinical Laboratory: An Introduction, *E. Clifford Toren, Jr. and Arthur A. Eggert*
9. The Chromatography of Hemoglobin, *Walter A. Schroeder and Titus H. J. Huisman*
10. Nonisotopic Alternatives to Radioimmunoassay: Principles and Applications, *edited by Lawrence A. Kaplan and Amadeo J. Pesce*
11. Biochemical Markers for Cancer, *edited by T. Ming Chu*
12. Clinical and Biochemical Luminescence, *edited by Larry J. Kricka and Timothy J. N. Carter*
13. Advanced Interpretation of Clinical Laboratory Data, *edited by Camille Heusghem, Adelin Albert, and Ellis S. Benson*

14. Practical Immunoassay: The State of the Art, *edited by Wilfrid R. Butt*

15. Instrument Evaluation in Biomedical Sciences, *James L. Driscoll, Benjamin J. Gudzinowicz, and Horace F. Martin*

16. Chemi- and Bioluminescence, *edited by John G. Burr*

17. Ligand-Binder Assays: Labels and Analytical Strategies, *Larry J. Kricka*

18. Human Prenatal Diagnosis, *edited by Karen Filkins and Joseph F. Russo*

19. Glycosylated Hemoglobins: Methods of Analysis and Clinical Applications, *E. C. Abraham*

20. Pathology of Unusual Malignant Cutaneous Tumors, *edited by Mark R. Wick*

21. Chorionic Villus Sampling: Fetal Diagnosis of Genetic Diseases in the First Trimester, *edited by Bruno Brambati, Giuseppe Simoni, and Sergio Fabro*

ADDITIONAL VOLUMES IN PREPARATION

Chorionic Villus Sampling

Fetal Diagnosis of Genetic Diseases in the First Trimester

edited by
Bruno Brambati
Giuseppe Simoni
First Institute of Obstetrics and Gynecology
University of Milan
Milan, Italy

Sergio Fabro
Columbia Hospital for Women
Georgetown University
Washington, D.C.

MARCEL DEKKER, INC. New York and Basel

Library of Congress Cataloging-in-Publication Data

Main entry under title:

Chorionic villus sampling.

(Clinical and biochemical analysis ; 21)
Includes index.
1. Chorionic villi--Biopsy. 2. Fetus--Abnormalities--Diagnosis. 3. Prenatal diagnosis. 4. Pregnancy--Trimester, First. I. Brambati, B. (Bruno) II. Simoni, G. (Giuseppe), [date] III. Fabro, Sergio. IV. Series. [DNLM: 1. Chorionic Villi--ultrastructure. 2. Genetic Screening--methods. 3. Pregnancy Trimester, First. 4. Prenatal Diagnosis--methods.
W1 CL 654 v.21 / WQ 209 C551]
RG628.3.C48C47 1986 618.3'2 85-27457
ISBN 0-8247-7360-8

MARCEL DEKKER, INC.
270 Madison Avenue, New York, New York 10016

Current printing (last digit):
10 9 8 7 6 5 4 3 2 1

PRINTED IN THE UNITED STATES OF AMERICA

In Memoriam

Dr. Sergio Fabro
a dedicated pioneer in the field of perinatal medicine
passed away during the final preparation of this volume.
He will be remembered fondly
by those of us who continue his work.

Foreword

Prenatal genetic diagnosis became a reality only as recently as the 1950s. Starting with the examination of amniotic fluid cells for the presence of a Barr body (for X-linked disorders), within a decade researchers had accomplished the first prenatal diagnosis of a chromosome abnormality and expanded the technique to include diagnosis of inborn errors of metabolism. The years since then have been devoted to assessing the safety of amniocentesis and refining laboratory techniques in order to decrease the time needed to make a diagnosis and to enhance the procedure's applicability to molecular DNA technology and chromosome banding. These continued endeavors soon led to the development of chorionic villus sampling, a procedure useful earlier in pregnancy, facilitating a more rapid diagnosis.

Though done under direct visualization in the 1960s, chorionic villus sampling has not been used with any frequency until this decade. In fact, the technique is so new that the existence of a text of this caliber is extraordinary. *Chorionic Villus Sampling: Fetal Diagnosis of Genetic Disorders in the First Trimester* offers the reader up-to-date information about all aspects of chorionic villus sampling. The editors have brought together experts from different fields to discuss techniques, usefulness, risks, social implications, and attendant ethical issues. The text is comprehensive, authoritative; the bibliographies are current and extensive. There is no doubt that this text will be invaluable to all individuals interested in prenatal genetic diagnosis and counseling, whether they be practitioners of the technical and laboratory aspects of chorionic villus sampling, students of the technique, or those concerned with its social and personal implications.

Gloria E. Sarto, M.D., Ph.D.
Professor of Obstetrics and Gynecology
University of Wisconsin Medical School
Milwaukee, Wisconsin

Preface

Prenatal diagnosis of genetic diseases is a comparatively young specialty; it attracted the attention of clinicians only in the last decade when it became apparent that amniocentesis during the second trimester was relatively safe and that it could be performed as an office procedure. There are problems with prenatal diagnosis during the second trimester of pregnancy. First, the procedure, although technically simple, is fraught with potential and significant medical complications. Furthermore, the time required to achieve a diagnostic karyotype of the amniotic fluid cells is approximately 2 to 3 weeks. Since amniocentesis can not be performed safely before 16 weeks of gestational age, interruption of pregnancy at 19–21 weeks represents a significant medical, social, and psychological problem for the mother. This is probably one of the reasons that significant research has been directed toward diagnosis during the first trimester using new, faster, cytogenetic techniques. As a result of these studies, the techniques originally used by Russian, Scandinavian, British, and Chinese investigators for obtaining fetal samples during the first trimester were developed into a reproducible method for chorionic villus sampling (CVS) by Bruno Brambati at the University of Milan. At the same institution, Giuseppe Simoni developed a cytogenetic technique for the analysis of trophoblastic tissue taken by CVS. The significant advantage of this technique was that the results could be known in few hours rather than in weeks, as with amniocentesis. By the spring of 1983 it was apparent that a method was available for prenatal diagnosis during the first trimester of pregnancy, since chorionic biopsy and cytogenetic analysis could yield reliable results as early as 8–10 weeks of gestation.

The purpose of this book is to outline the state-of-art techniques and to lend perspective to the most significant scientific, medical, ethical, and social problems in the rapidly developing field of prenatal diagnosis. Prenatal diagnosis during the first trimester by chorionic villus sampling has so many advantages that it is expected to represent the most important method for prenatal diagnosis in the near future. At present, different CVS techniques are being evaluated for accuracy and safety, and more than 9000 CVS procedures have been performed so far.

The well-qualified, international contributors to this book are pioneers and leaders in prenatal care.

Sergio Fabro

Contents

Contributors

Bruno Brambati, M.D., Perinatal Unit, First Institute of Obstetrics and Gynecology, University of Milan, Milan, Italy

Julianne Byrne, Ph.D.,* Department of Pathology, College of Physicians and Surgeons, Columbia University, New York, New York

Clara Camaschella, M.D., Medical Clinic A, Institute of Internal Medicine, University of Turin, Turin, Italy

Yves Dumez, M.D., University Clinic of Port-Royal, Paris, France

Sergio Fabro, M.D., Ph.D., Division of Maternal-Fetal Medicine, Columbia Hospital for Women, Georgetown University, Washington, D.C.

Maurizio Ferrari, M.D., Laboratory of Hematology, Istituti Clinici di Perfezionamento, Milan, Italy

Enrico Ferrazzi, M.D., Perinatal Unit, First Institute of Obstetrics and Gynecology, University of Milan, Milan, Italy

Gemino Fiorelli, M.D., Fourth Chair in Medical Pathology, Third Institute of Clinical Medicine, University of Milan, Milan, Italy

John C. Fletcher, Ph.D., Warren G. Magnuson Clinical Center, National Institutes of Health, Bethesda, Maryland

Hans Galjaard, M.D., Ph.D., Department of Cell Biology and Genetics, Erasmus University, and Department of Clinical Genetics, University Hospital, Rotterdam, The Netherlands

Michel Goossens, M.D., Department of Biochemistry and Genetics, Henri Mondor University Hospital, Créteil, France

Laird G. Jackson, M.D., Division of Medical Genetics, Department of Medicine, Jefferson Medical College, Thomas Jefferson University, Philadelphia, Pennsylvania

---

**Present affiliation*: Clinical Epidemiology Branch, National Cancer Institute, National Institutes of Health, Bethesda, Maryland

Willem J. Kleijer, Ph.D., Department of Cell Biology and Genetics, Erasmus University, and Department of Clinical Genetics, University Hospital, Rotterdam, The Netherlands

James L. Mills, M.D., Epidemiology Branch, National Institute of Child Health and Development, National Institutes of Health, Bethesda, Maryland

B. Modell, Ph.D., M.B.Chir., Faculty of Clinical Sciences, University College, London, England

John M. Old, Ph.D., Nuffield Department of Clinical Medicine, John Radcliffe Hospital, Oxford, England

Angelo Oldrini, M.D.,* Perinatal Unit, First Institute of Obstetrics and Gynecology, University of Milan, Milan, Italy

Eugene Pergament, M.D., Ph.D., Division of Medical Genetics, Michael Reese Hospital and Medical Center, Chicago, Illinois

Lorenza Romitti, Ph.D., Laboratory of Cytogenetics, First Institute of Obstetrics and Gynecology, University of Milan, Milan, Italy

Giuseppe Saglio, M.D., Medical Clinic A, Institute of Internal Medicine, University of Turin, Turin, Italy

Maurizio Sampietro, M.D., Fourth Chair in Medical Pathology, Third Institute of Clinical Medicine, University of Milan, Milan, Italy

Anthony R. Scialli, M.D., Reproductive Toxicology Center, Columbia Hospital for Women, Georgetown University, Washington, D.C.

Anna Serra, M.B., Medical Clinic A, Institute of Internal Medicine, University of Turin, Turin, Italy

Giuseppe Simoni, Ph.D., Laboratory of Cytogenetics, First Institute of Obstetrics and Gynecology, University of Milan, Milan, Italy

Joe Leigh Simpson, M.D., Section of Human Genetics, Northwestern University Medical School, Chicago, Illinois

Silvana Tedeschi, M.B., Laboratory of Hematology, Istituti Clinici di Perfezionamento, Milan, Italy

Gianluigi Terzoli, Ph.D., Laboratory of Cytogenetics, First Institute of Obstetrics and Gynecology, University of Milan, Milan, Italy

---

**Present affiliation*: Third Institute of Obstetrics and Gynecology, University of Milan, Milan, Italy

Yury Verlinsky, Ph.D., Division of Medical Genetics, Michael Reese Hospital and Medical Center, Chicago, Illinois

Dorothy Warburton, Ph.D., Departments of Pediatrics and Human Genetics and Development, College of Physicians and Surgeons, Columbia University, New York, New York

1

Fetal Diagnosis in the First Trimester: Introduction and Historical Perspectives

B. MODELL
Faculty of Clinical Sciences, University College, London, England

Chorionic villus sampling is an example of an obvious approach that was bound to be developed but had to await the appropriate technical and social developments.

The technique is founded first and foremost on the classic descriptions of human embryonic development, especially the contributions of Hertig and Rock (1941, 1945, 1948a,b, 1949) and on Boyd and Hamilton's (1970) comprehensive and beautiful work on the development of the human placenta. Fetal diagnosis itself was made possible by work arising from the seminal observations on the biochemical basis of metabolic disease (Garrod, 1923), from the demonstration of the chromosomal basis of Down's syndrome (Lejeune et al., 1959), and from the introduction of ultrasound into obstetric diagnosis (Donald et al., 1958). Amniocentesis was first used in the early 1950s for the spectroscopic analysis of bilirubin breakdown products in the third trimester of pregnancy in order to provide guidance in the management of rhesus isoimmunization (Bevis, 1956). Direct karyotyping of human chorionic villi was first used in cytogenetic epidemiological studies of early abortion material (Yamamoto et al., 1975). The integration of these methods for the genetic diagnosis of the fetus began with hemophilia, when the Barr bodies of amniotic fluid cells were used for fetal sexing (Serr et al., 1955; Fuchs and Riis, 1956). However, it was not until 1966 that amniocytes were successfully cultured and karyotyped for fetal diagnosis (Steele and

Breg, 1966). The approach was rapidly extended to intrauterine diagnosis of chromosomal disorders (Jacobson and Bata, 1967) and metabolic disorders (Nadler, 1968), and by 1970, this technique began to be used widely to avoid genetic disease. The application of ultrasound progressed hand-in-hand with the extension of amniocentesis, and the fetal diagnosis of neural tube defects by ultrasound alone or by amniotic fluid α-fetoprotein estimation was introduced in 1972 (Brock and Sutcliffe, 1972; Campbell et al., 1972). Finally, mid-trimester fetal blood sampling and fetoscopy were introduced in 1974, mainly for the diagnosis of the hemoglobinopathies (Hobbins and Mahoney, 1974). Over the last 15 years, the methods involved have been carefully assessed and have been shown to be safe and reliable in expert hands (e.g., Ferguson-Smith, 1983; Rodeck and Nicolaides, 1984). Figure 1 shows examples of the way that the demand for fetal diagnosis has risen in recent years in many places.

The most important factors influencing the development of fetal diagnosis are not technical but social, namely, the changing complex of attitudes to the control of human reproduction. Selective abortion of congenitally abnormal fetuses has naturally been associated with social tensions from the beginning because many individuals, both doctors and patients, find this to be an unacceptable solution; although in many societies termination of pregnancy because of a risk of serious disease in the fetus has been legal for a long time. For instance, many pregnancies have been terminated since the relationship between maternal rubella infection and multiple congenital abnormalities in the fetus has been understood (Gregg et al., 1945). On a more general plane, the extension of industrialization necessarily entrains a widespread change of attitude concerning the control of human reproduction because increased per capita consumption and extended education combine with decreased infant and childhood mortality and longer adult survival to make each child a greater economic as well as emotional investment. Family planning, therefore, becomes simultaneously more necessary and more realistic, and there is a steady global trend to smaller family size. This necessarily involves widespread use of contraception and the availability of early abortion as a backup resource. However, unless these changes in public attitudes are recognized by the law, it is very difficult to develop or perform fetal diagnosis, even when it is permissible in theory. For instance, in most of Italy, the present widespread interest in the prevention of thalassemia had to wait for liberalization of the abortion law in 1977. In any given country, the fact that there is, in general, an

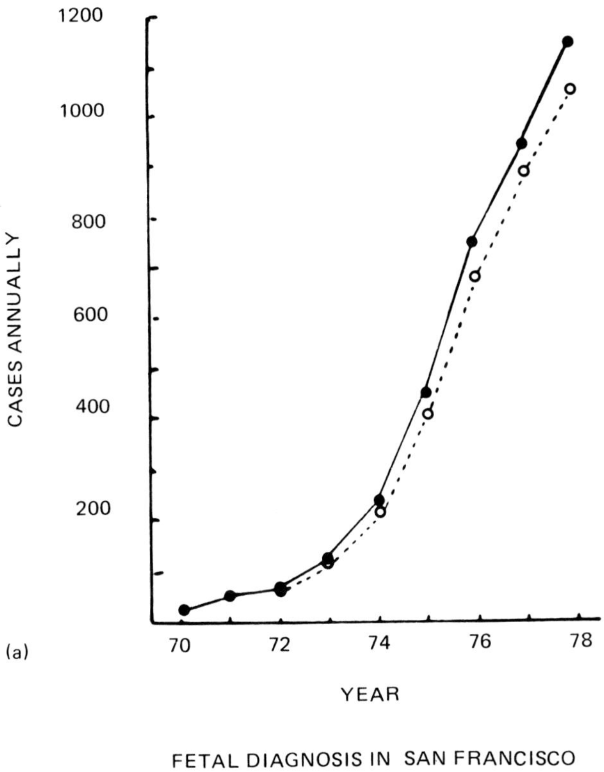

Figure 1 Examples of increasing demand for fetal diagnosis in different places. (a) Fetal diagnosis at the University of California Genetics Clinic in San Francisco. Closed circles represent total cases, open circles cases for chromosomal indications. After Golbus et al. (1979). (b) The increasing rate of amniocentesis in Denmark. From WHO (1984) with permission. (c) Global figures for fetal diagnosis of the hemoglobinopathies (Alter, Registry of prenatal diagnosis of the hemoglobinopathies, unpublished data).

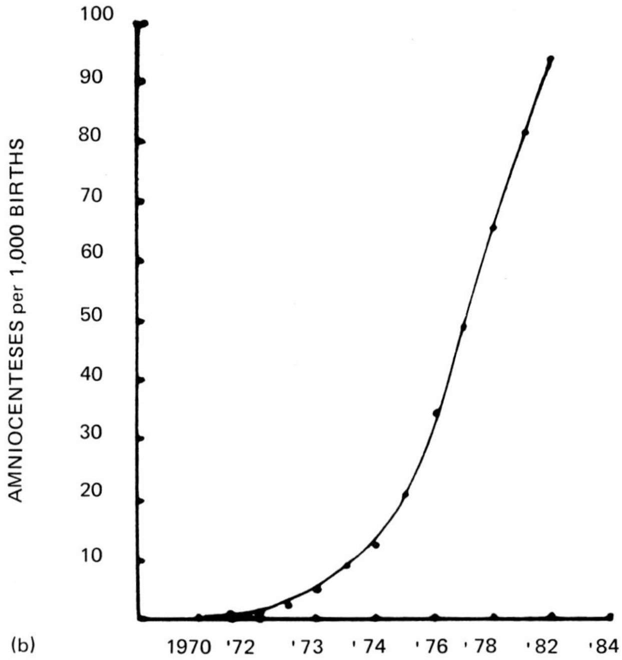

(b)

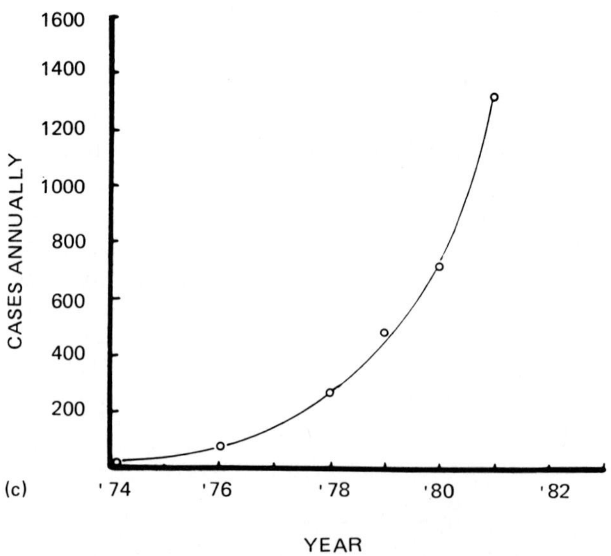

(c)

FETAL DIAGNOSIS FOR THE HEMOGLOBINOPATHIES

(GLOBAL FIGURES)

inverse relationship between the proportion of women bearing children after 35 years of age and the availability of fetal diagnosis is an interesting expression of the relationship between industrialization and the planning of human reproduction.

The influence of social pressures on the development of fetal diagnosis for hereditary disease varies with the time, place, nature of the local genetic problems, religious and social attitudes, level of economic development, activities of pressure groups, and extent and nature of media exposure. All these elements interact with technological factors in determining when and where new developments will take place, and all have played a part in the introduction of earlier fetal diagnosis.

Figure 1 shows, by analogy with bacterial cultures, that 1966–1973 was the "incubation period" for the development of fetal diagnosis, followed by a log growth phase. In this phase, the social and ethical issues related to the acceptance of selective midtrimester abortion had to be sorted out, not least within the medical profession itself. This has required slow and careful work by the geneticists, obstetricians, and pediatricians directly in contact with the mothers at risk and therefore best able to express their needs, and this issue has been at least as important as the more easily documented technical work on the safety and reliability of the fetal diagnostic procedures. The significance of this social groundwork for opening the way to further developments must not be underestimated. Mid-trimester amniocentesis is now well established on a sound basis of experience; it is well integrated into clinical practice; and it is widely accepted by mothers who are aware that they are at increased genetic risk. Its main limitation now is that its availability and its value are still not sufficiently known among the general population. Fetal diagnosis of the hemoglobinopathies is following a similar growth pattern 8 years later, while the curve for ultrasound diagnosis may be just about to take off.

Representative rates of abnormalities diagnosed (and therefore rates of abortion) associated with the different indications for fetal diagnosis are illustrated in Table 1 (from the report of the United Kingdom Clinical Genetic Society, 1978). The majority of fetal diagnoses undertaken are for chromosomal disorders; where the group at risk is large, the risk of mid-trimester abortion is low (about 3%), and the recurrence risk is small. Diagnoses for the higher risk conditions such as sex-linked and metabolic diseases are still a small minority, and few centers terminate many pregnancies for these indications. The exception is fetal diagnosis for the hemoglobinopathies; many high risk cases are concentrated at a few specialist centers where 25% of all presenting pregnancies are

Table 1 Fetal Abnormality Detection Rate According to Indication

	Number of pregnancies	Percent abnormal[a]
Previous neural tube defect	4460	3.0
Maternal age 40 years and over	2926	3.6
Maternal age 35–39 years	2858	1.4
Previous trisomy-21	1202	1.2
Parental chromosomal translocation	135	8.9
Parental chromosomal mosaicism	14	0
Previous autosomal aneuploidy excluding trisomy-21	188	0
Previous sex chromosome aneuploidy	18	0
Family history of Down's syndrome	557	0.4
Fetal sexing for X-linked disease	140	35.0[b]
Metabolic disorder (autosomal recessive or x-linked)	183	24.0
High maternal serum AFP[c]	364	21.4
Family history of neural tube defect	458	1.5
Maternal anxiety	471	0.6
Others	547	3.1
Secondary to excluding neural tube defect	(4786)	0.38
Secondary to excluding chromosomal aberrations	(2025)	0.64
	14,521	3.7

[a]For specific test.
[b]Male fetus.
[c]Cut-off points variable from 95 to 99 percentile.

teminated in the mid-trimester, thus, the limitations of the approach are perceived particularly acutely.

Several important disadvantages are associated with the classic methods of fetal diagnosis and have tended, among other things, to limit its application to the developed countries only. These include the lateness and relative obstetric sophistication of the termination of pregnancy when indicated, the cost and other considerations related to the need for tissue culture, the limited spectrum of diseases that are diagnosable at present, and the relatively long time taken to reach a diagnosis. Any new developments that would allow earlier and more rapid diagnosis, extend its range, and simplify the obstetric and laboratory aspects would greatly extend its applicability. Although it is highly likely that first-trimester diagnosis would allow great progress in all these areas, even when it began to seem technically feasible, there were difficulties in introducing it into clinical practice.

Safety is a key consideration in all medical procedures, but it is vitally important in preventive diagnostic techniques that invade a normal life process in order to screen for the abnormal, especially when the outcome involves the entire life of a human being, as in fetal diagnosis. Therefore, once a safe and reliable approach has been perfected, people become very wedded to it, and it can be very difficult to introduce change, except at the fringes where for one reason or another the established methods prove less satisfactory or the social pressures are greater. In the United States, in particular, legislation against using fetal material for research has ensured that any work done in this area is conducted under unusual stress and has inhibited the development of improved techniques for fetal diagnosis.

These considerations explain why the technique of chorionic villus sampling was developed more or less independently in several different countries for a variety of different specific purposes, by genetic groups with no contact and little, if any, awareness of each other.

Historically, techniques for placental biopsy were developed for the rapid diagnosis of hydatidiform mole, transcervically (Acosta-Sison, 1958) and transabdominally (Alvarez, 1966), but the approach was superseded by other methods. Placenta biopsy was also investigated as a diagnostic aid for placental pathology, but was abandoned because small samples proved to be unrepresentative of the whole placenta. These limitations do not, however, affect its value for genetic diagnosis.

Hahneman and Mohr (1968), started work on transcervical first trimester chorionic villus sampling for genetic diagnosis in the late 1960s in Denmark. Their rationale was that mid-trimester abortion is particularly unsuitable for women at high genetic risk, and they wished to develop an earlier approach for the diagnosis of sex-linked and metabolic diseases. In the absence of real-time ultrasound, the procedure had to be guided by direct vision, using a special fiber-optic hysteroscope inside a 4 mm-diameter metal tube with an oval 4 mm-long side hole. The instrument was inserted through the cervix and passed through the decidual covering of the ovum, and the chorion and chorionic villi were identified by direct vision. Tissue was pulled into the side hole by suction, and cut off by advancing a cylindrical knife blade within the outer tube. They reported their preliminary results in 1969, and in 1974 summarized their observations in 95 pregnancies, 67 sampled under anesthesia immediately prior to termination of pregnancy, and 28 sampled in "ambulant" patients from 1 to 8 days prior to therapeutic abortion. Naturally many problems were encountered in this initial attempt (Table 2). A clear view could be obtained in less than half the cases (a difficulty later resolved by others by instilling fluid through the viewing instrument). Useful samples were obtained in 80% of cases, but the chorionic and amniotic membranes were often pulled in and cut with the knife, leading to direct puncture of the sac in 8 cases and to amniotic biopsy in 18 more, both complications probably incompatible with normal continuation of the pregnancy. (This difficulty has been overcome by avoiding the use of cutting biopsy instruments.) It was noted that even when these complications had occurred, spontaneous abortion did not necessarily follow within 1-week waiting period, but it was felt that only about 50% of pregnancies sampled would have been able to continue normally if not interrupted. Initial difficulties in culturing the chorionic tissue for karyotyping were successfully overcome in the later cases. Sexing proved accurate, but two trisomies and two mosaics found among the 34 karyotyped samples highlighted the difficulty of interpreting spontaneous abortion after the procedure. Many of these difficulties could have been overcome if real-time ultrasound had been available, but the work was discontinued at the time because of the greater ease and safety of amniocentesis.

Chorionic villus sampling was started in China in about 1970. Karyotyping was not widely available, but examination of the Barr bodies was possible. Because of the stresses imposed by the intensive population control program, many women wanted fetal sexing to guarantee male offspring. The lateness of amniocentesis makes it particularly unsuitable for sex choice, so the objective was to develop an earlier technique to help these women. The report from Anshan (1975) is apparently representative of more widespread activity. Using a "blind" technique with a graduated metal cannula and introducer (Fig. 2), they obtained smears containing enough syncytial cells and villus branches for fetal sexing on Papanicolaou stains by the presence or absence of Barr bodies, in 99 out of 100 cases. The results were 90% accurate. Thirty pregnancies were terminated because the results showed a fetus of the

Table 2 Early Attempts at Chorionic Villus Biopsy Several Days prior to Elective Abortion

Reference	Patients (N)	Causes of fetal losses (N)	Pregnancy possibly would have continued	Successful biopsy	Successful culture
Hahnemann and Mohr (1969) and Hahnemann (1974)	28	Immediate punctures of sac (3) Spontaneous abortions[a] (3) Missed abortions[b] (4)	18	14	13
Kullander and Sandahl (1973)	39	Intrauterine gonococcal infections (2)	?37	39	19

[a]In one, no fetus (mother 41 years); one trisomy C; one normal male karyotype.
[b]Two normal female karyotypes; two no karyotype obtained.
Source: WHO (1984).

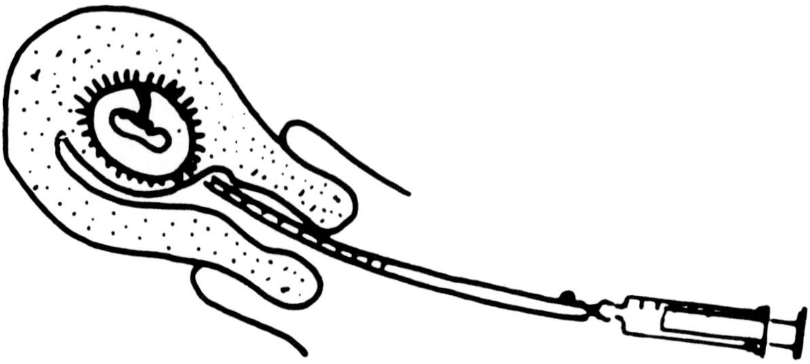

Figure 2 The Chinese approach to blind chorionic villus sampling. The instrument was a graduated metal introducer, and no attempt was made to place it where the chorionic villi are thickest. After Anshan (1975).

unwanted sex, and 4 of the 70 continuing pregnancies (6%) aborted spontaneously 3 to 7 weeks after sampling. Sixty-six normal babies were delivered at term. This was the first series including pregnancies that continued normally after the diagnostic procedure; however, even though it was reported in English in the *Chinese Medical Journal*, the work did not become widely known until subsequent developments underlined its importance retrospectively. The Chinese data on gestational age at sampling and the number of attempts required (Tables 3 and 4 and Fig. 3) prove in retrospect to be fairly typical, as does the delay

Table 3 Some Details of Blind Chorionic Villus Sampling in 100 Pregnancies in China

Procedures (N)	Patients (N)	Possible complications	Patients (N)
1	73	Blood present	86
2	24	Blood-stained fluid	11
3	3	Amniotic fluid	3
Fail	1		
Total	100		

Source: Anshan (1975).

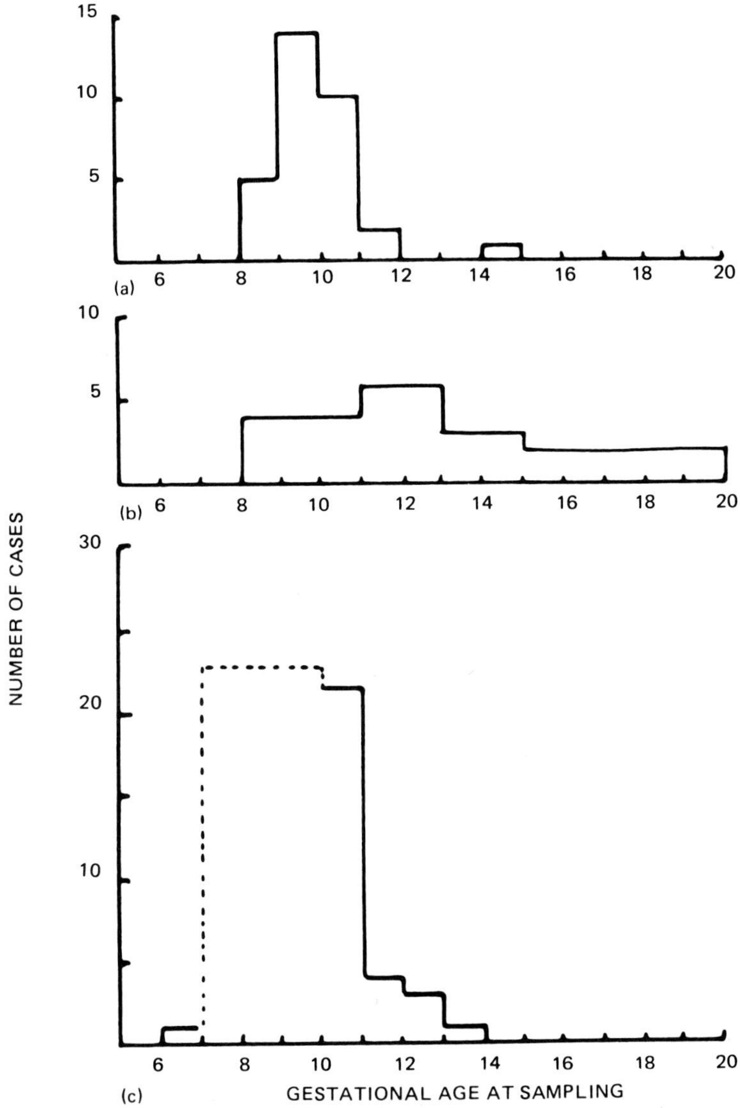

Figure 3 Gestational age at chorionic villus sampling. (a) The experimental series of Hahnemann (1974). Most cases were less than 11 weeks gestation. (b) The experimental series of Kullander and Sandahl (1973). (c) The diagnostic series from Anshan (1975). Dotted lines represent imprecision in reporting the precise gestational age at sampling. In both (a) and (c) gestational age at sampling corresponds fairly well with the present known optimum time.

Table 4 Details of Four Spontaneous Abortions

Gestational age at sampling (week)[a]	Comment	Time of spontaneous abortion (days)
11	Bled + 24 days	>28
10	—	>40
9½	Sac perforated	> 4
12½	Bled postoperatively	>20—Infection

[a]For gestation age at sampling see Fig. 3.
Source: Anshan (1975).

before spontaneous abortion in the four cases reported. However, the outcome (Table 5) made it clear that widespread action of this kind in China at this time could lead to imbalance of the sex ratio with undesirable social consequences, and the approach was rejected as a solution for the tensions arising from social policy. It is now being modified and reapplied for the fetal diagnosis of genetic disease, primarily for the diagnosis of the hemoglobinopathies by gene mapping. However, the shortage of ultrasound facilities complicates the evaluation of safety, because anembryonic pregnancies and missed abortions cannot be excluded.

In 1973, Kullander and Sandahl (from Sweden) reported their experience of experimental chorionic villus sampling under direct vision from 39 pregnancies 3 to 18 days prior to therapeutic abortion at the gestational ages indicated in Figure 3. They obtained suitable material and a successful culture in 50% of the cases using a 5 mm-diameter fiber optic "endocervicoscope" with a biopsy forceps attachment. Their procedure caused no ruptures of the amniotic sac or bleeding, but two women developed a gonococcal amnionitis. They also attempted diagnostic sampling in two wanted pregnancies with threatened abortion, one of which subsequently continued to term. These promising results were not followed up at the time, no doubt once again because of the speed with which amniocentesis was becoming established.

Rhine and Milunsky raised the issue again in the United States in 1979. They suggested a very gentle approach by simply washing out the uterine cavity with a saline solution and culturing the cells obtained. The fact that their first promising results could not be confirmed (Goldberg et al., 1980) made it clear that a more invasive approach was needed, but the

Table 5 Outcome of Chorionic Villus Sampling for Sex Selection in China

Prediction		Abortion			Delivery		
Sex	No.	Induced (%)	Spontaneous	Continuing pregnancies	Male	Female	Diagnostic error (%)
Male	53	1	2	50	47	3	6
Female	46	29	1	16	3	13	19
Unknown	1	0	1	0	0	0	0
Total	100	30	4	66	50	16	9

Source: Anshan (1975).

social pressures in the United Sates were antagonistic to the development of new fetal diagnostic techniques.

In the meantime, workers in the Soviet Union had been trying consistently to develop an earlier approach, and Kazy et al. (1982) reported their experimental work and first diagnostic cases in 1982. Their series included 165 cases. All sampling was done between 6 and 12 weeks of pregnancy, and the procedure was developed in four stages. In stage 1, the chorionic villi were located under direct vision by an embryo fetoscope 1.7 mm in diameter, and samples were taken with a biopsy forceps in 55 anesthetized patients undergoing induced abortion. In stage 2 (45 anaesthetized patients undergoing abortion), a real-time ultrasound machine was used instead of the fetoscope to locate the placenta and guide the biopsy forceps (Fig. 4). In stage 3, sampling was done in 39 patients 5 to 10 days prior to therapeutic abortion. The final step was

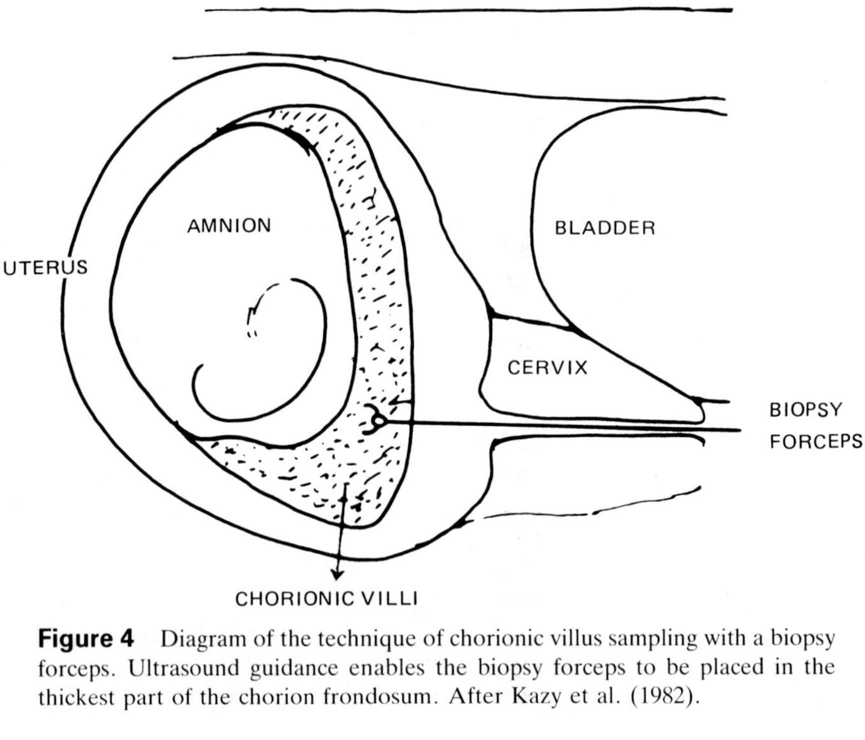

Figure 4 Diagram of the technique of chorionic villus sampling with a biopsy forceps. Ultrasound guidance enables the biopsy forceps to be placed in the thickest part of the chorion frondosum. After Kazy et al. (1982).

diagnostic sampling in 26 wanted pregnancies at high genetic risk (mostly severe X-linked conditions). Chorionic villi were obtained in all cases, but in a minority only at the second or third attempt. Fetal sex determination was by direct examination of the X and Y chromatin and proved correct in all cases. The activity of several enzymes of lysosomal origin was also assayed to obtain baseline levels. Eleven of these 26 pregnancies were terminated because the fetus was male and at risk for sex-linked disorder; two were terminated at the mother's request; and 13 continued uneventfully to term and ended with the delivery of normal infants. There were no unscheduled fetal losses. The paper was particularly important because it reported sampling for genetic diagnosis and the normal continuation of pregnancies in which an unaffected fetus had been identified. Its effect was highly reassuring to other groups already engaged in developing a similar approach elsewhere.

Work on first-trimester diagnosis in the United Kingdom had been stimulated by the need for a better solution for mothers at risk for having children with thalassemia major, many of whom were having to undergo repeated mid-trimester fetal blood sampling. Earlier diagnosis seemed particularly necessary because of the social and religious attitudes of some ethnic groups at risk. For instance, British Muslims originating from Pakistan are as distressed as anyone else by having children suffering from thalassemia major, but most find mid-trimester diagnosis and abortion unacceptable. However, they expressed a lively interest in the possibility of first trimester diagnosis. As it became clear that the new developments in gene mapping would permit the diagnosis of hemoglobinopathies using DNA from any nucleated cells originating from the zygote, it was felt that the most useful immediate application of the new technology might be to permit earlier diagnosis of genetic disease. Preliminary studies drawing attention to the fact that DNA from chorionic villi could be used for genetic diagnosis (Williamson et al., 1981) and could be obtained free from maternal contamination (Elles et al., 1983), generated more widespread interest. However, this potential could be realized only if a safe and simple obstetric method for obtaining chorionic villi were developed.

Simplicity was a priority in the obstetric approach because of the hope that the new method for diagnosing hemoglobinopathies would be useful in developing countries. It was felt that an ultrasound-guided transcervical approach using a soft plastic catheter with a formable metal introducer to adapt to the shape of the uterus and to increase ultrasound visibility might be the simplest. The instrument should be neither so large nor so small as to be able to traumatize the soft uterine tissue. The resulting (Portex) 1.5 mm-diameter catheter is shown in Figure 5 (Old et al., 1982; Ward et al., 1983). The method of sampling was developed at medical termination of pregnancy in the operating theater, by recording the success rate in obtaining chorionic villus samples: first blind (36% success), then with ultrasound guidance (65% success), and then with a microscope on the spot to check that villi were present (90% success). The first three diagnostic cases combining chorionic villus sampling with gene mapping were reported by Old and co-workers in 1982. They were used at once as a basis for further development in the United States (Pergament et al., 1983) and gave an additional boost to the developing international interest in the procedure. Numerous other initiatives have since been made in the United Kingdom.

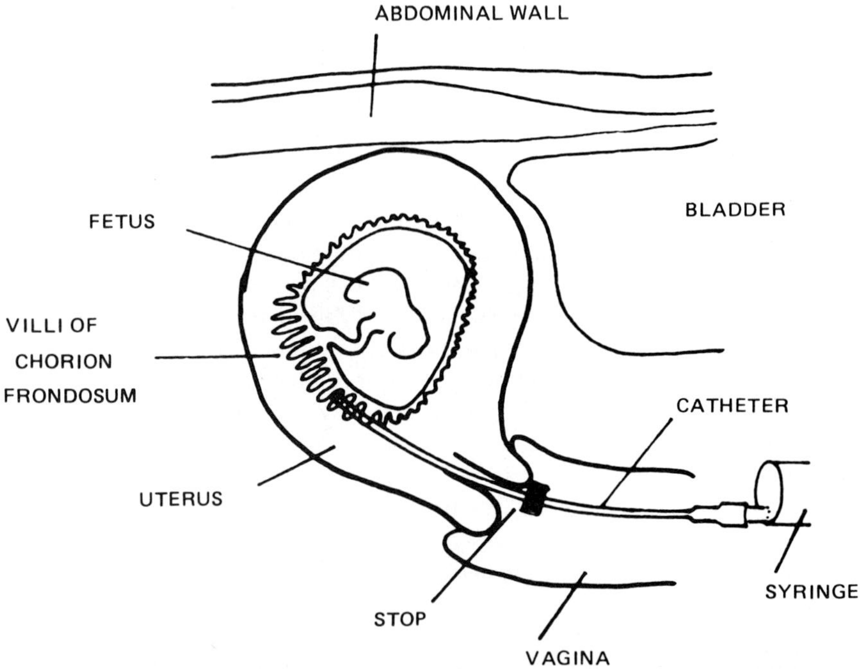

Figure 5 Diagram of chorionic villus sampling using the Portex catheter. As with sampling by biopsy forceps, ultrasound guidance enables the instrument to be placed in the thickest part of the chorion frondosum. From Old et al. (1982) with permission.

In France, experimental sampling was started using direct vision (Kaplan et al., 1983), but the group moved on to diagnostic sampling using biopsy forceps under ultrasound guidance for the diagnosis of sickle cell disease, once again a genetic problem of ethnic groups where mid-trimester termination of pregnancy is not generally accepted (Goossens et al., 1983).

Simultaneously, in Italy, Brambati and Simoni and their co-workers were building up a massive experimental experience. They compared the ease and success of three approaches, viz. transcervical fetoscopic sampling and, aspiration sampling without and aspiration sampling with ultrasound guidance, and they concluded that transcervical ultrasound-guided aspiration was the most satisfactory approach in their hands (Simoni et al. 1983) (Table 6). They particularly concentrated on its application for cytogenetic analysis and found that it was possible to achieve rapid diagnosis, even within hours of sampling, by applying a direct method for chromosome preparation (Brambati and Simoni, 1983; Simoni et al., 1983). This method had been developed for rapid cytogenetic study of mouse embryo membranes (Evans et al., 1972) and adapted for the study of human abortion material (Yamamoto et al., 1975). After these rigorous initial studies, they applied the approach for diagnostic karyotyping to a large group of women, mainly of advanced maternal age, and found a minimum of complications among the pregnancies continuing to term. Their work, reported elsewhere in this

Table 6 Success of Different Experimental Approaches to Chorionic Villus Sampling

Method	Number of cases	Success No.(%)	Perforation of sac No.	Bleeding No.(%)	Postoperative infection
Fetoscopy (direct vision)	62	42(76)	0	12(20)	1
Abbott cannula (blind)	159	102(64)	4	14(10)	0
Portex cannula					
blind	48	32(66)	1	6(12)	0
ultrasound	103	99(96)	0	5(5)	0

Source: WHO (1984).

treatise, shows conclusively that it should be possible to transfer mid-trimester cytogenetic diagnosis to the first trimester, and consequently has implications for every group currently engaged in fetal diagnosis. Not surprisingly, the approach was followed up extremely rapidly in the United States and other European centers. At this point, it also attracted the attention of the Hereditary Diseases Program of the World Health Organization, because of the importance of setting up reliable monitoring of diagnostic accuracy and obstetric risk from the outset (WHO, 1983). Consequently, the international registry, started on an informal basis by Dr. Laird Jackson throught the *CVS Newsletter,** has received WHO sponsorship. This coordinated effort has already made it clear that first trimester fetal diagnosis can be achieved with enough safety and reliability to enter clinical practice for the control of genetic disease, but that the necessary level of safety can be achieved only by expert groups with appropriate equipment and training and with sufficient practice. It is the purpose of this treatise to outline subsequent developments.

Considerably more work will be needed at every level, but it seems realistic to hope that the procedure may be brought to the same degree of safety and reliability that has been attained by anniocentesis. As the extent of the future usefulness of first trimest diagnosis depends on its obstetric risk, plans are being made for more formal international coordinated data collection. However, the only truly reliable way to evaluate risk will be through a randomized, controlled trial of the outcome after chorionic villus sampling compared with the outcome after amniocentesis for mothers of advanced maternal age. Such careful evaluation is particularly needed in view of the diversity of obstetric approaches that are currently being developed.

REFERENCES

Acosta-Sison H. (1958). Diagnosis of hydatidiform mole. *Obstet. Gynaecol. 12*:205–208.

Alvarez H. (1966). Diagnosis of hydatidiform mole by transabdominal placental biopsy. *Am. J. Obstet.* and *Gynecol. 95*:538.

Anshan 1975). Fetal sex prediction by sex chomatin of chorionic villi cells during early pregnancy. *Chin. Med. J. 1*:117–126.

*Dr. Laird Jackson, Division of Medical Genetics, Thomas Jefferson University, Eleventh and Walnut Streets, Philadelphia, Pennsylvania 19107, U.S.A.

Bevis, D. C. A., (1956), Amniotic fluid: Measurement of pigment by spectrophotometry. J. Obstet. Gynecol. Brit. Emp., 63:68.

Boyd, J. D. and Hamilton, W. J. (1970). *The Human Placenta.* 2nd ed. Heffer, Cambridge.

Brambati, B. and Simoni, G. (1983). Diagnosis of fetal trisomy, 21 in first trimester. *Lancet i*:586.

Brock, D. J. H., and Sutcliffe, R. G. (1972). α-Fetoprotein in the antenatal diagnosis of anencephaly and spina bifida. *Lancet 2*:197–199.

Campbell, S., Johnstone, F. D., Holt, E. M., and May, P. (1972). Anencephaly. Early ultrasonic diagnosis and management. *Lancet 1*: 1226–1227.

Clinical Genetics Society Working Party (1978). Prenatal diagnosis in relation to genetic counselling. *Bulletin Eugenics Soc Suppl.* No. 3.

Donald, I., Mac-Vicar, J., and Brown, T. G. (1958). Investigation of abdominal masses by pulsed ultrasound. *Lancet i*:1188–1195.

Elles, R. G., Williamson, R., Niazi, M., Coleman, D. V., and Horwell, D. (1983). Absence of maternal contamination of chorionic villi used for fetal gene analysis. *N. Engl. J. Med. 308*:1433–1435.

Evans, E. P., Burtenshaw, M. D., and Ford, C. E. (1972). Chromosomes of mouse embryos and newborn young: Preparation from membranes and tail tips. *Stain Technol. 47*:229–234.

Ferguson-Smith, M. A. (ed.) (1983). Early prenatal diagnosis. *Brit. Med. Bull. 39*:00–0000.

Fuchs, F. and Riis, P. (1956). Antenatal sex determination. *Nature (London) 177*:330.

Garrod, A. E. (1923). *Inborn Errors of Metabolism* 2nd ed. Oxford University Press, Oxford.

Golbus, M. S., Longhman, W. D., Epstein C. J., Halbasch, G., Stephens, J. D., and Hall, B. D. (1979). Prenatal Genetic diagnosis in 3000 amniocenteses. *N. Engl J. Med. 300*:157–163.

Goldberg, M. F., Chen, A. T. L., Young, W. A., and Reidy, J. A. (1980). First trimester fetal chromosome diagnosis using endocervical lavage: A negative evaluation. *Am. J. Obstet. Gynecol. 138*: 435–440.

Goossens, M., Dumez, Y., Kaplan, L. *et al.* (1983). Prenatal diagnosis of sickle-cell anemia in the first trimester of pregnancy. *N. Engl. J. Med 309*:831–833.

Gregg, N. M., Beavis, W. R., Heseltine, M., Macklin, A. E., and Vickery, D. (1945). Occurrence of congenital defects in children following maternal rubella during pregnancy. *Med. J. Austral. 2*:122–126.

Hahnemann, N. (1974). Early prenatal diagnosis: A study of biopsy techniques and cell culturing from extra-embryonic membranes. *Clin. Genet. 6*:294–306.

Hahnemann, N. and Mohr, J. (1968). Genetic diagnosis in the embryo by means of biopsy from extra-embryonic membranes. *Hull.* Eur. *Soc. Human Genet. 2*:23.

Hertig, A. T. and Rock, J. (1941). *Carnegie Contrib. Embryol. 29* (No. 184):127–156.

Hertig, A. T. and Rock, J. (1945). *Carnegie Contrib. Embryol. 31* (No. 200):65–84.

Hertig, A. T. and Rock, J. (1948a). *Am. J. Obstet. Gynecol. 55*:6–17.

Hertig, A. T. and Rock, J. (1948b). *Am. J. Obstet. Gynecol. 55*:440–4520.

Hertig, A. T. and Rock, J. (1949). *Am J. Obstet. Gynecol. 58*:968–993.

Hobbins, J. C. and Mahoney, M. J. (1974). In utero diagnosis of hemoglobinopathies. Technic for obtaining fetal blood. *N. Engl. J. Med. 290*:1065–1067.

Jacobson, C. B. and Barter, R. H. (1967). Intrauterine diagnosis and management of genetic defects. *Am. J. Obstet. Gynecol. 99*:795–805.

Kaplan, L., Dumez, Y., and Goossens, M. (1983). A method for fetal tissue sampling by chorion biopsy: A new approach to first trimester prenatal detection of abnormal genes. *I.R.C.S. Med. Sci. 11*: 85–86.

Kazy, Z., Rozovsky, I. S., and Bakharev, V. A. (1982). Chorion biopsy in early pregnancy: A method of early prenatal diagnosis for inherited disorders. *Prenatal Diag. 2*:39–45.

Kullander, S. and Sandahl, B. (1973). Fetal chromosome analysis after transcervical placental biopsies in early pregnancy. *Acta Obstet. Gynecol. Scand. 52*:355.

Lejeune, J., Turnpin, R., and Gautier, M. (1959). Le Mongolisime; Premier example d'aberration autosomique humain. *Ann. Genet. 1*:41.

Nadler, H. L. (1968). Antenatal detection of hereditary disorders. *Pediatrics 42*:912–918.

Old, J. M., Ward, R. H. T., Petrou, M., Karagozlu, F., Modell, B., and Weatherall, D. J. (1982). First trimester fetal diagnosis for haemoglobinopathies: Three cases. *Lancet ii*:1413–1416.

Pergament, E., Ginsberg, N., Verlinsky, Y., Cadkin, A., Chu, A. and Trinka, L. (1983). Prenatal Tay-Sachs diagnosis by chorionic villus sampling. *Lancet ii*:26.

Rhine, S. A. and Milunsky, A. (1979). Utilization of trophoblast for early prenatal diagnosis. In (ed). *Genetic Disorders and the Fetus,* A. Milunsky Plenum, New York.

Rodeck, C. and Nicolaides, M. (eds.). (1984). *Fetal Diagnosis.* Royal College of Obstetrics and Gynaecology, London.

Serr, D. M., Sachs, L. and Danon, M. (1955). Diagnosis of sex before birth using cells from the amniotic fluid. *Bull. Res. Coun. Isr. 5B*:137.

Simoni, G., Brambati, B., Danesino, C. et al. (1983). Efficient direct chromosome analyses and enzyme determinations from chorionic villi samples in the first trimester of pregnancy. *Human Genet. 63*:349–357.

Steele, M. W., and Breg, W. R., Jr. (1966). Chromosome analysis of human amniotic fluid cells. *Lancet 1*:383–385.

Ward, R. H. T., Modell, B., Petrou, M., Karagozlu, F., and Douratsos, E.

(1983). A method of chorionic villus sampling in the first trimester of pregnancy under real-time ultrasonic guidance. *Brit. Med. J. 286*:1542–1544.

Williamson, R., Eskdale, J., Colemand, D. V., Niazi, M., Loeffler, F. E., and Modell, B. (1981). Direct gene analysis of chorionic villi: A possible technique for first-trimester antenatal diagnosis of haemoglobinopathies. *Lancet ii*:1125–1127.

WHO, (1983). Report of a WHO Working Group on fetal diagnosis of hereditary diseases. Geneva, 14–15 April 1983. Unpublished WHO Document HMG/WG/83.2.

WHO, (1984). Report of a WHO/SERONO meeting on Prespectives in Fetal Diagnosis.

Yamamoto, M., and Fujimori, R., Ito, T., Kamimura, K., and Watanabe, G. (1975). Chromosome studies in 500 induced abortions. *Human Gene. 29*:9–14.

2

Estimates of the Prevalence of Chromosome Anomalies Expected in Chorionic Villus Sampling Procedures

DOROTHY WARBURTON and JULIANNE BYRNE*
College of Physicians and Surgeons, Columbia University, New York, New York

INTRODUCTION

Sampling of first-trimester pregnancies through chorionic villus biopsy will result in expected rates of chromosome anomalies that are quite different from those seen at amniocentesis at a gestational age of 16 weeks. Most chromosome anomalies are associated with a severe degree of developmental arrest or disorganization in the development of the embryo and lead to inevitable spontaneous abortion of the pregnancy, usually before the sixteenth week. Of all chromosome anomalies detected in a study of spontaneous abortion in New York City (Warburton et al., 1980), 87% were aborted before 16 weeks, and only 13% were aborted between 16 and 28 weeks. The modal gestational age at which chromosome anomalies were aborted was 11–12 weeks (Warburton et al., 1985). Therefore, most chromosomally abnormal pregnancies will still be in progress when chorionic villus sampling is done.

During the sampling procedure, ultrasound is routinely used to ensure that the procedure is carried out only on pregnancies where an apparently living embryo of appropriate size for gestational age is present. This will significantly reduce the rate of chromosome anomalies expected to be

**Present affiliation*: Clinical Epidemiology Branch, National Cancer Institute, National Institutes of Health, Bethesda, Maryland

detected. Only those pregnancies in which the development of the conceptus is apparently proceeding normally will be sampled. The rate of detected chromosome anomalies is still expected to be higher than that found at amniocentesis, even for pregnancies at risk only because of maternal age. This chapter will attempt to make some predictions about the size of this rate based on data from studies of spontaneous and induced abortions.

In this chapter we will use the work "disorganization" to describe conceptuses consisting of empty sacs, tiny embryos lacking the usual anatomic landmarks, and larger embryos whose size and appearance are markedly incompatible for their gestational age (Byrne, 1983; Byrne et al., 1985). We have classified fetuses with focal malformations among the apparently normal pregnancies, since the malformations would likely not be apparent on ultrasound so early in pregnancy.

METHODS AND RESULTS

The estimates to be derived in this chapter are based on data collected as part of the New York City Spontaneous Abortion Study. This is an epidemiological, cytogenetic, and pathological study of spontaneous fetal loss occurring before 28 completed weeks of pregnancy. Pathological examinations were conducted on about 3500 aborted products of conception between January 1977 and August 1981. Cytogenetic examinations were carried out on all aborted fetal tissues where possible.

For purposes of this discussion, it is useful to think of the relationship between disorganization of the embryo and the presence of chromosome anomalies in terms of a fourfold table (Table 1). All of the disorganized embryos (b+d) will spontaneously abort, although they would not be included in any chorionic villus sample where ultrasound was used to determine fetal "normality." A portion of anatomically normal embryos (a+c) will also spontaneously abort. It is those embryos that are anatomically apparently normal but chromosomally abnormal (cell c on Table 1) that would be diagnosed at chorionic sampling, and these pregnancies would then be terminated electively.

Estimates of the prevalence of chromosome abnormalities among all pregnancies at weeks 5 to 12 of gestation are provided by Yamamoto et al. (1975, 1976) on induced abortions, These may be considered to be a random sample of all pregnancies at a given gestational and maternal age, at least with respect to the presence of chromosome abnormalities. In this series, the overall rate of chromosome abnormalities detected between 5

Table 1 Estimated Prevalence of Normal and Abnormal Pregnancies at Any Gestation[a]

	Anatomy		
Chromosomes	Normal	Disorganized	
Normal	a	b	a+b
Abnormal	c	d	c+d
Total	a+c	b+d	N

[a]Of 1000 pregnancies at week 4, number surviving (N). French and Bierman (1962). Proportion of chromosome anomalies present at each week of gestational age [(c + d)/N]. Yamamoto et al. (1976). b, c, d = Estimates from New York City Spontaneous Abortion Study. a = N - (b + c + d).

and 12 weeks was 7.3%. The rate was 10.7% at 5–6 weeks and decreased to 7.4% at 7–8 weeks, 7.2% at 9–10 weeks, and 4.8% at 11–12 weeks.

We do not have data on the anatomical distribution of human embryos at each week of gestational age; however, we do have such data for those human conceptuses that spontaneously abort from our own cytogenetic and pathological study of miscarriages in New York City. In this study (Byrne et al., 1985), spontaneous abortions were classified according to 17 morphological categories. By 8 weeks of gestational age, or 6 weeks of developmental age, the earliest time at which a chorionic villus biopsy is usually done, the fetus should at least have a crown–rump length of 20 mm (Moore, 1971). Anything below this would be considered either abnormally delayed in development or too early a gestational age for the procedure.

A total of 509 chromosomally abnormal specimens were studied in the sample investigated morphologically in our study; of these, 468 were classified as having a "disorganized" morphology, and 41 were apparently anatomically normal. The assumption is made that all or almost all specimens with disorganized morphology will have aborted by 28 weeks gestational age, the time at which we stopped collecting specimens. Any pregnancy that aborted at week x was necessarily present at all prior weeks. Thus, those 509 specimens were all present at 4 weeks, and a decreasing proportion were present at all succeeding weeks (Table 2).

It is usually estimated that about 5% of chromosomally abnormal recognized pregnancies survive into the third trimester. These will not be disorganized, and one can assume that they will appear normal on first-trimester ultrasound. Therefore, we must add these 27 survivors to the 509 spontaneous abortions with chromosomal abnormalities, giving a total of 536 chromosomally normal pregnancies at week 4. This is shown in Table 3. At 6 weeks, the proportion of chromosomally abnormal pregnancies that will appear disorganized is high, 87.2%. As gestation increases, more and more of these are eliminated by spontaneous abortion, leaving 75.3% at the beginning of the thirteenth week, and zero by the twenty-eight week.

If we want to estimate the proportion of all pregnancies that will be morphologically normal but chromosomally abnormal, we must know the proportion of all pregnancies that are chromosomally abnormal for each gestational age and the proportion of all pregnancies that are aborted at each gestational interval. The first data come from a study of first-trimester induced abortions (Yamamoto et al. 1976), and for the

Table 2 Numbers of Chromosomally Abnormal Specimens Aborted at Each Gestational Age

Gestational age (weeks)	Disorganized (N)	Anatomically normal (N)
4–5	3	0
6	6	0
7	3	2
8	23	2
9	22	8
10	68	0
11	89	0
12	89	2
13–28	165	27
Total	468	41

Table 3 Estimated Prevalence of the Proportion of Chromosomally Abnormal, Anatomically Disorganized Pregnancies at the Beginning of Each Gestational Interval

Gestational age (weeks)	Anatomy: Disorganized (N)	Anatomy: Normal (N)	Disorganized (%)
6	465	68	87.2
7	459	67	87.1
8	456	66	87.4
9	433	64	87.1
10	411	56	88.0
11	343	56	86.0
12	254	56	81.9
13–25	165	54	75.3
16–19	60	47	56.1
20–23	17	43	28.3
24–27	4	35	10.3
28+	0	27	

second we have used the estimates of French and Bierman (1962) based on a prospective study of pregnancy loss in Hawaii. Thus, if we begin with 1000 pregnancies at week 4, we will have 892 remaining by week 8. Of these, 7.4% are expected to have abnormal chromosomes.

The relative proportion of anatomically normal and disorganized pregnancies among those with chromosome abnormalities is given by our previous estimates on Table 1, based on our spontaneous abortion data and corrected for those pregnancies that survive to term. For example, for week 8, shown in Table 4, we have 7.4% × 892 = 66 chromosomally abnormal pregnancies, and 87.1% of these are disorganized. We now have the quantities N, c, and d, and by subtraction (a+b) in our fourfold table. The proportion of disorganized conceptuses that are chromosomally normal, b, can be obtained from our spontaneous abortion data as well, using the ratio of chromosomally normal to abnormal abortuses among all those that are disorganized. The quantity, a, is obtained by subtracting (b+c+d) from N.

Table 4 Estimated Numbers of Conceptuses Present at 8 Weeks, Surviving from a Cohort of 1000 Pregnancies Present at Week 4

	Anatomy		
Chromosomes	Normal	Disorganized	Total
Normal	762	64	826
Abnormal	8	58	66
Total	770[a]	122	892

[a]8/770 = 1.0%—Proportion of all anatomically normal pregnancies that have abnormal chromosomes

Table 5 Estimated Prevalence of Chromosome Anomalies among Anatomically Normal Pregnancies at the Beginning of Each Week of Gestation

Gestation (weeks)	Percentage
6	2.0
7	1.2
8	1.0
9	1.1
10	0.9
11	0.8
12	0.9

Thus, at the beginning of the eighth week, from a cohort of 1000 pregnancies present at week 4, 108 have aborted, leaving 892 still present. Of these, 122 should appear abnormal on ultrasound, consisting either of a very small embryo or no embryo at all, and no detectable beating heart. Of the remaining 770 pregnancies that will appear to be developing normally, we estimate that 8 (or 1%) will have chromosome anomalies. The proportion [∂] of apparently normal pregnancies that actually have chromosome anomalies, or the expected yield of the screening procedures, is calculated in this manner, and the results [∂] shown in

Table 5 for weeks 6–12 of gestation. It can be seen that the proportion of chromosome anomalies among anatomically normal pregnancies falls from around 2% at week 6 to 0.9% at week 12 of gestation.

DISCUSSION

The estimates in Table 5 can be criticized on several grounds. First, it is difficult to know how some of the specimens in our spontaneous abortion series would have been interpreted on ultrasound. Misclassification errors may presumably occur in both directions, i.e., a pregnancy that is disorganized but has a beating heart may be interpreted as normal, while one that is normal may be interpreted as abnormal because of small size or incorrect dating of pregnancy. In addition, our assumption that a disorganized conceptus aborted at 15 weeks will be recognized as disorganized at 8 weeks will be subject to some error.

A bigger problem is the effect of the maternal age distribution on the expected frequency of chromosomal anomalies. Women being screened by chorionic villus sampling will generally be those of advanced maternal age (except where there is some other high-risk situation where our estimates are not applicable). Our series of women having spontaneous abortions, from which the karyotype–morphology correlations were derived, are older than the general population, but not as old as women having prenatal diagnosis because of risks associated with advanced maternal age. However, analysis of our data indicates that maternal age does not affect the proportions of chromosomally abnormal specimens that are anatomically normal or disorganized. At each gestational age, these proportions are the same for women over 35 and women under 35. However, older women have, over all gestations, about twice as many abortions in which the fetus measures over 30 mm and has a chromosome anomaly.

Available data do not permit us to calculate Table 5 for different maternal age classes. Some idea of the changes due to maternal age in the proportion of chromosomally abnormal conceptions can be obtained from the data of Yamamoto et al. (1975) on induced abortions. They provide a figure of 20% for the rate of chromosome anomalies in women over 39 at weeks 5–12 of gestation. Recently Warburton et al. (1985) have estimated the proportion of chromosome abnormalities among recognized conceptions in women of various maternal age classes; estimates are of the same order of magnitude, i.e., about 20–25% in women over 35. If we recalculate Table 5 using these estimates, we will arrive at a rate of chromosome anomalies among anatomically normal specimens of 12% at 5 weeks and 2% at 12 weeks. It is interesting that the rate of 2% at 12 weeks is the same as the 2% rate of chromosome anomalies found at amniocentesis at 16 weeks in women over 35 (Golbus et al., 1979).

We urge caution in using these estimates because of the large number of assumptions involved in their calculations. However, we feel that they are useful as a starting point in working toward more precise estimates of chromosome anomalies likely to be detected in early pregnancy screening.

ACKNOWLEDGMENTS

This work was supported in part by grants from the National Institutes of Health (1 RO1-HD-12207, 5 RO1-DA-02090, RO1-HD-15909, 5 T32-HD-07040).

REFERENCES

Byrne J. (1983). Birth defects original article series 19 (2). *Fetal Pathology Laboratory Manual.*

Byrne J., Warburton D., Kline J., Blanc, W., and Stein Z. (1985). Morphology of early fetal deaths and their chromosomal characteristics. *Teratology*, in press.

French, F. E., and Bierman, J. M. (1962). Probabilities of fetal mortality. *Pub. Health Rep. 77*:835–847.

Golbus, M. S., Loughman, W. D., Epstein, C. J., Halbasch, G., Stephens, J. D., and Hall, B. D. (1979). Prenatal genetic diagnosis in 3000 amniocenteses. *New Engl. J. Med. 300*:157–163.

Moore, K. L. (1971). *The Developing Human*, W. B. Saunders, Philadelphia.

Warburton, D., Stein, Z., Kline, J., and Susser, M. (1980). Chromosome abnormalities in spontaneous abortion: Data from the New York City Study. In *Human Embryonic and Fetal Death* (I. H. Porter and E. B. Hook, eds.). Academic Press, New York.

Warburton, D., Kline, J., Stein, Z., and Strobino, B. (1985). Cytogenetic abnormalities in spontaneous abortions of recognized conceptions. In *Perinatal Genetics: Diagnosis and Management.* (A. Willey and I. H. Porter, eds.). Academic Press, New York.

Yamamoto, M., Fujimori, R., Ito, T., Kamimura, K., and Watanabe, G. (1975). Chromosome studies in 500 induced abortions. *Human Genet. 29*:9–14.

Yamamoto, M., Ito, T., and Watanabe, G. (1976). Eine weitere chromosomenanalyse bei kunstlichen aborten. *Human Genet. 34*:69–71.

3

Development of the Human Conceptus: Membranes and Placentation During the First Trimester

SERGIO FABRO
Columbia Hospital for Women, Georgetown University, Washington, D.C.

INTRODUCTION

The purpose of this chapter is not to present a comprehensive review of the developmental processes that take place in the human conceptus during the first trimester of pregnancy, but rather to give an account of the development of its external anatomical structures. A firm understanding of this process is a prerequisite for performing chorionic villous sampling (CVS).

For a comprehensive review of human embryology during the first trimester, the reader is referred to a number of available authoritative books (Arey, 1965; Hamilton et al., 1972; Langman, 1981; Moore, 1982). This chapter will focus on the gross anatomical features of the human conceptus with its membranes from the fifth to the twelfth week of gestation.

PRENATAL PERIODS, LENGTH OF PREGNANCY, AND ESTIMATION OF CONCEPTUS AGE

Human prenatal development is usually divided into three main periods: (1) The *pre-embryonic period* is the period culminating in implantation and elaboration of the blastocyst before the establishment of an intraembryonic circulation. During this time, approximately the first 3 weeks of prenatal life (third to fifth menstrual weeks), fetal membranes are established and germ layers are laid down in the embryonic disc. (2) In the *embryonic period*, which extends from the beginning of the fourth week to the end of the eigth week (sixth to tenth menstrual weeks), there is rapid growth and differentiation of all the main organs and systems of the body and the establishment of major features of external body form. (3) The *fetal period* extends from the eleventh menstrual week until birth.

There are different methods for definition of embryonic age. *Menstrual or gestational age* uses day 1 as the first day of the last menstrual period; this age is normally 14 ± 2 days longer than the ovulation age. (2) *Ovulation age* extends from the time at which the mature egg leaves the ovary during the process of ovulation. (3) *Coital age* can be about 2 days less than the ovulation age. (4) *Fertilization age* is from the time of union of sperm and egg; this can be up to 4 days less than the coital age. Unless specifically indicated, the menstrual age is used throughout this chapter.

Age determination of the embryo or fetus by these measurements are notoriously variable, and other, direct measurements of the conceptus are also employed. Thus, (1) *Crown–rump length*, (the measurement from the vertex of the skull to the breech) and (2) *crown–heel length* are most common, although (3) *neck–rump length* (often used in embryos that are markedly flexed) and (4) *foot length*, which is usually not obtainable in embryos with a crown–rump length less than 30 mm, are also used. In Figure 1, crown–rump lengths of human embryos as reported in the literature are compared with crown–rump lengths obtained by ultrasonography at different weeks of pregnancy.

THE FIRST MONTH OF PREGNANCY

The First and Second Week (1–14 Days)

This period extends from the beginning of the last menstrual period to fertilization, the actual beginning of pregnancy. Since menstrual age is used, during the first and second week of gestational age the woman is not pregnant. During this time, the uterine endometrium undergoes the proliferative changes that are characteristic of the preovulatory period. At the end of the second week, ovulation takes place and, after coitus, fertilization occurs usually in the distal one-third of the Fallopian tube.

The Third Week (15–21 Days)

The third week may be characterized as encompassing the preimplantation stages of pregnancy. After fertilization, the zygote undergoes

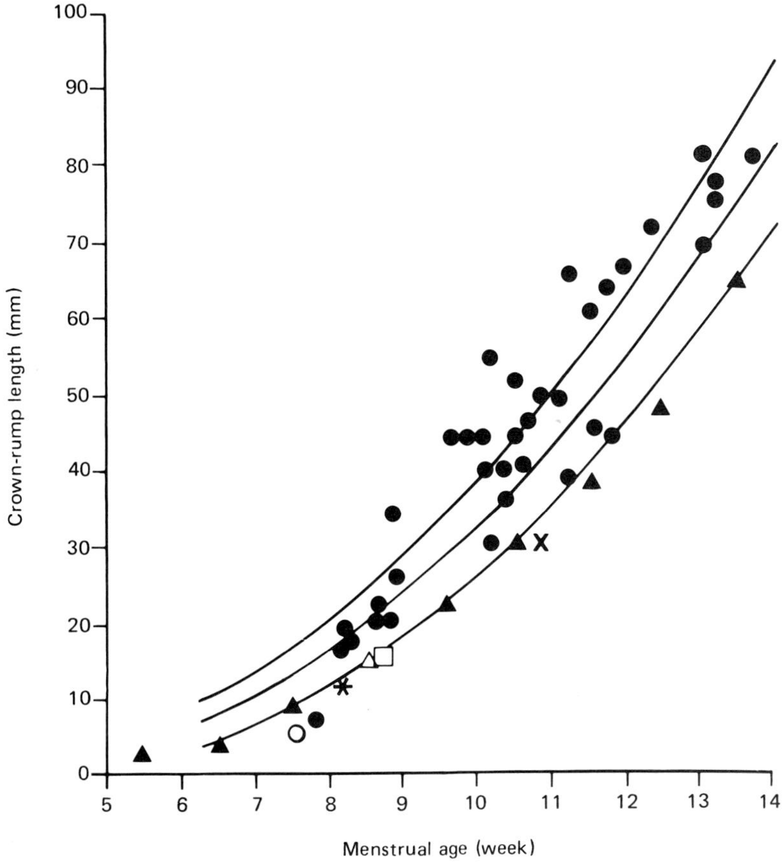

Figure 1 Comparison of crown–rump lengths of embryos obtained by direct measurements (data points) and mean ± 2 standard deviations of crown–rump lengths obtained by sonography (lines) at different menstrual ages. Sonographic measurements from Robinson et al. (1975). Direct measurements from Hamilton et al. (1972) and Pijnenborg et al. (1980).

cleavage and reaches the morula stage while traveling from the distal to proximal end of the Fallopian tube. The morula enters the uterine cavity at about 4 days after fertilization and rapidly becomes a blastocyst (Fig. 2). The blastocyst is a spherical structure limited by the trophoblast; it contains a fluid-filled cavity (blastocoele) and an undifferentiated inner cell mass, the embryoblast.

The blastocyst at the end of the third menstrual week begins to implant in the uterine mucosa about late in the sixth day after ovulation. The embryonic pole of the blastocysts always contacts first and initiates implantation.

At the time of implantation, the uterine mucosa is at the twentieth day of a normal menstrual cycle. It is thought that the rich vascularization, edema, and secretion of mucus and glycogen from the secretory

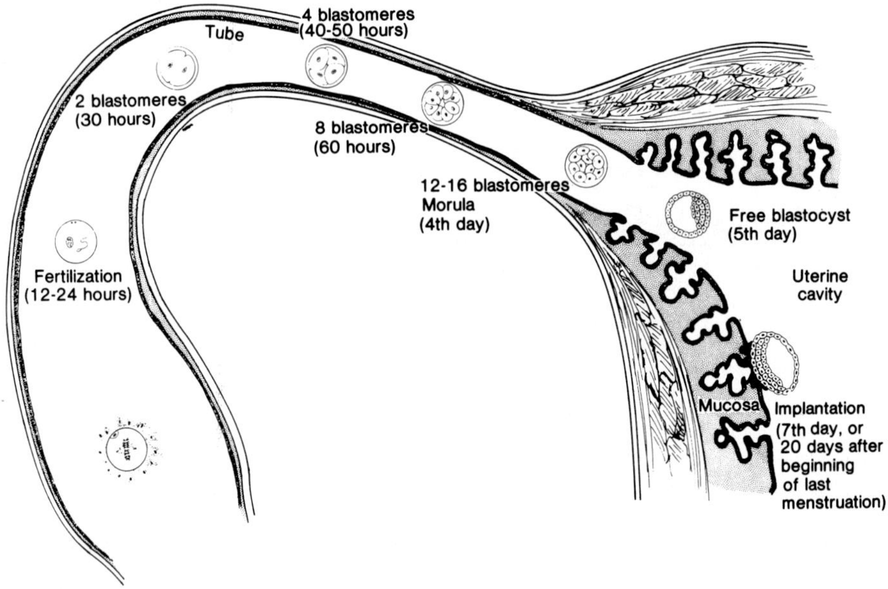

Figure 2 Schematic representation of the preimplantation stages of human pregnancy.

endometrium favors implantation, with penetration and invasion promoted by lytic activity of the syncytiotrophoblast.

The Fourth Week (22–28 Days)

The conceptus enters the fourth week in the blastocyst stage. During this week, an *embryonic disc* is formed from the embryoblast when the endoderm and then the ectoderm undergo successive differentiation from this cellular mass, while the blastocyst invades the uterine mucosa. Toward the end of that week (28 days), the primitive streak appears, indicating the beginning of gastrulation and of the presomite period. With the development of intraembryonic endoderm, a layer of mesotheloidlike cells (Heuser's membrane) marks the establishment of the *primitive yolk sac*.

As implantation occurs, the unilaminar blastocyst is transformed into bilaminar then a trilaminar blastocyst, made up of an outer layer of trophoblastic ectoderm and an inner layer of extraembryonic mesoderm. They layers together constitute the chorion, and the blastocyst becomes known as the chorionic vesicle.

At eight days after ovulation age (day 22, menstrual age) and before the endoderm has completely formed the primitive yolk sac, a second and initially very much smaller cleft, (*the amniotic cavity*) forms between the cells of the inner cell mass (the embryonic ectoderm) and covering trophoblast (Fig. 3). Later, the roof of the amniotic cavity is composed of cells delaminated from the trophoblast, giving rise to a single layer of flattened cells, *the amnion*. The region of mesodermal attachment of amnion and embryonic primordium to the trophoblast, after the appearance of the extraembryonic coelom, is the precursor of the *connecting stalk*. The extraembryonic coelom is established as a cleft between chorionic mesoderm and amnion or yolk sac mesoderm.

The trophoblast, primitive yok sac, amnion, and connecting stalk are the primary fetal membranes, and the formation of the embryonic disc marks the definitive segregation of embryonic body material from that of the membranes. During this time, there is a significant growth of the gestational sac as well as the establishment of the villi, the essential structure of the definitive placenta.

The chorion undergoes intense growth and differentiation during the fourth, fifth, and sixth menstrual weeks (from day 9 to day 25, ovulation age). The gestational sac grows from an average outside diameter of 0.5 mm at 9 days (23 menstrual days) to 1.1 mm at 13 days (27 menstrual

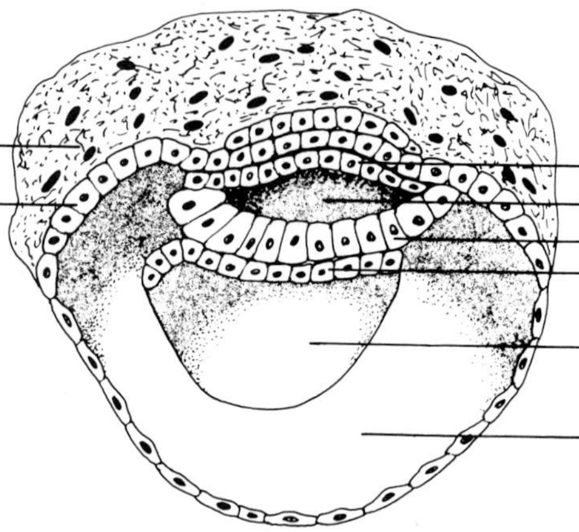

Figure 3 Early developmental features of the human conceptus at the beginning of the fourth menstrual week.

days). During this time, there is a rapid growth of the gestational sac and its villi, and the essential structures of the definitive placenta are established. The human blastocyst (chorionic vesicle) by the eleventh or twelfth day after ovulation (25 or 26 days after the beginning of the last menstrual period) is completely embedded in the stroma of endometrium. At about 13 days after ovulation, the primary villi begin to appear in the form of syncytial branches separated by lacunae (intervillous spaces).

THE SECOND MONTH OF PREGNANCY

The Fifth Week (29–35 Days)

It is during this week that a woman with normal cycle will notice the lack of her menses. The conceptus during the fifth week undergoes changes characteristic of the so-called *presomite period*.

This period extends from the time of appearance of the primitive streak (28–29 days, 14–15 days ovulation age) until the differentiation of the first pair of somites (34 days, 20 days ovulation age).

The conceptus at the beginning of the fifth week consists of a bilaminar disc of ectoderm and endoderm lying between the amniotic and the yolk sac cavities (Fig. 4). At this stage, none of the characteristic features of the human body, such as head, neck, trunk, or limbs, are present. The embryo is indeed a disc. With further growth, the embryonic disc increases in size, elongates, and changes its shape, become first oval and then pear-shaped due to mesoderm formation. At the same time, the embryonic disc develops head and tail folds and bulges into the amniotic cavity. Gastrulation then rapidly occurs, resulting in the formation of the third germ layer, *the mesoderm*, and the *notochord*. Thus, at the end of gastrulation, the three germ layers are in place. The notochord serves, in a way, as the primary skeleton of the three-layered embryo.

The gestational sac also increases in size, and significant changes take place in the chorion. At the beginning of the fifth menstrual week (about 15 days ovulation age), the villi acquire a central loose mesenchymal core that grows within the cytotrophoblast in its extension toward the decidua. Thus, the secondary villi are established as a part of each cell column with its outer covering of syncytiotrophoblast. As the cell columns progress, they open maternal vessels whose blood spreads out in the intervillous

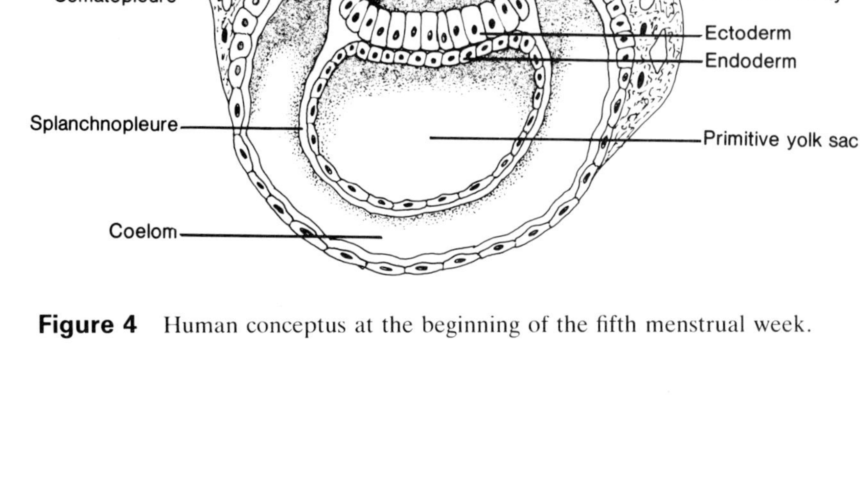

Figure 4 Human conceptus at the beginning of the fifth menstrual week.

spaces. This is the beginning of the maternal placental circulation. At about 32 days (18 days ovulation age) the villi are formed by a mesenchymal core surrounded by a double layer of cyto- and syncytiotrophoblast. In the middle of the villus mesenchyme, vascular islets appear and coalesce, anticipating service to the future fetal circulation. In contrast, the lacunae, now intervillous spaces, are already sites of intense maternal circulation. At the end of the fifth menstrual week (about 21 days ovulation age) the intravillus vascular network connects with the umbilical–allantoic vessels, and the fetal component of the placental circulation is established.

The development of an arterial–capillary–venous system within the core of each villus transforms it into a tertiary villus. The terms primary, secondary, and tertiary, when applied to the chorionic villi, do not apply to the tips of the villi, which remain trophoblastic in character and constitute the so-called *cytotrophoblastic cell column* and *cytotrophoblastic shell*. During the fifth menstrual week, the villi are found around the whole periphery of the chorionic sac. From the caudal part of the yolk sac, a small, hollow, endodermal outgrowth—the allantois or allantoenteric diverticulum—extends into the body stalk, paralleled by fetal vessels that link with chorionic vessels noted above. The amniotic cavity enlarges, carried along by the edges of the embryonic disc during cephalocaudal flexion.

The Sixth Week (36–42 Days)

This week is characterized by the formation of the somites. The *somite period* extends approximately from day 34 to day 44 menstrual age (20–30 days ovulation age).

During the fifth week, the paraxial mesoderm becomes divided successively into symmetrically arranged paired blocks called *somites*. The somites increase in number as development progresses, new ones being added caudally until, generally, 42 to 44 pairs are formed. The somites are conspicuous features of embryos in this period, and they are the bases from which the greater part of the axial skeleton and musculature develop.

Embryos during the somite period show features of the head fold that will eventually result in the formation of the face and neck. These features are the five ectodermal grooves, which are lateral to the embryonic pharynx and separated by four elevations called the first (mandibular), second (hyoid), third, and fourth pharyngeal arches.

Frontonasal and maxillary prominences, flanking the developing eye, also appear during this period.

In an embryo with one pair of somites, the embryonic disc is elongated with the cephalic extremity of the neural plate broader and more elevated. The primitive streak is still a conspicuous feature at the caudal end of the disc. By the 7-somite stage (36 days), the lateral boundaries of the neural groove have become obvious neural folds and, at the level of the fourth to seventh somites, have fused dorsally to enclose a neural canal. In a 10-somite embryo (37 days), the closure of the neural folds have progressed cranially in front of the somite region to the area that will become the mesencephalon (midbrain); the unclosed cranial and caudal ends of the developing neural tube are now known as the anterior (cranial) and posterior (caudal) neuropores. The head fold is much more marked, and, underlying it, the mandibular process of the first arch can be seen on either side. The pericardium appears as a bulge ventrolateral to each mandibular process. The head region shows certain marked features: the maxillary and mandibular processes and the hyoid.

In late somite embryos (e.g., 25 and 28 somites) both neuropores are completely closed. The whole embryo is more elongated and markedly curved, with the attachments of the amnion and yolk sac relatively much reduced on the ventral aspect so that an umbilicus and umbilical cord can now be recognized. By the 28-somite stage (30 days), the otic depression has separated from the surface ectoderm to form the otic vesicle. The two olfactory placodes are now present as localized thickenings of the ectoderm on the ventrolateral aspects of the head above the stomodeum. The attenuated tail, with its somites curled ventrally and forward to the region of the umbilical cord, is a feature of these stages.

The amniotic cavity enlarges at the expense of the extraembryonic coelom that becomes smaller. The primitive yolk sac constricts; it appears attached to the primitive gut by the future vitelline duct. The allantois progresses in the connecting stalk, along with the umbilical–allantoic vessels. The chorionic villi are being actively formed around the whole periphery of the chorion sac.

The Seventh Week (43–49 Days)

At the beginning of the seventh week, the head and trunk regions are well established. The head is markedly flexed on the trunk at the cervical flexure. The optic and otic vesicles as well as the roof plate of the rhombencephalon (hindbrain) are seen. An olfactory pit is also present.

Somites, although no longer conspicuous as surface contours, continue to be formed until the 11-mm stage. Paired, paddle-shaped fore- and hindlimb buds appear.

The yolk sac is constricted by the development of the umbilical region; it appears attached to the primitive gut by the constricted part that will be the vitelline duct. The amniotic cavity enlarges at the expense of the extraembryonic coelom that becomes relatively smaller. At this time (5-mm crown–rump length embryo), the amniotic cavity is larger than the yolk sac (Fig. 5).

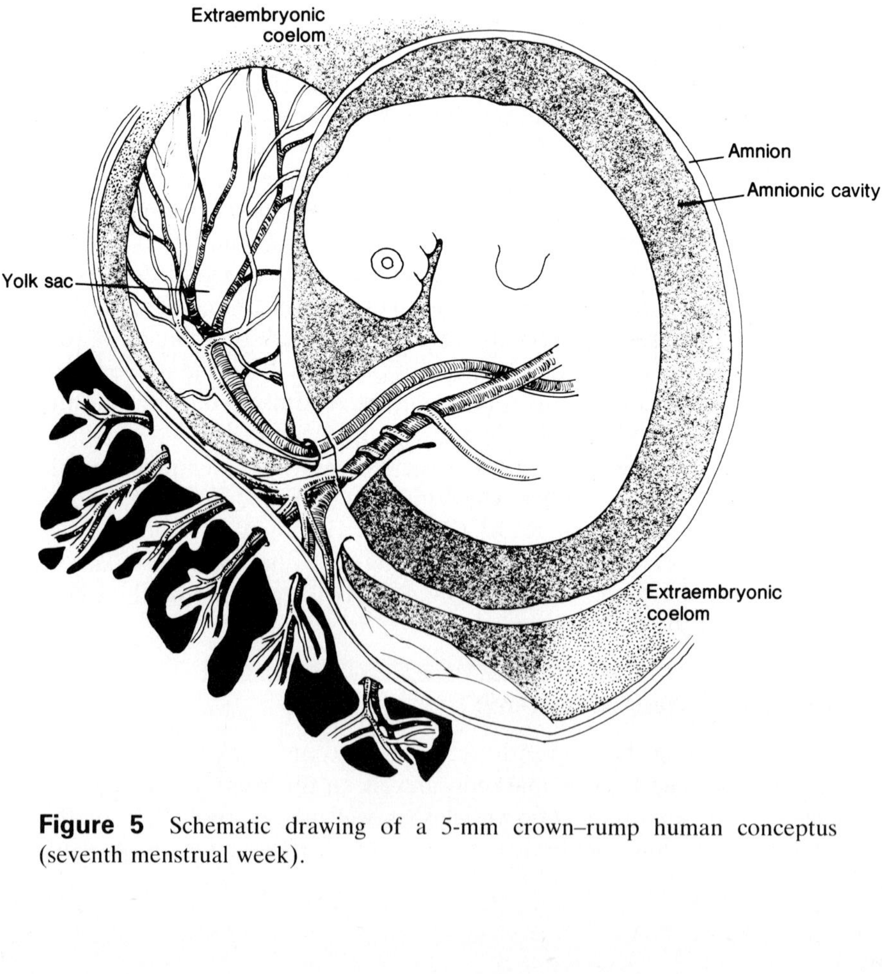

Figure 5 Schematic drawing of a 5-mm crown–rump human conceptus (seventh menstrual week).

The Eighth Week (50–56 Days)

The external appearance of embryos of about 10-mm crown–rump length (51 day menstrual age, 37 day ovulation age) has much changed (Fig. 6). For example, the maxillary process on each side has extended forward beneath the corresponding optic vesicle and is fusing with the lateral surface of the lateral nasal processes. The upper limb buds are now subdivided into arm, forearm, and hand while the hindlimb bud still retains its primitive paddle shape. The tail is undergoing retrogressive changes.

In slightly older embryos, the size of the head is markedly increased, and the appearance of obvious forebrain vesicles are easily recognizable.

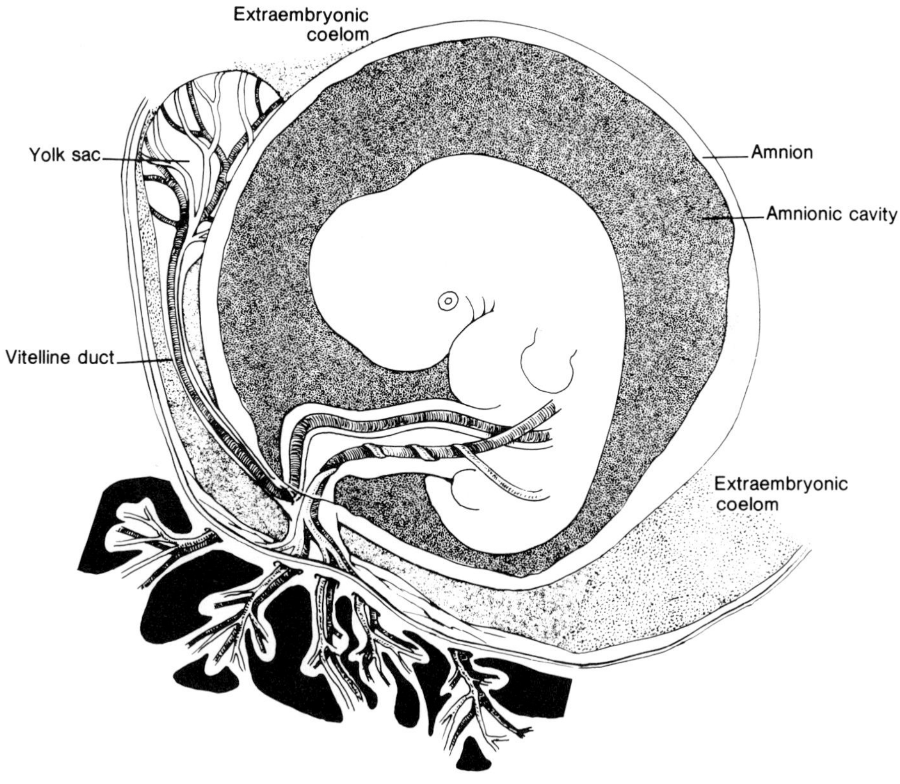

Figure 6 Schematic drawing of a 10-mm crown–rump length human conceptus (eighth menstrual week).

The hand now shows the outlines of the future digits. The hindlimb bud has divided into thigh, leg, and foot regions. Cephalic to the attachment of the umbilical cord, there is a swelling that defines the liver and the pericardial area through which the beating heart can be seen.

In embryos of 9 to 10-mm crown–rump length, the yolk sac attached to the umbilical region by the vitelline duct is smaller than the amniotic cavity, which has increased markedly in size. The umbilical cord is thick and short (about 1 cm in length). The chorion is covered with villi. Although they are visible over the entire surface of the gestational sac, they begin to be thinner and less developed under the decidua capsularis.

THE THIRD MONTH OF PREGNANCY

The Ninth Week (57–63 Days)

By the forty-sixth day ovulation age (60 days menstrual age), when the embryo is about 17 mm (crown–rump length), the head region has increased even further in size and is less flexed. Eyelids are forming, and the external ear is established around the external auditory meatus. The digits of the hands are separating, but those of each foot still appear as united rays.

The yolk sac is in the extraembryonic space between the expanding amnion and the chorionic plate of the developing placenta. With the development of the anterior abdominal wall, the region of umbilical attachment contracts, decreasing the diameter of the umbilical cord. The chorionic villi adjacent to the decidua basalis constitute the chorion frondosum.

The Tenth Week (64–70 Days)

At the end of the tenth week, embryos (about 30-mm crown–rump length) have assumed a human appearance. The neck region is established; the eyelids and the external ears are obvious; the umbilical cord is relatively thinner and is now attached on the less protuberant ventral abdominal wall. The digits of both hands and feet are clearly defined. The tail has now almost completely disappeared. The intramesenchyal segment of the allantois has disappeared. The umbilical vessels continue their development. The extraembryonic coelom, effaced by the enlargement of the amniotic cavity, is obliterated. Eventually it will disappear when the amnion will fuse with the chorion. The chorionic villi of the chorion levae are rare and atrophic. The mature chorion–

allantoid placenta is formed in relation to the decidua basalis. The gestational sac is now about 5 cm in diameter.

The Eleventh and Twelfth Week

From this period to birth, the human conceptus is referred to as a fetus. The distinction between embryo and fetus is arbitrary, but is useful in that it emphasizes the possession by the conceptus of an unmistakably human appearance. The term fetus is commonly used for a conceptus of 30-mm or greater crown–rump (69 to 74 days from the beginning of the last period, 55 to 60 days ovulation age).

During this time, the fetus grows rapidly, nearly doubling its length in the next 4 weeks (11–14 weeks menstrual age), and most of the parts of the body reach their definitive fetal positions. Early during this time, vibrissal hairs appear in the eyebrow region, the upper lip, and the carpal and tarsal regions. At 50-mm crown–rump length, it is possible to identify the sex of a fetus by external inspection.

ACKNOWLEDGMENTS

I would like to acknowledge and thank Dr. Frank Allan for his helpful suggestions and critical review of the manuscript.

REFERENCES

Arey, B. L. (1965). *Developmental Anatomy*, 7th ed., Saunders, Philadelphia.

Boue, A., Henrion, R., and David G. (1979). Development Prenatal Normal et Pathologique. In *Pediatrie* (R. Debre and P. Royer, eds.), 341. Collection Medicochirurgicale. Flammarion Medicine-Sciences, Paris.

Hamilton, W. J., Boyd, J. D., Mossman, H. W. (1972) *Human Embryology*, 4th ed. William and Wilkins, Baltimore.

Langman, J. (1981) *Medical Embryology*, 4th ed. William and Wilkins, Baltimore.

Moore, K. L. (1982) *The Developing Human*, 2nd ed. W. B. Saunders, Philadelphia.

Pijnenborg, R., Dixon, G., Robertson, W. B., and Brosens, I. (1980). Trophoblastic invasion of human decidua from 8 to 18 weeks of pregnancy. *Placenta*, *1*:3–19.

Robinson, H. P. and Fleming, J. E. E. (1975). A critical evaluation of sonar crown-rump length measurements. *Br. J. Obstet. Cynaecol. 82*:702.

4

Ultrasonic Evaluation of the Pregnant Uterus in the First Trimester

BRUNO BRAMBATI, ANGELO OLDRINI,* and ENRICO FERRAZZI
First Institute of Obstetrics and Gynecology, University of Milan, Milan, Italy

Reliable sonographic imaging procedures and measurements for assessing fetal well-being and for guiding the sampling device had to be developed for the application for chorionic villus sampling (CVS) techniques to first-trimester fetal diagnosis.

The substance of this chapter is the role of first-trimester sonography in evaluating ovular development and in permitting safe and successful sampling.

ULTRASOUND EQUIPMENT AND METHODOLOGY

To guarantee an accurate evaluation of the intrauterine anatomy and reliable guidance of the thin aspiration device, a machine with a high-resolution scanner should be used. A first-choice transducer should have the highest frequency to be able to read the region of interest, following the general rule that the higher the frequency, the better the axial and lateral resolution. The disadvantage of higher-frequency transducers is that the sound is more strongly attenuated. However, despite the reduced penetration, all the antiverted uteri can be effectively examined at 5 MHz rather than at the conventional 3.5 MHz, clearly

**Present affiliation*: Third Institute of Obstetrics and Gynecology, University of Milan, Milan, Italy

providing better resolution. Moreover, in the second and third month of pregnancy, the uterus is generally situated from 5 to 10 cm from the maternal surface and therefore in the range corresponding to the focal zone of a 5-MHz transducer. In cases of retroverted uteri, a preliminary examination could be made using a 3.5-MHz transducer with a full bladder. Nevertheless, at the time of sampling, the traction of the cervix by a tenaculum usually allows the rotation of the uterus, and one can operate under standard conditions.

Although to date a lot of relatively short, linear transducers are available, their straight construction does not always allow an easy fit to the maternal abdominal surface and makes it difficult to angle the beam to visualize both the cervical canal and the inferior part of the uterus. Because of the small contact surface and the shape of the scanning plane, a mechanical sector scanner prevents these inconveniences, permitting easy handling of the transducer in all the scanning sections with a "state-of-the-art" visualization of the whole anatomical system involved in chorionic villi sampling (CVS) (Fig. 1).

The full bladder technique was rejected in this study, since it can cause undesired distortion of the uterine content, which is precisely the object of the examination (1). In fact, the contact surface of the sector scanner allows the bowels to be squeezed away from the uterus with just slight pressure on the abdomen. On the other hand, when the bowels were covering the uterus, we learned the poor efficacy of the full bladder in pushing the bowels away from the fundus. Therefore, a partially empty bladder was the standard condition both for ultrasound monitoring of the early pregnancy and for ultrasound guidance of CVS, with obvious advantages for the patient.

Presently all the ultrasonic examinations are performed by an ATL MK 300 I ultrasound system provided with a mechanical rotating 5-MHz scanner characterized by a focal depth of 2 to 7 cm and a scanning angle of 90°. The digital caliper's steps are 1 mm. The intrauterine structures we systematically investigated in the first trimester of pregnancy included gestational sac; amniotic membrane; amniotic space and extraembryonic coelom; embryo-fetus, including an approximate heart activity and trunk movements evaluation; yolk sac; umbilical cord; nonechogenic areas; and multiple pregnancy (Fig. 2).

Gestational sac volume and crown–rump length were measured according to standard procedures as proposed by Robinson (2) and Robinson and Fleming (3), respectively. The gestational sac volume was used to monitor the very early stages of the first-trimester development

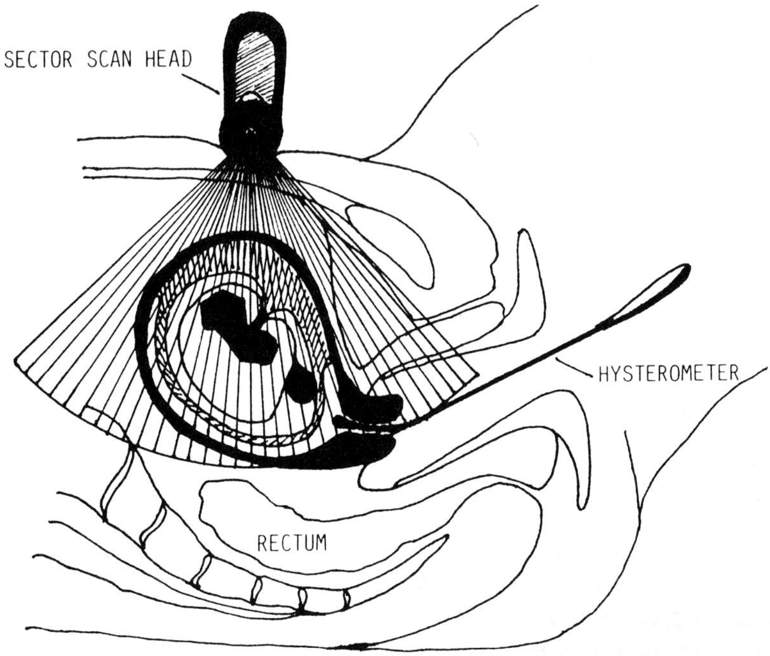

Figure 1 Diagram of a pregnancy at 8–9 weeks. The 90° scanning angle allows visualization of the uterus and cervix at the same time, while the depth of scan fits well with the length of the focal zone.

until the visualization of a viable embryo, while crown–rump length was used to estimate the gestational age and the growth of the embryo-fetus until the thirteenth week. Diagnosis of missed abortion was made when (a) the gestational sac volume did not double every 7 days from the fifth to the seventh week, (b) when an embryonic structure, of at least 5 to 10 mm, according to the quality of reflected echoes, was clearly visualizable and no heart activity detectable. In those cases in which the gestational sac reached a volume of 5 ml (corresponding to the gestational age of 6 +2SD at the sixth week) and in which no embryonic structures were visualizable, a diagnosis of blighted ovum was assumed.

The yolk sac demonstrated itself to be a structure that is not always spheric and, on the ultrasonic display, frequently appeared as an elliptical surface. For this reason, the sonographic measurements reported were the mean value of two orthogonal diameters, the longest and the shortest

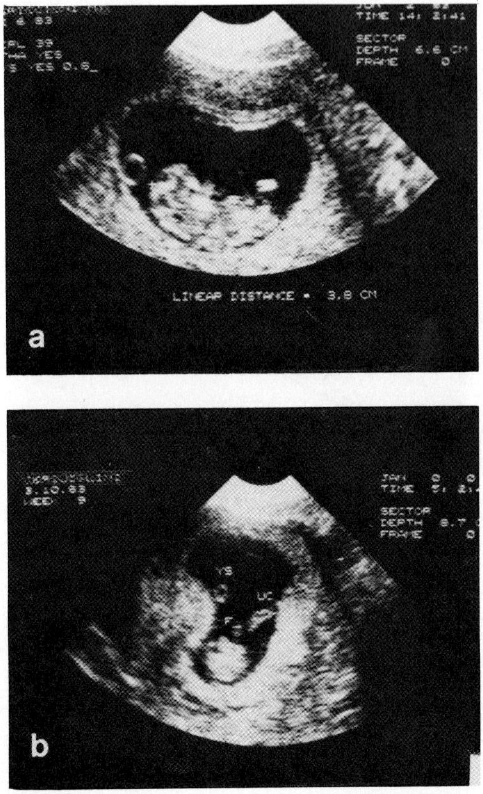

Figure 2 Anatomic details of the gestational sac of sonographic interest in CVS. (a) Ten-week-old embryo and yolk sac, (b) Umbilical cord insertion and chorion frondosum site. (c) Yolk sac and yolk duct from the site of umbilical cord insertion. (d) Amniotic membrane at 9 weeks of gestation.

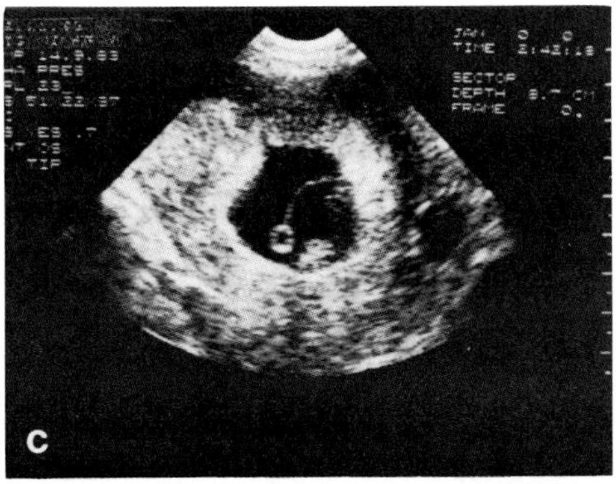
TIME
SECTOR
DEPTH
FRAME

c

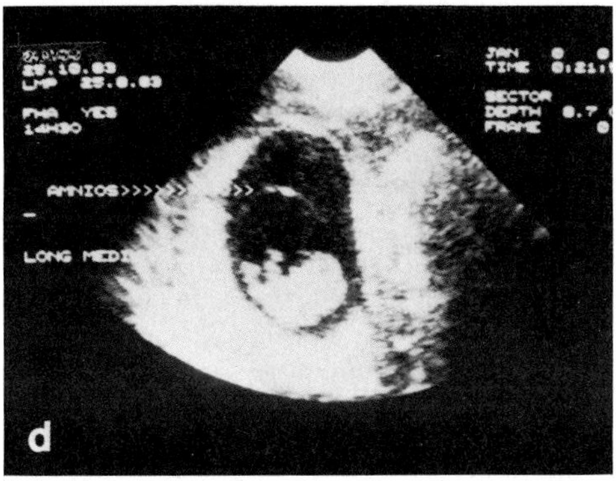
JAN
TIME
SECTOR
DEPTH
FRAME
FHA YES
AMNIOS>>>
LONG MEDI

d

one, respectively. When the yolk sac circumference was not completely outlined, the measurements of the diameter was judged to be unreliable and was rejected.

The chorion frondosum site was defined as the thickest iperechogenic site of the gestational sac. At the time of CVS, the umbilical cord insertion was used as a point of reference to interpret the sonographic features related to the ovular insertion. The microscopic control of the aspirated specimens assured a retrospective confirmation. The umbilical cord was identified by three parallel and strongly echogenic lines, corresponding to the three umbilical vessels, frequently characterized by rhythmical movements. The diameter values were calculated as the mean of several measurements obtained as the orthogonal distance between the two peripheral lines.

In cases where a nonechogenic space was evident between chorion and decidua parietalis, its extension was semiquantitatively evaluated only from its thickness and its relationship with the different parts of the sac. Amniotic membranes were detected, but the amniotic space and the extraembryonic coelom were not quantitated in any way. Fetal heart activity and fetal movements were also observed but not utilized for any specific analysis.

THE ROLE OF THE ULTRASOUND IN CHORIONIC VILLUS SAMPLING

The use of the ultrasound in CVS by transvaginal aspiration is an absolute necessity, and the importance of the quality of the ultransonic apparatus to the safety and efficacy of the procedure was confirmed by experience at the most active diagnostic centers (4). In the Milan Mangiagalli Center, on 103 experimental cases and on 250 diagnostic cases, no gestational sac perforations were suspected, and a successful sampling rate of over 97% was reported (5).

The major criteria to assure a correct approach to CVS by an aspiration catheter and to guarantee the highest reliability in sampling included: (a) identification of placental site by detecting the umbilical cord insertion; (b) visualization of the cervical canal and localization of the internal cervical os by the combined use of hysterometer and ultrasound, allowing evaluation of the best way to reach the placenta; and (c) continous monitoring of the end of the aspiration catheter.

Although the placenta localization can be accurately determined in nearly 100% of the cases during the second and the third trimester (6) it was found that this was not so for the first trimester. In the early stage of gestation, decidua and chorionic villi form a strong reflecting zone surrounding the gestational sac, which is visible in all the scanning sections. As pregnancy progresses, chorion laeve regresses while chorion frondosum thickness continues to increase, facilitating the ultrasonographic identification of the placental site. However, until 11-12 weeks, in a consistent number of cases, it is likely that the strong reaction of decidua parietalis and/or individual unfavorable echogenic conditions make the placental implantation area detection difficult or unreliable. In all these cases, the identification of the umbilical cord insertion is essential to localize a suitable area for CVS. This is particularly relevant for a twin pregnancy with fused placentas: the sampling should be performed in two placental areas lying just below the umbilical cord insertion of each fetus, respectively (Fig. 3) (7).

The evaluation of the relationship of the cervical canal and the internal cervical os with the sampling site revealed a very useful step for bending the catheter properly before introducing it into the uterine cavity. Too acute an angle between the cervical axis and the intrauterine cervical os could prevent any sampling attempt (Fig. 4).

The perforation of the ovular sac is a potential danger of the aspiration technique and was observed in a very small number of cases in which poor ultrasonic visualization was available (4). In our experimental study, although the ovular sac was demonstrated to be highly resistent, a wrong movement of few millimeters could threaten the membranes' integrity (Fig. 5). A good coordination between ultrasonographer and the physician performing the CVS is mandatory to avoid complications and to assure a highly successful sampling rate.

PATIENTS

There was an investigation of 286 candidates for CVS in the first trimester. The first ultrasonic control was obtained no earlier than the sixth week. A viable pregnancy was diagnosed in 250 cases. These patients had CVS, and then serial controls were performed for a total of 1150 examinations before the thirteenth week. After fetal diagnosis, voluntary abortion was requested in 23 cases. Of 227 pregnancies intended to continue, nine aborted spontaneously, 93 delivered viable babies, and 125 are progressing. The birth weight in 85 cases was between the nintieth and the tenth precentile, in two cases above the nintieth percentile, and in six cases below the tenth percentile. Missed abortion before CVS occurred in 36 cases, in 19 of which no embryonic/fetal structures were visualized. Blighted ovum was diagnosed in ten cases.

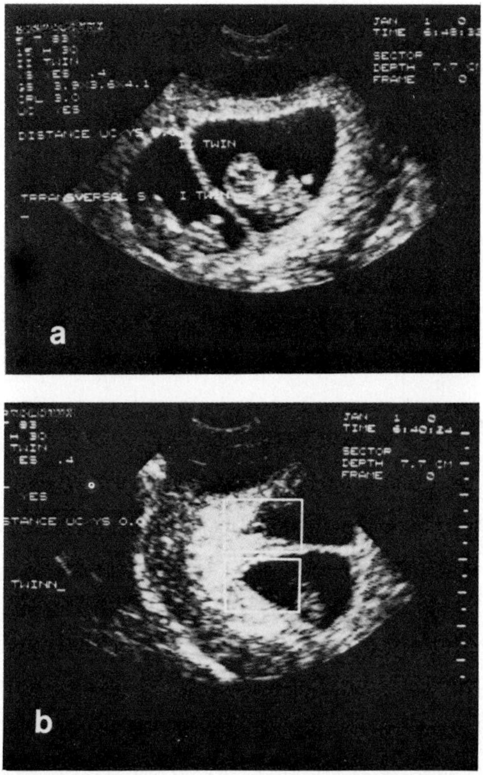

Figure 3 (a) Twin pregnancy at 10 weeks with fused placentas. (b) Areas inside squares are represented in detail in (c) and (d) where umbilical cord insertions of two fetuses are clearly recognizable (arrows).

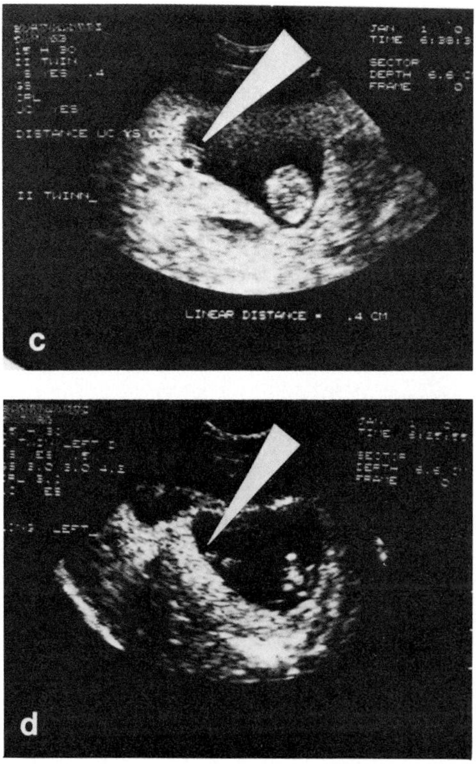
TIME
SECTOR
DEPTH
FRAME
II TWINN_
LINEAR DISTANCE = .4 CM
c
d

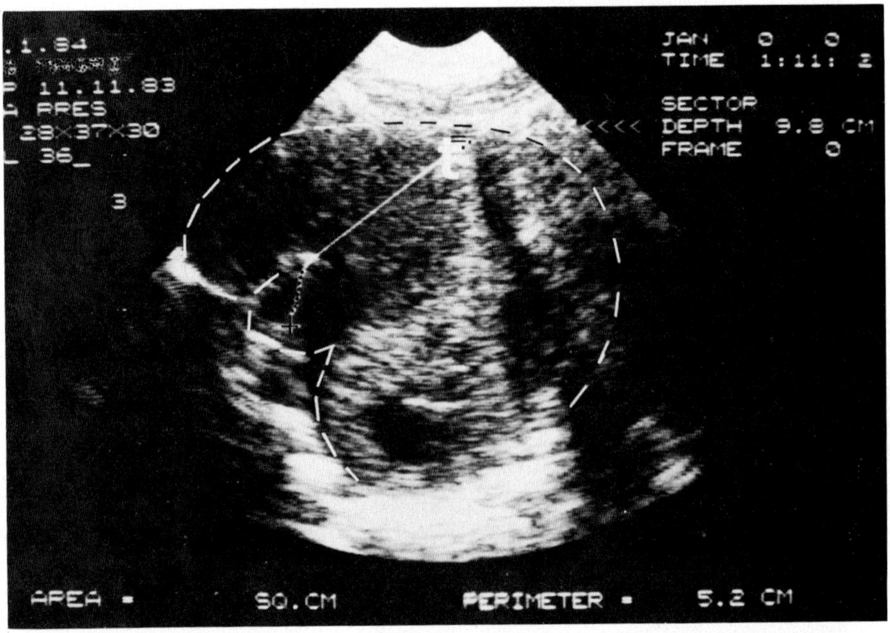

Figure 4 Pregnancy at 10 weeks with a very pronounced retroflexion of the uterus. The catheter could not be appropriately bent to aspirate safely at the placental site. The cervical canal is represented by a white line. t, internal cervical os.

A SONOGRAPHIC APPROACH TO THE ANATOMY OF THE FIRST TRIMESTER

The sonographic monitoring of the fetus in the second and third trimester has demonstrated to be an efficacious guarantee of a reliable prognosis. In the first trimester, the prognostic value of ultrasound examination of the uterine content has still to be demonstrated. In an effort to approach this problem, we have evaluated a number of sonographic anatomic characteristics for assessing both fetal well-being and intrauterine modifications that could appear following CVS.

Gestational Sac

In our series, the absolute and serial values of the gestational sac, calculated for uncomplicated pregnancies delivering normal babies, fit

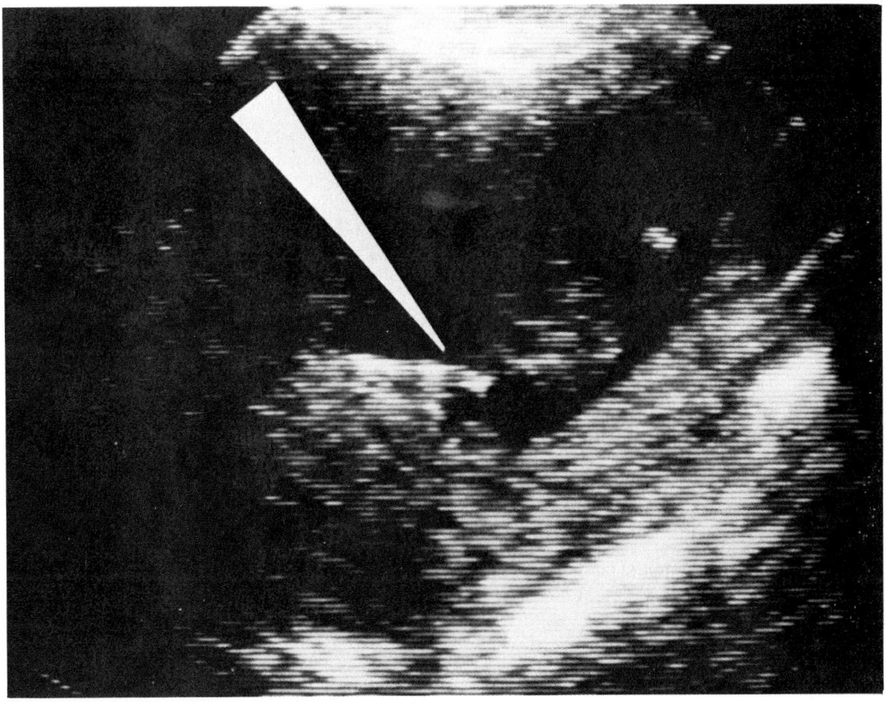

Figure 5 An uncontrolled movement of the catheter is threatening the ovular sac integrity.

well within the normal standards reported by Robinson (2). All but two pregnancies bearing chromosomally abnormal fetuses had either single values in the normal ranges or serial determinations paralleling the normal trend (Fig. 6). In two cases with trisomy 16 and trisomy 14, respectively, the sac volume had a value slightly below the inferior limit. Fetal demise was observed 1 week after sampling, just before selective abortion, in the case with trisomy 14. At this time, the sac volume was significantly increased. In the cases in which a diagnosis of missed abortion or blighted ovum was made, heterogeneous occurrences were observed: single values within or outside the normal limits or serial values below or above normal (Fig. 7). In the six cases in which a small-for-date-baby was born, no abnormal gestation sac in the first trimester was observed.

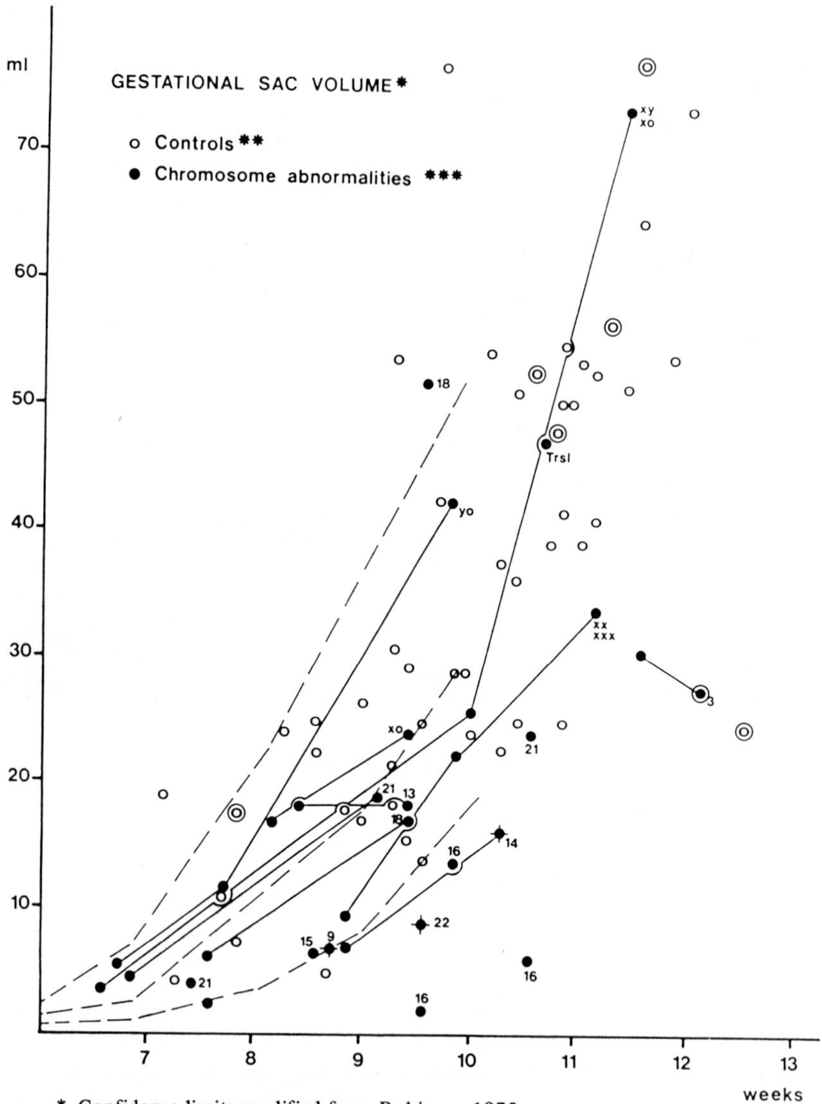

* Confidence limits modified from Robinson 1975

** Normal karyotyping normal pregnancies

*** Crossed dots stand for missed abortions

Circled dots stand for cases with uncertain dates

Figure 6 Gestation sac volume distribution in normal and chromosomally abnormal fetuses.

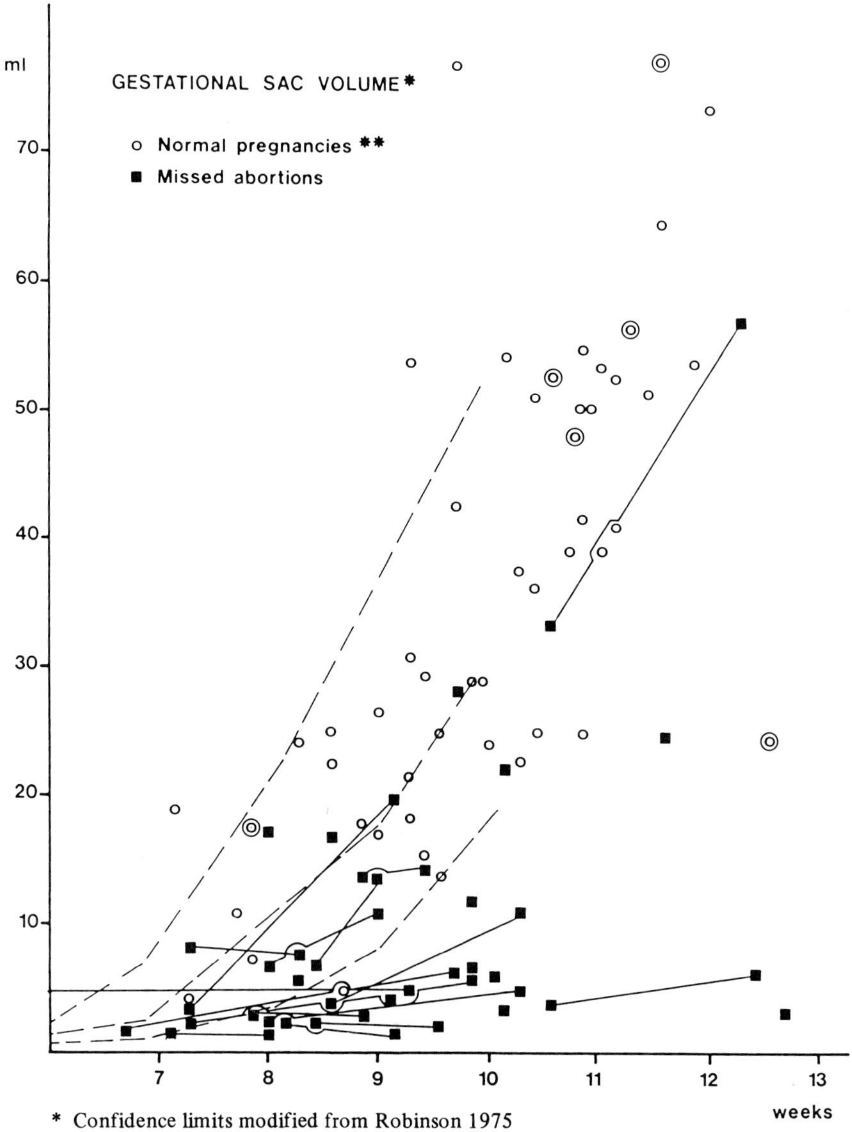

* Confidence limits modified from Robinson 1975

** Normal karyotyping normal pregnancies

Circled dots stand for cases with uncertain dates

Figure 7 Gestation sac volume distribution in cases of missed abortion and anembryonic ovum.

Crown–Rump Length

The individual and serial measurements performed in the uncomplicated cases were in agreement with normal limits (3). The living fetuses with abnormal karyotype were not differentiated from the normal population. Only one trisomy 14 fetus had a crown–rump length value just below the lower limit (Fig. 8). In the three fetuses affected by mucopolysaccaridosis, trisomy 3, and at risk for Duchenne muscular dystrophy, respectively, the abnormally low values can be explained by the unreliability of the last menstrual period (LMP) with a likely late fertilization. Maternal complications in the second and third trimester and intrauterine growth retardation (IUGR) were not preceded by abnormal crown–rump length values in the first trimester. In all the cases in which a diagnosis of missed abortion was made, crown–rump length overlapped or was beyond the inferior limit after the first ultrasound control (Fig. 9). No specific features in fetal heart activity or fetal movements could be identified in cases with chromosomal abnormalities or fetal complications later in pregnancy.

Yolk Sac

The measurements of the yolk sac were related to crown–rump length (Fig. 10). Although a marked variability was present among the individual values, the scattergram suggested an increase in size up to about 11 weeks. (The mean values and ranges of yolk sac diameter are reported in Table 1.) This tendency was apparently confirmed in the small number of cases in which serial values were available. In 18% of 200

Table 1 Mean Values and Ranges of Yolk Sac Diameter in Normal Pregnancies

Gestational age (weeks)	No. of Cases	Yolk sac diameter (mm)	
		Mean	Range
7	6	4.3	4–6
8	16	5.1	3–7
9	19	5.3	4–6
10	18	5.5	4–7
11	8	5.4	4–6

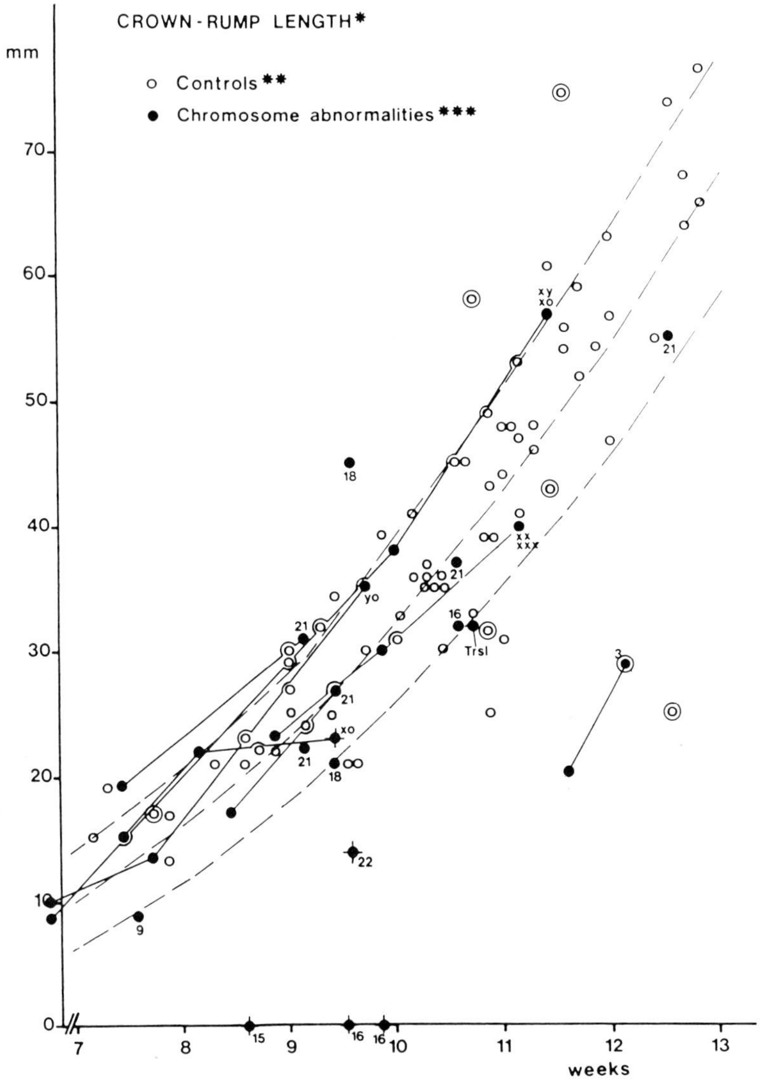

* Confidence limits modified from Robinson 1975

** Normal karyotyping normal pregnancies

*** Crossed dots stand for missed abortions
Circled dots stand for cases with uncertain dates

Figure 8 Crown–rump length distribution in normal and chromosomally abnormal fetuses.

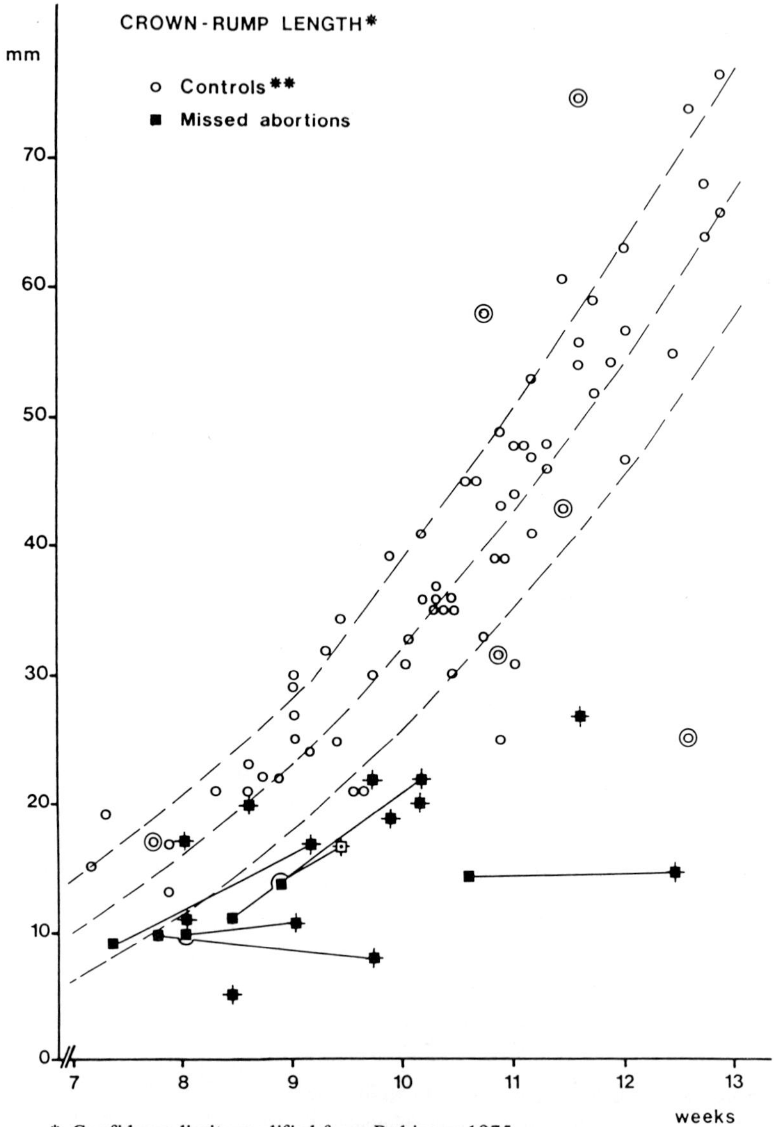

* Confidence limits modified from Robinson 1975

** Normal karyotyping normal pregnancies

Circled dots stand for cases with uncertain dates

Figure 9 Crown–rump length distribution in cases of missed abortion.

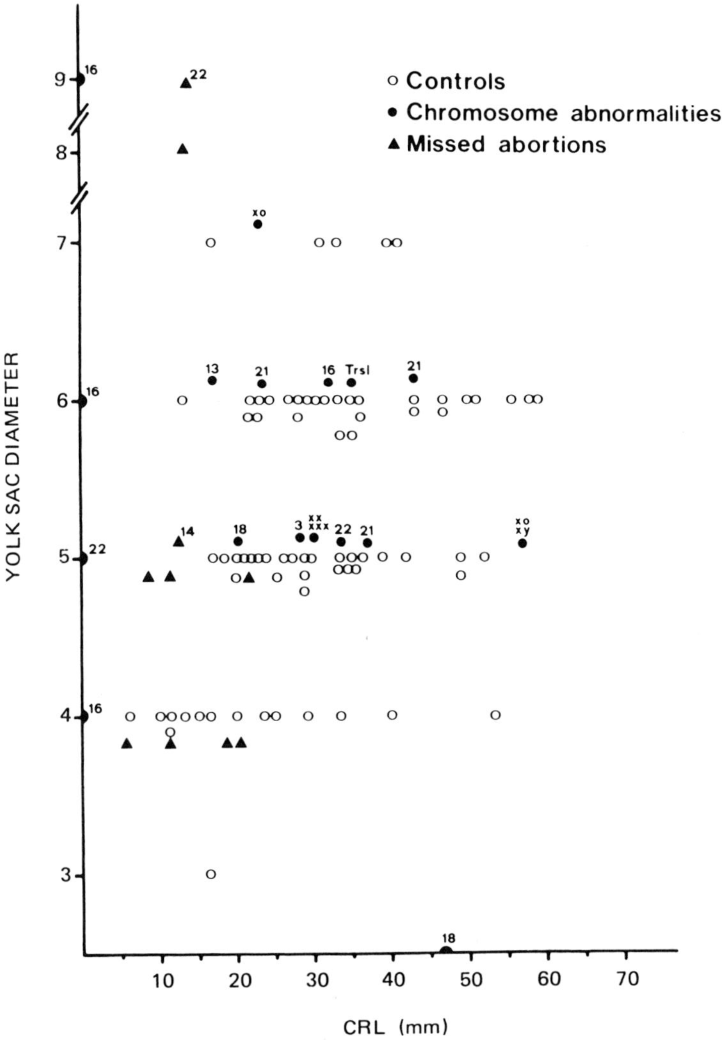

Figure 10 Yolk sac diameter distribution in normal and chromosomally abnormal fetuses, in missed abortion, and in blighted ova.

cases, the yolk sac failed to be visualized at the time of CVS, which ranged from 8 to 12 weeks. However, the failure rate fell to 7% when serial examinations for each case before and after CVS were considered. The thin wall of YS is barely echogenic and easily disappears when masked by fetal and/or maternal parts. In the pregnancies with "absence" of yolk sac, no abnormalities in the fetus at birth or in progressing pregnancies occurred. In the pregnancies associated with a chromosomally abnormal but living fetus, the yolk sac value did not differ from those found in the unaffected fetuses.

In six cases in which the embryo was not echographically visualizable, a yolk-sac-like structure was observed. On four occasions, karyotyping was successful. In three cases a trisomy 16 and in one case a trisomy 22 were diagnosed. Both these anomalies were also found in cases of missed abortion. Of 20 embryonic deaths, diagnosed by sonography (crown–rump length $\geqslant$ 5 mm and fetal heart activity absent) yolk sac was visualized only in ten, and, in four of these, the diameter was clearly exceeding the normal values.

Umbilical Cord

Between the eighth and the twelfth week, the umbilical cord insertion to the placenta was identified in 93% of 200 cases. The measurement of the diameter was obtained in nearly all the cases, and ranged from 2 to 5 mm. No specific trends were recognizable when the diameter values were plotted against the week of gestation (Fig. 11), even though the values of 2 and 5 mm were observed only before 9 weeks and after 10 weeks, respectively. The relatively poor precision of the calipers used on the sonographic display could be partly responsible for the broad distribution of the values, with both umbilical cord and yolk sac measurements, which could mask specific patterns.

Amniotic Sac and Extraembryonic Coelom

The relationship between the amniotic cavity and the extraembryonic coelom was observed and described, but no reliable measurements could be made. At 7 and 8 weeks, the extraembryonic coelom appeared very expanded, exceeding or equaling the amniotic sac. The amniotic space steadily enlarged, and the extraembryonic coelom was reduced to a thin layer or disappeared at about 12 weeks (Fig. 12). The amniotic sac was generally observed as a distended membrane, since it was sometimes detected to be clearly floating (Fig. 12c).

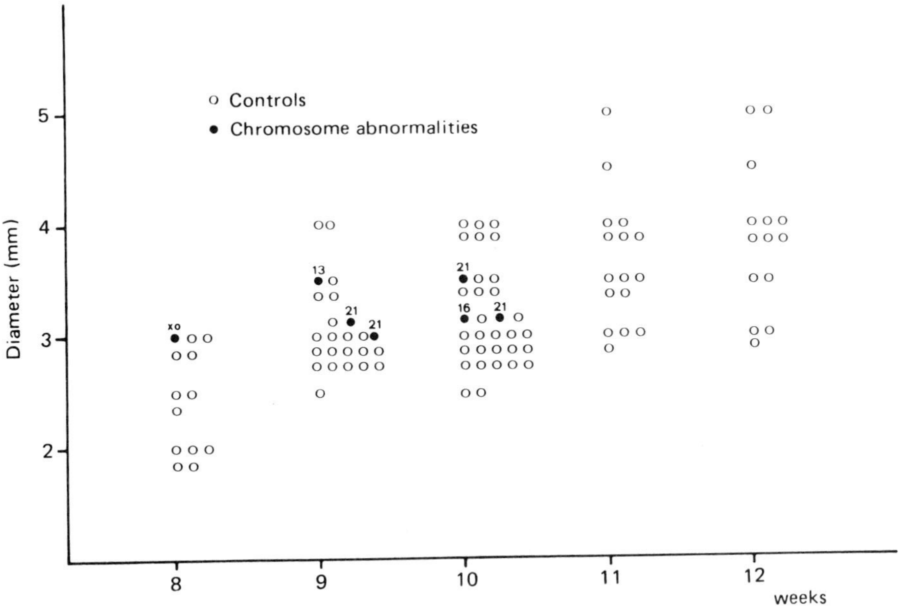

Figure 11 Umbilical cord diameter distribution in normal and chromosomally abnormal fetuses.

Multiple Pregnancy

A twin pregnancy with viable fetuses was recognized in 4 out of 250 candidates for CVS. This indicates a rate of 1.6%. A fifth case was probably present in a patient in whom a large nonechogenic space was observed next to a normal embryonic sac and was interpreted to be a second empty sac. In this case, a previous ultrasonic control made elsewhere and an abnormally high human chorionic gonadotropin value seemed consistent with a twin pregnancy. The patient was referred for ultrasonic study because of persistent bleeding. Another case of monovular twinning was suggested by a blighted ovum containing two yolk-sac-like structures, both 8 mm in diameter, observed in a patient at the ninth week.

The number of twin pregnancies reported in this study indicates a rate ranging between 1.6 and 2.2%, which fits well within the estimates of the frequency of twinning in the west European countries (8). Thus, the higher incidence of multiple human conceptions with a high rate of early

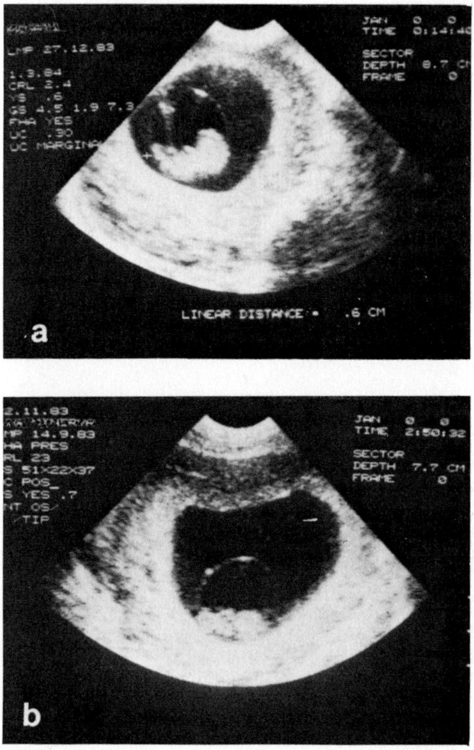

Figure 12 (a) and (b) Amniotic sac at 9 weeks. (c) Floating amniotic membrane at 10 weeks. (d) Extraembryonic coelom at 11 weeks. The YS appears to be compressed between amnion and chorion.

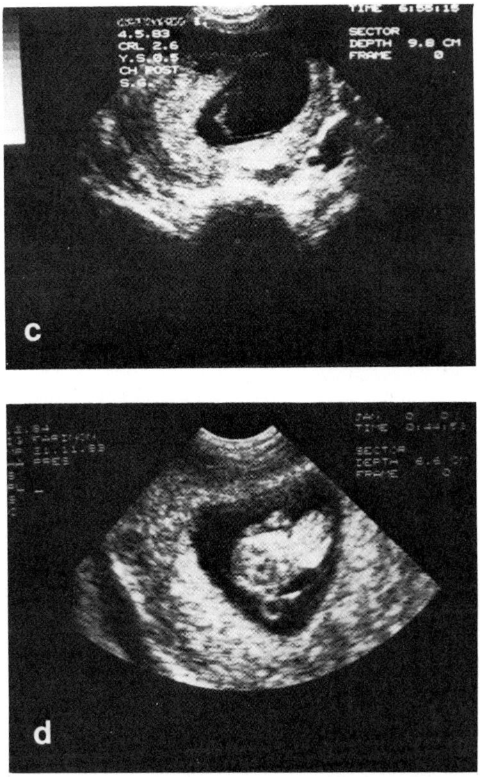
4.5.83
CRL 2.6
Y.S.0.5
CH POST
S.G.
SECTOR
DEPTH 9.8 CM
FRAME 0
c
d

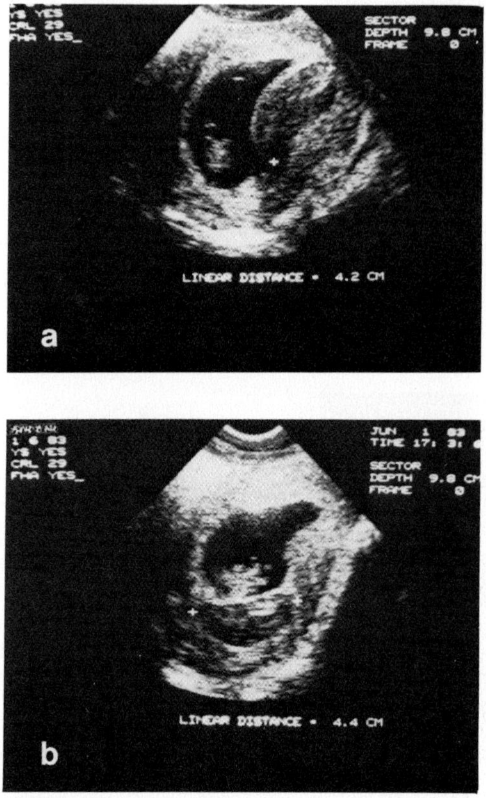

Figure 13 Evolution of intrauterine hematoma observed after CVS (time) in a pregnancy at 9 weeks. (a) 17:00:39, intrauterine hematoma of the right lateral wall, maximum width 24 mm (probable volume 17 ml). (b) At 17:03:06, the hematoma has dropped during real-time observation to the inferior pole of the gestational sac. (c) and (d) After 18 hr, marked reduction of the volume of the hematoma represented in transverse and longitudinal planes, respectively.

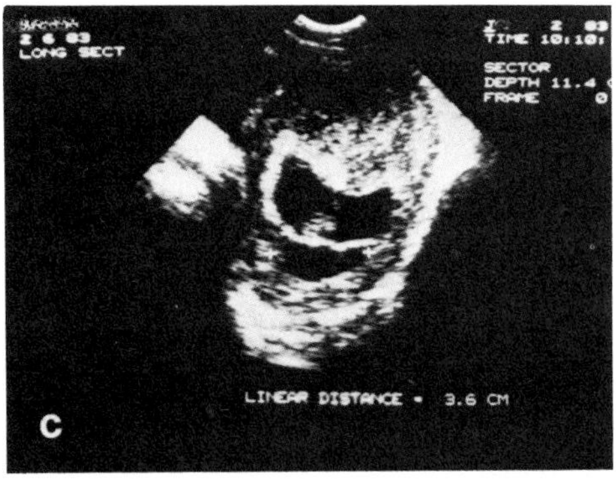
LONG SECT
SECTOR
FRAME
LINEAR DISTANCE = 3.6 CM
c

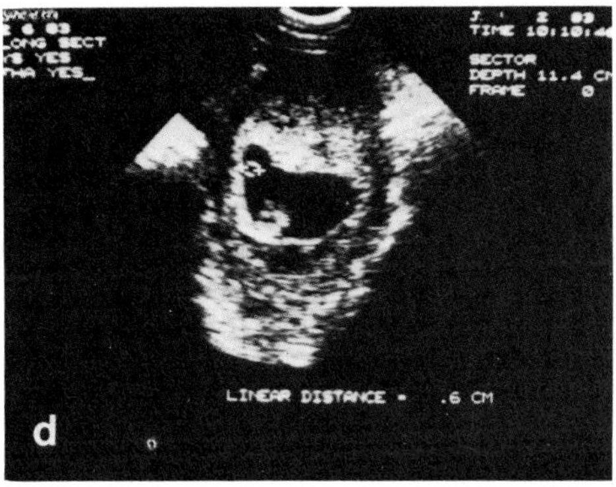
SECTOR
DEPTH 11.4
FRAME
LINEAR DISTANCE = .6 CM
d

disappearance of one fetus that was previously reported using ultrasound were not confirmed (9). This discrepancy could be partially related to misinterpretation of the intrauterine anatomy, probably occurring when low-quality sonographic apparatus is used and/or no pathological evidence is available. One obvious explanation of our underestimation could arise from too few pregnancies being used as controls before the seventh week, although in the previous sonographic studies the occurrence of the vanishing twin was reported from the seventh to the twelfth week (9).

Sonographic Features of Complications after CVS

In our CVS patients we have investigated the presence of nonechogenic areas during routine sonographic controls and monitored vaginal bleeding following CVS. The patients were requested to contact one of us without delay on the appearance of bleeding and inform us about its development. The frequency of sonographic controls done depended on the clinical situation. Vaginal bleeding occurred within 2 weeks after sampling in 34 of 250 cases. In 28 of these cases, vaginal bleeding stopped within a few days. In six cases, the bleeding persisted past day 15 post-CVS. Nonechogenic areas were detected in 17 cases of the former group and in no cases of the latter group.

The bleeding was a likely consequence of decidual lesions or small chorion frondosum abruption that could follow traumatic movements of the aspiration system before, during, and after aspiration. Hematoma was recognized as an extraplacental area with increased transonicity (Figs. 13 and 14), and the relatively low percentage of cases (50%) in which hematoma was detected probably depends on the amount of blood lost and retained in the uterine cavity.

In two patients in which a selective abortion was made the day after CVS because a male fetus at risk for X-linked disease was diagnosed, blood clots of about 1.0×0.5×0.5 ml were present in the material evacuated, and apparently localized in the margin of placenta, but were not visualized during the sonographic control preceding abortion. The inability of sonography to demonstrate very small fresh clots does not seem a real clinical shortcoming. In fact, in the cases in which bleeding was apparently not related to abnormal sonographic features, a normal outcome of pregnancy was always observed. Moreover, in the cases with postsampling intrauterine hematoma, it was still useful to exclude the abruption of the placenta and, by evaluating its volume, to formulate a prognosis. With regard to this, when an approximate evaluation of the

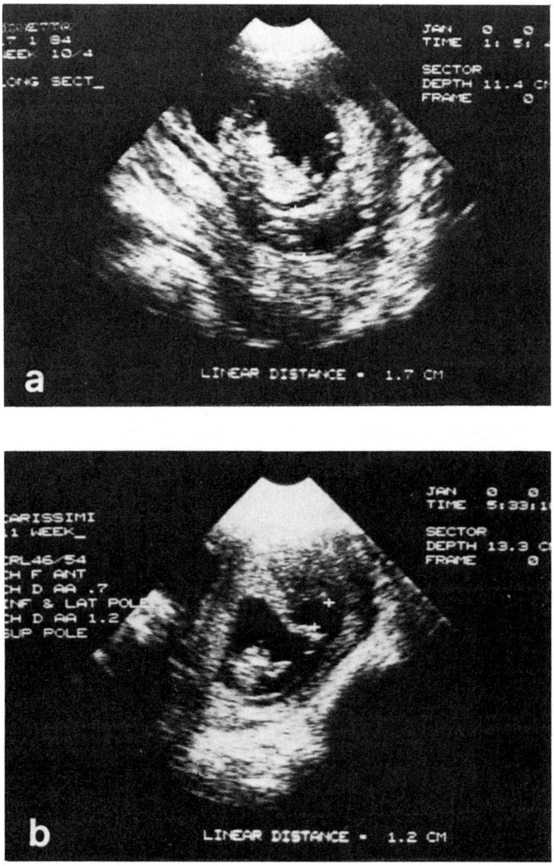

Figure 14 Hematomas observed 1 hr after CVS. (a) Large intrauterine hematoma of the anterior wall and inferior pole, maximum width 17 mm (probable volume 20 ml) in a pregnancy at 10 weeks. (b) Intrauterine hematoma of the posterior wall and superior pole, maximum width 24 mm (probable volume 12 ml) in a pregnancy at 11 weeks. Part of the clot is still fluid and dropping to the inferior pole.

hematoma volume was attempted, it was always found to be far lower than 60 ml, which should be considered a bad prognostic factor for the progress of pregnancy (10). Moreover, retrospectively, we observed that all the cases in which hematoma was present, characterized by a thickness ranging from 3 to 24 mm, no maternal or fetal complications were seen in the course of pregnancy. Thus, while awaiting more extensive data and looking for a more precise sonographic evaluation of the hematoma volume and a better characterization of the vaginal bleeding and intrauterine nonechogenic area, we would like to point out the usefulness of our criteria for a first clinical approach in monitoring CVS patients.

CONCLUSIONS

No relationship between ovular components studied and either fetal chromosomal disorders or poor gestation evolution were discovered. The crown–rump length and gestational sac abnormal values detected in the two cases with chromosomally abnormal fetuses could be the effect of a measurement error or due to the wide individual biological variations. Moreover, no specific ultrasonic trends characterize the different types of chromosomal anomalies, whose values seem to be randomly distributed within the normal limits. In the case in which fetal loss occurred following CVS and a chromosomally normal fetus was diagnosed, no data were available to consider whether fetal loss was a spontaneous or induced occurrence. Moreover, the individual and serial ultrasonic measurements before and after CVS were constantly normal. The unusually large yolk sac observed in cases of missed abortion seems to be a specific but late sign of a pregnancy that has already stopped. Moreover, the yolk-sac-like structures observed in the case of blighted ovum were interpreted to be cystic forms and were considered to be part of an amniotic cyst abortus in which embryo, cord, yolk sac, and amnion are absent and one or more cystic structures are attached to the inner surface of the chorionic membrane (11).

From this experience, it could be concluded that ultrasound investigation in the first trimester of pregnancy is unable to anticipate the clinical outcome. In addition, normal ultrasonic findings cannot rule out the possibility of a chromosomal fetal abnormality or adverse pregnancy evolution. The apparently low prognostic value of ultrasound could be related to the high biological diversification of the pathological events in early pregnancy. Therefore, more extensive study is necessary to give significant data on ultrasonic capability for assessing abnormal ovular features. In this respect, a strict and intensive sonographic protocol for monitoring the pregnancies entering a CVS study is obligatory to guarantee a reliable investigation. Fetal heart activity and fetal movements, if accurately detected, should also be studied to evaluate their predictive value. Additionally, the combined use of ultrasound and biochemical parameters, namely, the pregnancy-associated plasma protein A, could provide a higher efficacy in detecting and understanding abnormal conditions (12).

ACKNOWLEDGMENT

This research was supported by a grant from the Associazione Italiana per lo Studio, la Prevenzione e la Terapia delle Malformazioni, Milan, Italy.

REFERENCES

1. Nelson, P., Bowie, J. D., and Rosenberg, E. R. (1983). Early intrauterine pregnancy or decidual cast: An anatomic–sonographic approach. *J. Ultra sound Med.* *2*:543 547.
2. Robinson, H. P. (1975). Gestation sac volumes as determined by sonar in the first trimester of pregnancy. *Br. J. Obstet. Gynaecol.* *82*:100–107.
3. Robinson, H. P. and Fleming, J. E. E. (1975). A critical evaluation of sonar crown–rump length measurements. *Br. J. Obstet. Gynaecol.* *82*:702–710.
4. WHO, Working Group on First Trimester Fetal Diagnosis of Hereditary Diseases (1984). Geneva, 2–4 May 1984.
5. Brambati, B., Simoni, G., Danesino, C., Oldrini, A., Ferrazzi, E., Romitti, L., Terzoli, G. L., Rossella, F., Ferrari, M., and Fraccaro, M. (1985). First trimester fetal diagnosis of genetic disorders. Clinical evaluation of 250 cases. *J. Med. Genet.* *22*:92–99.
6. Hobbins, J. C. and Winsberg, F. (1977). *Ultrasonography in Obstetrics and Gynecology*. pp. 1–174. Williams and Wilkins, Baltimore.
7. Brambati, B., Oldrini, A., Simoni, G., Terzoli, G. L., Romitti, L., Rossella, F., and Ferrari, M. (1984). First trimester fetal karyotyping in twin pregnancy. *J. Med. Genet.* *21*:58–60.
8. Buhner, M. G. (1960). The twinning rate in Europe and Africa. *Ann. Hum. Genet.* *24*:121–125.
9. Landy, H. J., Keith, L., and Keith, D. (1982). The vanishing twin. *Acta Genet. Med. Gemellol.* *31*:179–194.
10. Mantoni, M. and Perdersen, J. F. (1981). Ultrasound visualization of

intrauterine hematoma in threatened abortion. In *Recent Advances in Ultrasound Diagnosis*, A. Kuryak and A. Kratochwil (eds.), pp. 139–143. Excerpta Medica, Amsterdam.

11. Fantel, A. G., Shepard, T. H., Vadheim-Roth, C., Stephens, T. D., and Coleman, C. (1980). Embryonic and fetal phenotypes:Prevalence and other associated factors in a large study of spontaneous abortion. In *Human Embryonic and Fetal Death*, I. H. Porter and E. B. Hook (eds.), pp. 71–87. Academic Press, New York.
12. Westergaard, J. G., Sinosich, M. J., Bugge, M., Madsen, L. T., Teisner, B., and Grudzinskas, J. G. (1983). Pregnancy-associated plasma protein A in the prediction of early pregnancy failure. *Am. J. Obstet. Ginecol. 145*:67–69.

5

Methods of Chorionic Villus Sampling

BRUNO BRAMBATI and ANGELO OLDRINI*
First Institute of Obstetrics and Gynecology, University of Milan, Milan, Italy

Fetal diagnosis of genetic diseases in the first trimester requires obtaining new ovular tissue to analyze using appropriate sampling techniques. In fact, the traditional second-trimester diagnostic approach requiring amniotic fluid aspiration would be unsuitable in the first trimester for obvious reasons. First, in the earlier stages of pregnancy, the number of viable cells per milliliter of fluid is markedly reduced, and the total volume of amniotic fluid available is very limited (1). Second, until the twelfth week, a consistent extra-amniotic space (the extraembryonic coelom) still surrounds the amniotic sac, making aspiration of amniotic fluid through the amniotic membrane both unreliable and unsafe for fetal integrity. The chorionic villus was thought to be a suitable structure for sampling, being situated outside the gestational sac and having the same genetic characteristics as the fetus. Also, it could easily be attained by way of the cervical canal.

Owing to the poor resolution of ultrasonic apparatus available in the early 1970s, chorionic villus sampling (CVS) utilized direct endoscopic visualization.

Present affiliation: Third Institute of Obstetrics and Gynecology, University of Milan, Milan, Italy

HISTORY OF CHORIONIC VILLUS SAMPLING

Kullander and Sandhal, in 1973 (2), and Hahnemann, in 1974 (3), were the first to present experiences of chorionic tissue sampling in patients (before elective abortions) as an alternative to transabdominal amniocentesis. In both cases, a large endoscopic system was introduced into the uterine cavity through the cervical canal in order to select the biopsy site. Kullander and Sandhal (2) took chorionic tissue with biopsy forceps under direct visual control, while in Hahnemann's procedure (3), the optic lens was removed and the tissues selected, sucked, and then biopsied with a cylindrical knife. Although chorion was obtained in a very high percentage of cases, chromosome analysis was only successful in a small number of cultures (Table 1). In addition, some major complications, such as gestational sac perforation and acute infection, occurred, advising against the diagnostic application of the method. By this time, amniocentesis in the second trimester was demonstrated to be a highly safe and reliable procedure and was gaining world-wide usage.

In 1975, a Chinese group (4) described a blind aspiration technique of chorionic tissue sampling, for sex prediction in 100 pregnancies between the sixth and the fourteenth week . The apparatus consisted of a rigid metal cannula with an outer diameter of 3 mm and a thinner blunt internal tube 1 cm longer than the cannula. The cannula was inserted 6 to 9 cm from the external cervical os and stopped when a soft resistance was felt. The inner tube was then advanced 0.5–1.0 cm, and aspiration used a 5-ml syringe. Slight postprocedural bleeding was seen in six cases the day of the procedure or for a few days after, and in four of the 70 pregnancies intending to continue, fetal loss was observed. In three cases, the fetal loss was reported 20 to 40 days after CVS. In the fourth case, amniotic fluid was aspirated at sampling and a spontaneous abortion occurred 4 days later. Sixty-six patients delivered at term without maternal or fetal complications. The high efficiency and the very limited fetal hazard reported by the Chinese stimulated European groups to reevaluate the practicability of the transcervical approach. Technical innovations, such as miniaturized endoscopic systems and improved ultrasonic resolution, convinced researchers that the limitations reported in the previous Scandiavian experience could be resolved.

In 1982, Kazy et al. (5) reported experiences of chorion biopsy in 165 cases from the Soviet Union. In 100 cases, abortion was induced immediately after sampling: in 39 cases 5 – 10 days later; while in 26 patients, the biopsy was attempted for genetic reasons, and 13 of them

Table 1 Timetable of CVS Research and Technical Specifications

References	Sampling route	Sampling method	Cases (N)	Success rate(%)	Weight of the specimen (mg)	Complications
2	Transcervical	Endoscope and biopsy forceps	39	100	Not reported	Two infections
3	Transcervical	Endoscope and biopsy forceps	50	94	Not reported	Ovular sac perforations (8%)
4	Transcervical	Metallic cannula blind aspiration	100	100	Not reported	Three ovular sac perforations
5	Transcervical	Endoscope and biopsy forceps	55	100		None
		Ultrasound and biopsy forceps	110	100	10–25 mg	
7	Transcervical	Ultrasound and plastic catheter	66	66	10–75 μg DNA	One infection
8,9	Transcervical	Endoscope and biopsy forceps	13	100	2–5 μg DNA	None
		Ultrasound and silver cannula	40	90	10–30 mg	None
11	Transcervical	Endoscope and biopsy forceps	42	100	7–10 μg DNA	None
		Ultrasound and biopsy forceps	30	100	5–40 μg DNA	None
6	Transcervical	Plastic cannula blind aspiration	82	40	26–876 mg	Three ovular sac perforations
13	Transabdominal	Ultrasound and spinal needle	80	87	15–45 mg	None

had a selective abortion. Sonographic or endoscopic visualization of the placenta insertion preceded the sampling with a biopsy forceps. No maternal or ovular complications were observed, and of the 13 patients intending to continue their pregnancies, 11 delivered normal babies and the 2 others were progressing normally. The weight of chorionic specimens ranged between 10 and 25 mg. No comparisons of the efficiency of the two methods were made.

A blind transcervical approach was used in 82 patients by Howell et al. (6) in 1983 using a 16-gauge intravenous cannula attached to a 20-ml syringe. Chorionic villi were obtained from 40% of cases, and the weight of specimens seems largely to exceed the diagnostic needs, with a mean value of 190 mg and a range of 26 to 876 mg. Perforation of the gestational sac was observed in two cases during the first attempt and in one case during the second attempt.

A second British group (7) developed a new aspiration method consisting of the introduction of a very thin catheter into the uterine cavity through the cervical canal under continuous ultrasonic monitoring. An aluminum stylet assured that the system was both easily formed to the required shape and easily visualized for a safe and accurate positioning. In a series of 66 cases, a mean value of 66% successful sampling was obtained, which increased to 90% in the last group of 21 patients. One of the seven diagnostic cases included in the last group ended in missed abortion 2 days after CVS. An acute intrauterine infection was suspected as the cause of the fetal loss.

In 1983, Gosden et al. (8) reported a series of 13 experimental cases in which biopsies were taken from villi adjacent to the implantation site by needle aspiration or with biopsy forcepts under direct endoscopic vision. The endoscopic system, consisting in a 2.4×4.0 mm cannula housing a 2.2 mm fetoscope, was introduced under ultrasound guidance. The instillation of about 20 ml of warmed saline solution improved visualization. In spite of its 100% success rate in obtaining chorionic villi that was uncomtaminated by maternal tissue, this system was judged to be complex and to provide too small an amount of chorionic tissue. Thus, the same group experimented on 40 patients, eight patients for diagnostic reasons, using an aspiration approach consisting of a malleable silver cannula with a standard mucous extractor introduced under ultrasound guidance (9). A 90% sampling success rate with no maternal or fetal complications was observed.

An endoscopic biopsy system was also developed by Kaplan et al. (10). A 4-mm hysteroscope was transcervically introduced, and the uterine cavity was distended with CO_2 injected under low pressure. Biopsies were obtained under direct vision in 42 women before voluntary abortion between 7 and 10 weeks. A 100% success rate with no obstetrical complications was reported. Nevertheless, Goosens et al. (11) replaced this system by a simpler, new one consisting of a thin and rigid biopsy forceps introduced into the uterine cavity under ultrasonic visualization. The same operator should easily be able to handle the ultrasonic transducer to guide the biopsy forceps held by the second hand. This approach was evaluated in 30 women at 7 to 10 weeks immediately before voluntary abortion.

A modification of the direct vision technique was described by Gustavii in 1983 (12). Preliminary studies were done in 33 women about to undergo first-trimester abortion. A special cannula, 3.0×4.7 mm in cross section, housed a 1.7-mm diameter fetoscope and a biopsy forceps. Saline was continuously instilled through the cannula to distend the extra-ovular space and to have a clear view of the ovular surface. The amount of saline needed to distend the uterine cavity properly was about 150 ml, corresponding to 15–20 mm Hg. The endoscopic system was directed to the site where the ovular sac merges with the uterine wall. A piece of decidua was removed, and the instrument was introduced some centimeters into the placenta, allowing chorionic villi sampling uncontaminated by maternal tissue. This procedure is at present currently used by the author for diagnostic sampling.

The transabdominal assay was used by Smidt-Jensen et al. (13) in 80 women seeking legal abortion. Chorionic villi were aspirated in 70 of them, and the amount of chorionic tissue ranged from 15 to 45 mg. No signs of fetal wastage or placental damage were observed, and the preferred biopsy time was the ninth and tenth week of pregnancy. Using a linear ultrasound scanning head with a biopsy guide, a 1.2-mm guide needle was introduced to the outer limit of the placental echoes. Chorionic villi were aspirated with a 10-ml syringe attached to a thinner 0.7 mm needle, the tip of which penetrated into the thickness of the placenta. To obtain an adequate amount of chorionic tissue, the aspirating needle had to be introduced several times.

The practicality of four different sampling methods was evaluated by Simoni et al. (14) in 372 patients requiring legal abortion between 6 and 12 weeks. They compared the samplings obtained in 62 cases under direct endoscopic vision with a biopsy forceps; in 159 and 48 cases by a blind aspiration approach using two different cannulae, respectively; in 103 cases by the aspiration of chorionic tissue guided by ultrasound. In the first series, a multiple rod-lens Storz endoscope 2.4 mm in diameter and a 1.0-mm biopsy forceps housed in a cannula with a 3.3×4.7 mm cross section were used. In the second and third series, blind aspiration was attempted with a plastic intravenous cannula (Abbot-T 14G) 6.35 cm long and a flexible polyethylene catheter (Portex Ltd., England) 15.40 cm long and 1.5 mm in diameter with a solid and bendable aluminium obturator, respectively. In the fourth series, the same catheter as in the third series was introduced through the cervical canal under direct ultrasonic visualization. In the first three series, a sampling success rate of 64 to 76% was achieved, whereas with ultrasound guidance the success was nearly 100%, and in 80% of cases adequate tissue was obtained at the first attempt. Both blind sampling aspiration approaches were characterized by a high failure rate and were associated with ovular sac perforations. The endoscopic technique appeared to be a relatively complex and invasive technique providing a very limited amount of chorionic tissue (Table 2). A series of considerations, such as the very reduced diameter and the good echogenicity of the cannula, the possibility of fashioning the system to the desired shape allowing anatomy to be respected, and the simplicity and the high degree of efficacy, made the ultrasonic-guided aspiration method suitable for diagnostic sampling.

These conclusions were formulated in general agreement with the Ward's group experience (7). At nearly the same time, the University College Hospital group of London and Mangiagalli group of Milan were able to communicate their success in first-trimester diagnosis of hemoglobinopathies and chromosomal disorders, respectively (15,16).

Table 2 Successful Sampling Rate and Complications of Four Procedures[a]

	Cases (N)	Successful sampling (%)	Average weight of the sample (mg)	Ovular sac perforation
Series I	62	76	3	None
Series II	159	64	40	4
Series III	48	66	20	1
Series IV	103	96	25	None

[a]Series I, endoscope and biopsy forceps; Series II, blind aspiration by an intravenous cannula; Series III, blind aspiration by the Portex catheter; Series IV, Portex catheter guided by ultrasound.

Two others groups, at Jefferson University in Philadelphia (17) and at Reese Medical Center in Chicago (18), using the same sampling procedure as the two previous groups, reported shortly afterward on the feasibility of CVS for diagnosis in Tay-Sachs disease. Thus, first-trimester fetal diagnosis of genetic diseases became a real alternative to the second-trimester diagnostic methods (Table 3).

To date, four main methodological approaches to CVS are being used for diagnostic purposes (Fig. 1). In three of these methods, placenta is reached through the cervical canal and sampling is performed by aspiration with a flexible catheter under ultrasonic guidance (Fig. 1a), a rigid biopsy forceps guided by ultrasound (Fig. 1b), and a biopsy forceps under direct endoscopic vision (Fig. 1d), respectively. The fourth approach is transabdominal, and chorionic tissue is aspirated by a stainless steel needle guided by ultrasound (Fig. 1c). More than 80% of the world's diagnostic activity is performed with transcervical aspiration device, and the Portex system is the most common one in use to day. However, variations of the Ward–Brambati approach using different plastic or metallic catheters are being reported (Table 4).

Table 3 Approaches to Fetal Diagnosis

1. Amniocentesis
   a. Chromosomal disorders
   b. Metabolic disorders
   c. X-linked diseases
   d. Neural tube defects
2. Fetoscopy
   a. Visualization of structural abnormalities
   b. Fetal tissues biopsy
   c. Fetal blood sampling
3. Ultrasound
   a. Major structural defects
   b. Multiple pregnancy, fetal age, fetal growth, amniotic fluid volume
4. MS-AFP Screening
   a. Neural tube defects
5. Chorionic Villi Sampling in the First Trimester
   a. Hemoglobinopathies (15)
   b. Chromosomal disorders (16)
   c. Metabolic disorders (17, 18)

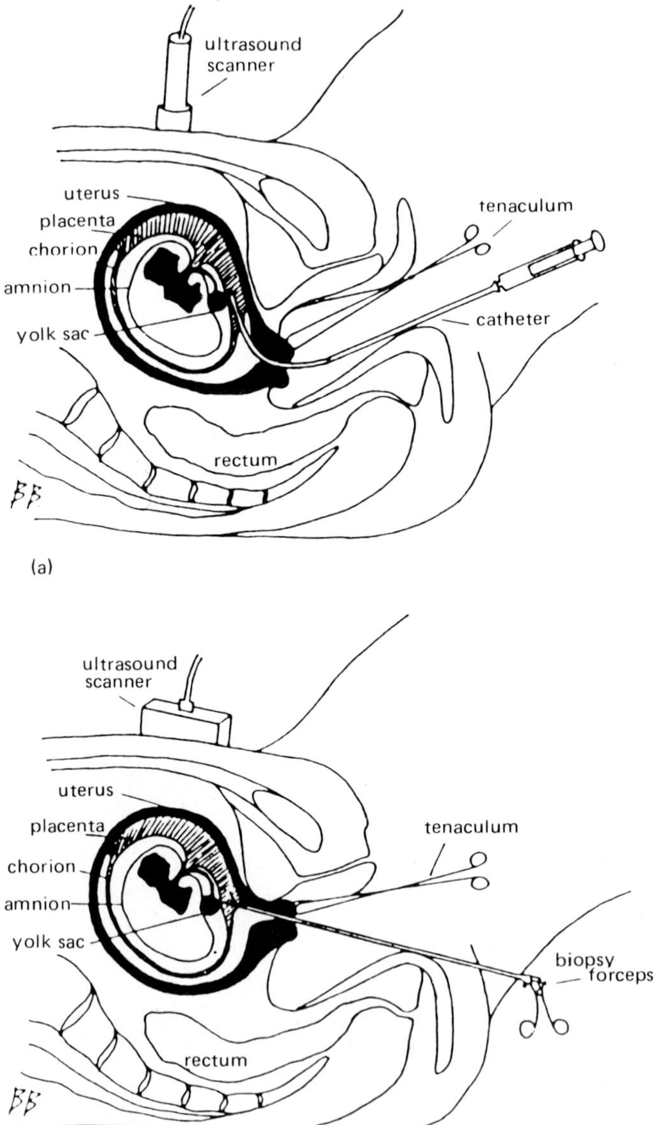

Figure 1 Chorionic villus sampling methods used in the diagnostic routine: (a) Ultrasound and plastic catheter. (b) Ultrasound and biopsy forceps. (c) Ultrasound and transabdominal needle aspiration. (d) Endoscopy and biopsy forceps.

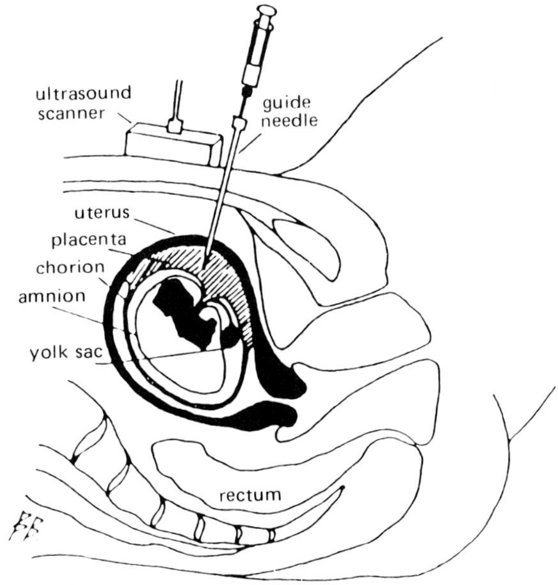
ultrasound
scanner
guide
needle
uterus
placenta
chorion
amnion
yolk sac
rectum

(c)

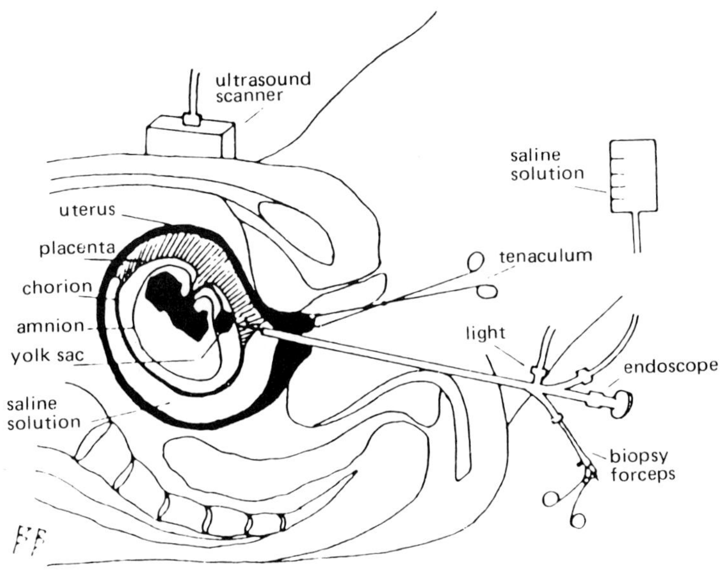
ultrasound
scanner
saline
solution
uterus
placenta
chorion
amnion
yolk sac
saline
solution
tenaculum
light
endoscope
biopsy
forceps

(d)

Table 4 The Main Chorionic Villi Sampling Procedures

Method	Sampling route	Sampling system	Diagnostic center
Biopsy forceps and endoscope	Transcervical	1.7-mm Endoscope in 3.0×4.7-mm cannula	Lund, Sweden
Biopsy forceps and ultrasound	Transcervical	2.0—2.4-mm Rigid biopsy forceps	Port Royal, Paris, France
Aspiration and ultrasound	Transabdominal	0.7-mm Needle in 1.2-mm guide needle	Aalborg, Denmark
	Transcervical	1.9-mm Polyethylene catheter and steel stylet	Yale University, New Haven, Connecticut
		1.5-mm Polyethylene catheter and steel stylet	Karolinska Institutet, Stockholm, Sweden
		3.0-mm Nylon catheter and steel stylet	Royal Victoria Hospital, Montreal, Canada
		1.6-mm Malleable silver cannula and steel stylet	King's Cross Hospital, London
		3.5-mm Polyethylene catheter and steel stylet	University of Szeged, Hungary
		1.45-mm Polyethylene catheter and bendable steel stylet	Mangiagalli Institute, Milan, Third Obstetrical Institute, Milan, Gaslini Institute, Genoa, Université Libre, Brussels, Belgium, Erasmus University, Rotterdam, Kennedy Institute, Copenhagen, University College Hospital, London, Jefferson University, Philadelphia, M. Reese Medical Center, Chicago, San Francisco, Athens,

METHODS AND TECHNIQUES FOR CHORIONIC VILLUS SAMPLING

Indications and Counseling

Although CVS has passed the initial stages of research, it clearly remains at an applied research phase, since we must have more extensive data in order to estimate diagnostic accuracy and sampling safety. This raises the important issue of the responsibility of the medical center in providing an adequately informed consent, emphasizing the possible risks involved in such recent technologies. The new diagnostic method should be offered to the highest-risk group of pregnant women, the characteristics of which depend on the sociocultural rules of each community. We decided to start offering the new test to pregnant women who (a) were 40 years old or more, (b) had a previous abnormal child, (c) were a carrier of X-linked diseases, (d) were at risk for autosomic recessive diseases, or (e) were seeking fetal diagnosis but did not accept the perspective of a second-trimester termination.

Ultrasound Equipment and Pregnancy Control

The smallness and location of the anatomical structures involved in CVS and the very thin aspiration device require sonographic apparatus with high-resolution and sector scanning characteristics. Sonographic control is a necessary tool for verifying the actual conditions of ovular development and for controlling the possible effects of the sampling procedure on uterine content integrity. For this purpose, a sonographic programme should be established before, during, and after CVS, including the investigation of fetal malformations and abnormal intrauterine growth later in pregnancy.

At the time of genetic counseling, generally 1 or 2 weeks before CVS, ultrasound evaluation of the uterine cavity should allow CVS to be scheduled for the most appropriate time and for incidental anomalies to be monitored. Missed abortion or blighted ovum was diagnosed in 15 to 20% of the patients asking for CVS between the sixth and the eightth week. Sonographic control at the time of sampling is necessary to confirm the viability of the pregnancy and to guarantee safe and reliable sampling. Ten to 15 days after sampling, a routine examination should monitor the early possible effects of the procedure, such as fetal demise and hematomas. Finally, neural tube defects and other major fetal abnormalities should be detected from 18 to 22 weeks, while fetal growth should be confirmed at 32–34 weeks. α-Fetoprotein (AFP) evaluation in maternal serum at 16–18 weeks would give further information about the risk of fetal abnormalities and/or poor intrauterine development.

Timing of CVS

The ninth and tenth gestational weeks are generally considered the most suitable for obtaining placental biopsies. Indeed, before the ninth week, the identification of the placental site frequently appears uncertain since the reduced thickness of the placenta cannot be differentiated from the strong echogenicity of the decidual hypertrophic tissue that surrounds the ovular sac together with the chorion laeve. Moreover, the umbilical cord insertion at this stage of pregnancy can rarely be identified. However, the identification of the endometrial canal, visible until 8–9 weeks as an elongated and thin space at increased transonicity, could help in the correct evaluation of the placental site. As the pregnancy advances, the gestational sac increases in size, occupying a greater proportion of the uterine cavity, and, from the tenth week, the decidua basalis and capsularis are generally fused. Therefore, late in the third month, it could be more difficult to separate the uterine wall from the ovular sac to attain placenta without increasing the risk of damaging membranes.

Chorionic Villus Sampling Room and Equipment

The operating room contains a visiting table and facilities for scrubbing. There is a sector scan machine (ATL MK I 300) with a 5-MHz transducer and a video tape recorder. An inverted microscope allows the immediate identification of the tissue sampled and the initial processing of the chorionic tissue. The sampling catheter used for experimental training and during the first half of the diagnostic activity consists of a soft polyethylene cannula, 1.5 mm in diameter and a 15.7 cm long, with a solid bendable aluminium obturator (Portex Ltd., England). More recently, a new Portex catheter, 21 cm long and 1.45 mm in diameter with a soft stainless steel obturator was introduced (Fig. 2). This catheter is still under development. The instrumentation for sampling includes a single toothed tenaculum, two sponge forceps, two 30-ml syringes with 4 ml of Hank's saline balanced solution with 1 mg/ml eparine, a Grave's speculum, a hysterometer, and one Portex catheter (Fig.3). The CVS team consists of one ultrasonographer, one sampler, and one operator for the microscopic identification of the sample.

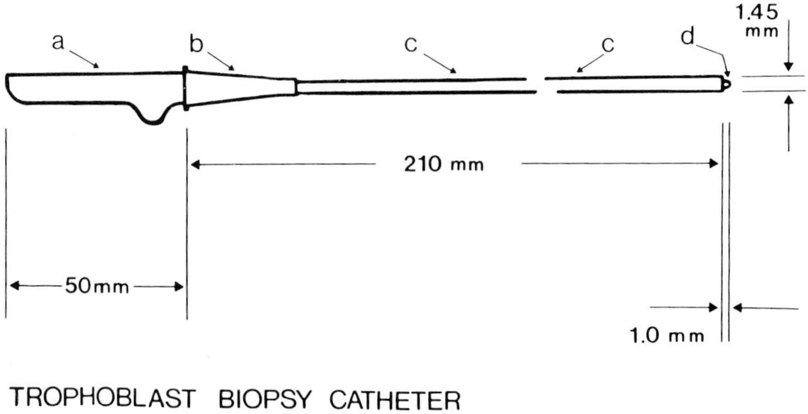

Figure 2 Technical characteristics of the aspiration system presently used at Mangiagalli Clinic of Milan (Portex, Ltd., England). a, handle; b, female leuer mount; c, catheter; d, stylet.

Technique for Chorionic Villus Sampling

Chorionic Villus Sampling is an outpatient procedure and does not require any preoperative preparation or postoperative care of the patient. It is necessary to have a strict protocol in the research phase to ensure reliable data collection by a stable working system. The first step of the procedure is an accurate sonographic study of the uterine content with the patient lying in a supine position with a partially empty bladder. The aim of the ultrasonic examination is to obtain ovular measurements and to recognize placental insertion with the help of the umbilical cord insertion. Then the patient is placed in the lithotomy position, and after an external genitalia toilet, the cervix is visualized with a speculum. The cervix and the vaginal fornix are cleaned with a broad spectrum antiseptic solution (Betadine solution), and the anterior lip of the cervix is grasped with a tenaculum. A swab is taken from the cervical external os to provide information about bacterial contamination. The use of the hysterometer with a rounded tip of about 3 mm allows painless, nontraumatic exploration of the cervical canal and allows the internal os to be fixed on the sonographic display (Fig. 4). Moreover, by means of this instrument, the uncontrolled movements that could be produced in evaluating a suitable way to get to the placenta should not threaten the membrane's

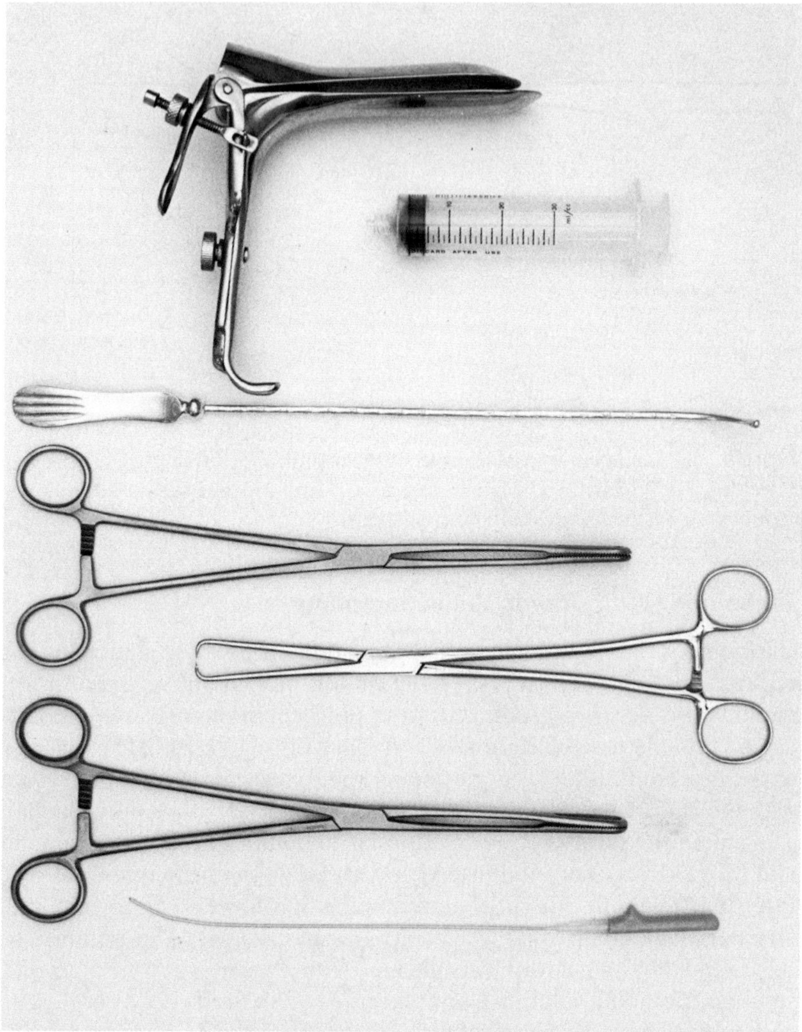

Figure 3 Instruments used for CVS. From top to bottom: Grave's speculum, 30-ml leuer-lock syringe, Portex catheter, sponge forceps, tenaculum, sponge forceps, and an hysterometer.

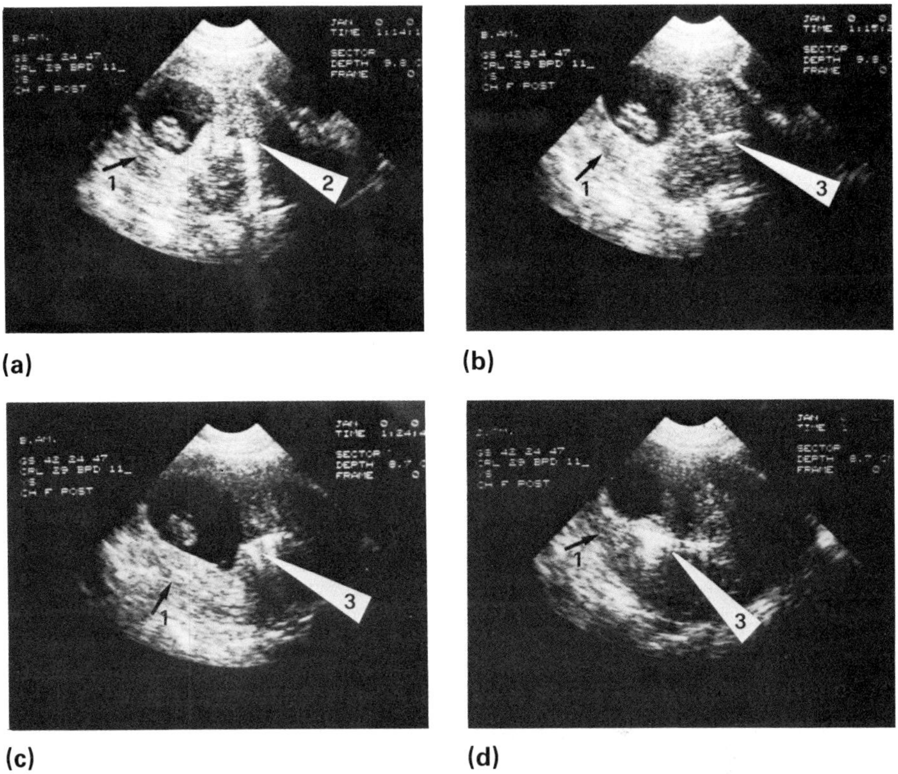

Figure 4 Sonographic control of CVS procedure: (a) The internal os is localized by the extremity of the hysterometer (arrow). (b) The aspiration device is stopped at the level of the internal os (arrow). (c) The catheter is pushed in a wrong direction threatening the gestational sac. (d) The extremity of the catheter is positioned next to the chorionic plate. 1, placenta; 2, hysterometer; 3, catheter.

integrity. The ultrasonographer should maintain the transducer steady on the longitudinal plane containing the internal os, awaiting the introduction of the catheter. The catheter is suitably curved following the angle between the placenta and the cervical canal. The catheter is slowly inserted through the cervical canal and stopped at the level of the internal os. From this point, any further movement should only be undertaken under continuous sonographic visualization to avoid damaging the ovular sac. The end of the catheter should deeply enter into the placenta to be positioned next to the chorionic plate. The obturator is then removed, and a 30-ml syringe containing Hank's medium with eparine is attached. The withdrawal of the obturator, carefully controlled on the sonographic display, should take place without disturbing the end of the catheter. The maneuver can be correctly executed by firmly fixing the hand holding the leuer mount of the catheter to the speculum. Five to 10 ml of negative pressure is applied one to three times, slowly removing the tip from the original site. Finally, the entire system is withdrawn under partial negative pressure. The contents of the syringe is immediately flushed into a 100-mm plastic petri dish containing about 10 ml of RPM-I medium without serum and examined under the inverted microscope for the presence of villous material.

Chorionic Villus Sampling Procedural Problems

In our experience, the sampling technique previously described gave a sampling success rate of 97–98% on more than 300 cases. This could be increased to nearly a 100% by careful patient selection. In fact, in most of the unsuccessful samplings, the failure to obtain chorionic tissue was probably a consequence of unsuitable anatomical conditions for this procedure. When the pregnancy is less than 8 weeks, the placental tissue can scarcely be outlined making CVS unreliable. Moreover, in cases of a retroflected or anteflected uterus, in which the angle between the cervical axis and the intrauterine canal to the placenta is unusually pronounced, the catheter cannot be adequately bent to reach the placenta without risk of ovular sac damage. Generally, to reduce the inconvenience of failing to obtain chorionic tissue because the placental site is not well characterized and clear identification of the cord insertion is not feasible, it seems appropriate to limit the sampling to the ninth and tenth week, or at least to delay the procedure for 1 or 2 weeks.

In cases in which the catheter cannot be curved to the shape needed to reach the sampling site, a transabdominal aspiration can be used as an alternative technique. In our experience, a 20-gauge spinal needle can be

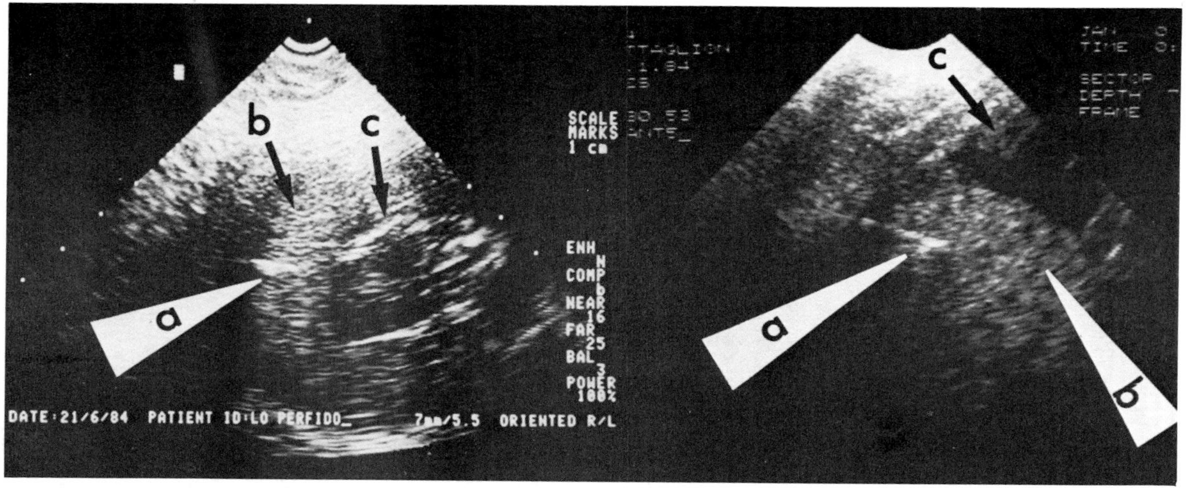

Figure 5 Chorionic villus sampling by transabdominal aspiration in two cases at 11 weeks. The 20-gauge spinal needle is clearly visible in the thickness of the placenta. a, Needle extremity; b, placenta; c, gestational sac.

introduced under ultrasound guidance, and chorionic tissue can be aspirated by exerting a vacuum of about 10 ml Hg with a 30-ml syringe (Fig. 5). Chorionic tissue was successfully aspirated in six cases at the first attempt. In another case, the puncture had to be repeated. The weight of chorionic villi ranged from 2 to 5 mg. The needle was introduced a short distance from a 5-MHz sector scan transducer, and the path of the needle was easily visualized. The very limited amount of tissue obtainable can be inadequate for specific studies and is barely sufficient for cytogenetic analysis. Hahnemann's approach (13) using a 1.2-mm guide needle allows several aspirations with a thinner needle and should prevent this problem, but it produces some uncertainty because of the unusual large diameter of the guide needle fixed into the uterine wall.

A second alternative procedure to consider is the transcervical use of a thin but rigid device such as biopsy forceps or a metallic cannula. In fact, the cervical–uterine angle could be significantly modified by a rigid instrument, and the placenta can then be easily reached. In two of our cases in which the bowels were covering the uterus, the latter approach was chosen and successfully used. (Fig. 6).

The discovery of twins with fused placentas at the time of CVS can complicate the obstetrical procedure (19). In order to ensure high reliability in pure tissue sampling from both twins, it is necessary to detect the umbilical cord insertion of each fetus and to guide the tip of the catheter into the proximity of the insertion point. If this precaution cannot be taken, there is a consistent probability of diagnosing only one twin, a situation that must be discussed with the patient before proceeding.

COMPLICATIONS FOLLOWING CVS

Although a fetal loss rate of 3.3% was roughly estimated by considering the first 500 cases, 269 of which were in progress, the follow-up of the first 200 cases in which the pregnancy was intended to continue gave a corrected rate of 5% (Table 5). Nevertheless, a randomized control study on an adequate number of cases must be carried out in order to produce meaningful risk data (21). A direct relationship between the sampling procedure and fetal loss can be postulated in only one out of the ten cases observed (Table 5). In this case, bleeding and uterine contractions were present on the third day after CVS, and a complete abortion took place on the tenth day (20). Furthermore, no particular patterns can be recognized in the distribution of fetal losses according to the time elapsed

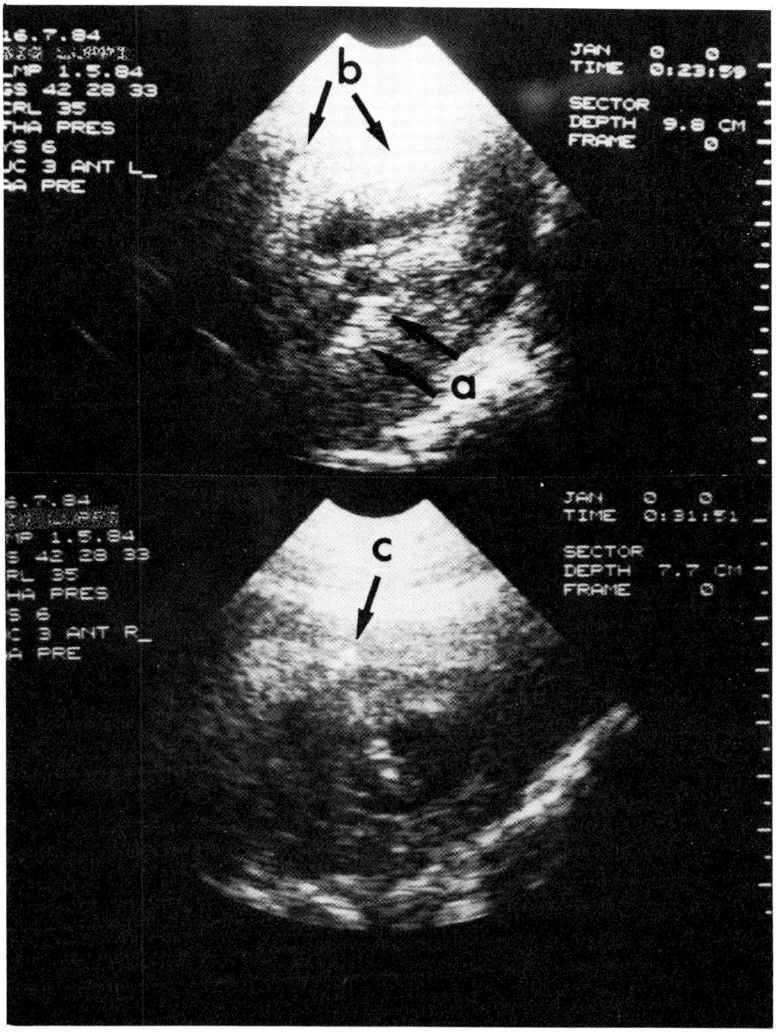

Figure 6 Chorionic villus sampling by biopsy forceps (tip 2.4 mm in diameter) in a case at 10 weeks. a, Cervical canal direction outlined by the hysterometer; b, placental site; c, tip of the biopsy forceps.

Table 5 Clinical Outcome of the First 200 Completed Pregnancies after CVS

Outcome	Number	
Twin pregnancies	3	
Failed sampling	5	
Repeated sampling	1	
Amniocentesis	6	
Fetal losses		
After 1 to 2 weeks	5	
After 3 to 6 weeks	2	(5.0%)
After 10 weeks	3	
Amniotic fluid leakage	4	
Bleeding before CVS	8	
Bleeding after CVS	40	(20%)
Intrauterine growth rate (weight < 10th percentile)	12	(6.0%)
Placenta previa	1	
Abruptio placentae	1	
Premature delivery	10	(5.0%)
Preeclampsia	4	
Essential hypertension	4	
Diabetes	2	
Malformations		
Major	1	
Minor	3	
ABO immunization	3	

Source: Data from the Mangiagalli Clinic of Milan.

after CVS, although 7 of 14 cases occurred in the 3 weeks following sampling (Fig. 7).

No acute infections could be detected in our experience, and, in the literature, there were only a very small number of cases in which fever, fetal demise, and/or spontaneous abortion were observed in the first days. These were a probable consequence of bacterial invasion following the introduction of the catheter (7 and L. Marsk, personal communica-

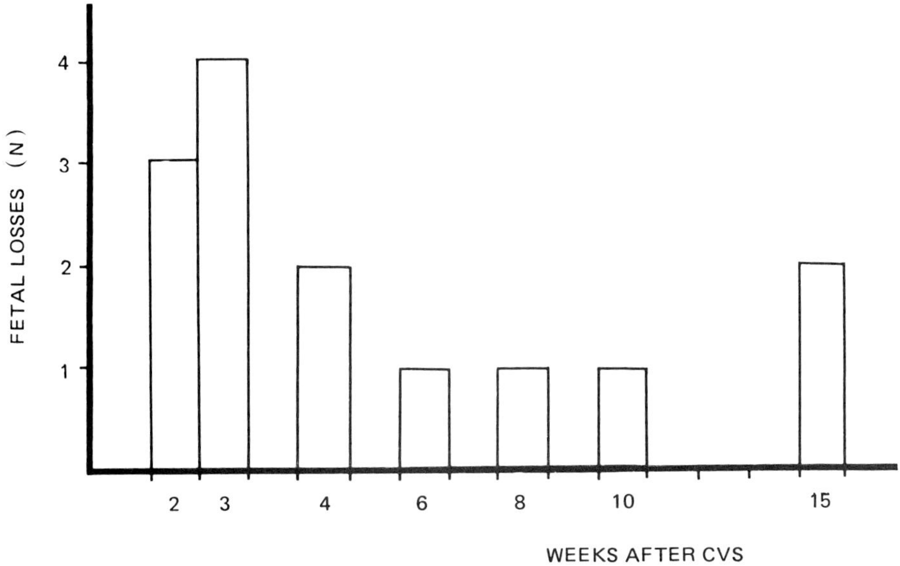

Figure 7 Number of fetal losses at each week of gestation after CVS.

tion). Another case of intrauterine infection in a patient with cervicitis was diagnosed some days after CVS and was successfully treated. The pregnancy progressed normally (E. Pergament, personal communication). Since acute intrauterine infection seems a very limited adverse consequence, bacterial transfer to the uterine cavity could play an unforeseen etiological role in later complications, including in utero fetal death.

Gestational sac perforation was rarely observed and was attributed to poor sonographic visualization of the catheter (B. Modell, personal communication). What probably happens is that an indentation of the chorion by the end of the catheter could cause a stripping of the membrane. The amnion could herniate through, with the possibility of a spontaneous rupture. Therefore, CVS can be implicated in the amniotic fluid leakage reported in four of our cases (Table 5), although there were no technical difficulties during sampling, and threatened abortion or premature labor were observed before the leakage.

The slight or moderate bleeding that occurred in 20% of cases (Table 5) during the days immediately following CVS was frequently undetectable by ultrasound and never threatened pregnancy development. Thus, it should be judged to be a harmless effect of the decidual trauma and/or placenta perforation.

Considering the clinical evidence for the first 200 completed pregnancies, no adverse findings ascribable to CVS could be ascertained in the mother and the fetus (Table 5). The premature delivery rate, the number of small-for-date babies, and maternal complications (such as preeclampsia and hypertension) do not exceed the expected figures (22), especially considering maternal age (75% of patients were 35 years old or more) and clinical characteristics. The three cases of first ABO isoimmunization in the third trimester lead us to consider feto-maternal transfusiuon to be a consequence of CVS. This possibility was demonstrated by a significant increase in the α-fetoprotein level in maternal serum after CVS in a consistent proportion of cases. A correlation with the weight of the specimen aspirated could also be demonstrated (B. Brambati, unpublished data).

CONTRAINDICATIONS TO CHORIONIC VILLUS SAMPLING

An absolute contraindication to CVS is a patient with an Rh isoimmunization because fetal bleeding in the maternal circulation could be sufficient to stimulate the maternal immunoresponse, worsening the prognosis of the pregnancy in the presence of a feto-maternal incompatibility. In the case of a Rh-negative woman at risk for Rh isoimmunization, 50 μg of immunoglobulins should be given.

Clinically evident vaginal infections should be specifically treated and, together with vaginal bleeding, are indications for deferring the sampling procedure.

Finally, a twin pregnancy with fused placentas should be a contraindication to CVS whenever the umbilical cord insertions are not identified.

REQUIREMENTS IN ESTABLISHING A CHORIONIC VILLUS SAMPLING PROGRAM

Having decided to mount a CVS program two major considerations have to be pointed out: (a) Personnel requirements: prior experience of the obstetrical team in ultrasonography and in second-trimester fetal sampling techniques is an advantage in understanding the procedural problems of CVS. Chorionic villus sampling in continuing pregnancies should be performed by physicians who have gained experience and demonstrated sufficient CVS skill with at least 50 women in whom pregnancy was terminated after CVS. Moreover, it would be expected that acquired skills could be maintained with an annual experience of 100 to 200 procedures, either research or diagnostic. Excellent ultrasound facilities should be available for the procedure. The most appropriate apparatus is a sector scan with a 5-MHz transducer. The CVS team must have sonographic expertise in recognizing the intrauterine anatomy of the first trimester. b)Post-operative follow-up: A high success rate in the follow-up has to be assured by an efficient secretarial service. Ultrasound monitoring, a reliable system of controlling selective and spontaneous abortions, and a pediatric checkup at 6 and 12 months are the necessary bases to provide information about CVS effects. Participation in the International Collaborative Study (21) is recommended to monitor international experience and to contribute to a relaible evaluation of the safety and accuracy of this new diagnostic approach.

ACKNOWLEDGMENT

This research was supported by a grant from the Associazione Italiana per lo Studio, la Prevenzione e la Terapia delle Malformazioni, Milan, Italy.

REFERENCES

1. Nelson, M. M. (1973). Antenatal sex determination. In *Antenatal Diagnosis of Genetic Disease*, A. E. H. Emery (ed.), pp. 58–68. Churchill Livingstone, Edinburgh.
2. Kullander, S. and Sandahl, B. (1973). Fetal chromosome analysis after transcervical placental biopsies during early pregnancy. *Acta Obstet. Gynecol. Scand. 52*:355–359.
3. Hahnemann, N. (1974). Early prenatal diagnosis: A study of biopsy techniques and cell culturing from extraembryonic membranes. *Clin. Genet. 6*:294–306.
4. Anshan, Department of Obstetrics and Gynecology, Tietung Hospital of Anshan Iron and Steel Co., Anshan, China (1975). Fetal sex prediction by sex chromatin of chorionic villi cells during early pregnancy. *Chin. Med. J. 1*:117–126.
5. Kazy, Z., Rozovsky, I. S., and Bakharev, V. A. (1982). Chorion biopsy in early pregnancy: A method of early prenatal diagnosis for inherited disorders. *Prenatal Diag. 2*:39–45.
6. Horwell, D. H., Loeffler, F. E., and Coleman, D. V. (1983). Assessment of a transcervical aspiration technique for chorionic villus biopsy in the first trimester of pregnancy. *Br. J. Obstet. Gynaecol. 90*:196–198.

7. Ward, R. H. T., Modell, B., Petrou, M., Karagozlu, F., and Douratsos, E. (1983). A method of chorionic villus sampling in the first trimester of pregnancy under real time ultrasonic guidance. *Br. Med. J. 286*:1542–1544.
8. Gosden, J. R., Mitchell, A. R., Gosden, C. M., Rodeck, C. H., and Morsman, J. M. (1983). Direct vision chorion biopsy and chromosome-specific DNA probes for determination of fetal sex in first trimester prenatal diagnosis. *Lancet ii*:1416:1419.
9. Rodeck, C. H., Morsman, J. M., Nicolaides, K. H., McKenzie, C. M., Gosden, C. M., and Gosden, J. R. (1983). A single-operator technique for first trimester chorion biopsy. *Lancet ii*:1340–1341.
10. Kaplan, L., Dumez, Y., and Goosens, M. (1983). A method for fetal tissue sampling by chorion biopsy: a new approach to first trimester prenatal detection of abnormal genes. *IRCS Med. Sci. 11*:85–86.
11. Goosens, M., Dumez, Y., Kaplan, L., Lupker, M., Chabret, C., Henrion, R., and Rosa, J. (1983). Prenatal diagnosis of sickle cell anemia in the first trimester of pregnancy. *N. Engl. J. Med. 309*:831–833.
12. Gustavii, B. (1983). First trimester chromosomal analysis of chorionic villi obtained by direct vision technique. *Lancet ii*:507–508.
13. Smidt-Jensen, S., Hahnemann, N., Jensen, P. K. A., and Therkelsen, A. J. (1984). Experience with transabdominal fine needle biopsy from chorionic villi in the first trimester—An alternative to amniocentesis. *Nordic Meeting on Medical Genetics*, February 17–19, 1984, Helsinki.
14. Simoni, G., Brambati, B., Danesino, C., Rossella, F., Terzoli, G.L., Ferrari, M., and Fraccaro, M. (1983). Efficient direct chroosome analyses and enzyme determinations from chorionic villi samples in the first trimester of pregnancy. *Human Genet. 63*:349–357.
15. Old, J. M., Ward, R. H. T., Karagozlu, F., Petrou, M., Modell, B., and Weatherall, D. J. (1982). First-trimester fetal diagnosis for haemoglobinopathies: Three cases. *Lancet ii*:1414–1416.
16. Brambati, B. and Simoni, G. (1983). Fetal diagnosis of trisomy 21 in the first trimester of pregnancy. *Lancet i*:586.
17. Grebner, E. E., Wapner, R. J., Barr, M. A., and Jackson, L. (1983). Prenatal Tay-Sachs diagnosis by chorionic villi sampling. *Lancet ii*:286–287.
18. Pergament, E., Ginsburg, N., Verlinsky, Y., Cadkin, A., Chu, A., and Trnka, L. (1983). Prenatal Tay-Sachs diagnosis by chorionic villus sampling. *Lancet ii*:26.
19. Brambati, B., Oldrini, A., Simoni, G., Terzoli, G. L., Romitti, L., Rossella, F., and Ferrari, M. (1984). First trimester fetal karyotyping in twin pregnancy. *J. Med. Genet. 21*:58–60.
20. Brambati, B., Simoni, G., Danesino, C., Oldrini, A., Ferrazzi, E., Romitti, L. Terzoli, G. L., Rossella, F., Ferrari, M., and Fraccaro, M. (1985). First trimester fetal diagnosis of genetic disorders. Clinical evaluation of 250 cases. *J. Med. Genet. 22*:92–99.

21. WHO Working Group on First Trimester Fetal Diagnosis of Hereditary Diseases (1984). Geneva, 2–4 May 1984.
22. Bossi, A., Caccamo, M. L., De Scrilli, A. M., Milani, S. (1980). Weight of the Italian newborn infants (from the 32nd to the 43rd week of gestation). *I. J. Ped.* 6:153–170.

6

Fetal Karyotyping by Direct Chromosome Preparation

GIUSEPPE SIMONI, GIANLUIGI TERZOLI, and LORENZA ROMITTI
First Institute of Obstetrics and Gynecology, University of Milan, Milan, Italy

INTRODUCTION

Through the development of obstetric techniques in obtaining first-trimester chorionic villi specimens, a new kind of fetal material has become available for prenatal diagnosis of genetic diseases. This stimulated investigators to develop, together with the biopsy procedures, diagnostic methods using chorionic villi. Fetal sex prediction by X and Y chromatin assays and trophoblast cell culture procedures for first-trimester fetal karyotyping has been described by several authors (Table 1). Studies on villi sampling and trophoblastic cell culture were reported in the early 1970s (Hahnemann, 1974; Kullander and Sandahl, 1973). However, while chorionic villi were successfully obtained trophoblastic cells showed a low growth potential under culture conditions and failed to grow in culture in nearly half of the samples.

In addition to this problem, the identification and selection of pure fetal material was not easy. It was soon realized that maternal cell contamination is a real problem when using chorionic villi, and this problem is greater than in amniotic fluid cell cultures. These technical difficulties slowed down the development of first-trimester chorionic villi sampling during the next several years. Moreover, the greater ease of performing amniocentesis and the success of amniotic fluid cell culture rapidly induced a wide application of second-trimester diagnosis in many countries. Thus, CVS investigations were confined to experimental purposes and were not used for diagnostic purposes.

Table 1 A Summary of the Experimental Studies of First-Trimester Trophoblast Cultures and Cytogenetic Analysis

References	Sex chromatin assays	Culture success	Direct chromosome analysis	Karyotype (M/F)	Comments
Kullander and Sandahl (1973)	—	20/39	—	12/7	Mixed XX and XY mitoses in one case
Hahnemann (1974)	—	34/63	—	16/18	Inclusive of cultures from villi, amnion, and decidua
Rhine et al. (1975)	31/36	—	—	—	Disagreement in five cases
Anshan (1975)	99/100	—	—	—	Disagreement in six cases
Rhine et al. (1977)	—	30/34	—	1/16	? (Not controlled)
Goldberg et al. (1980)	—	9/12	—	0/9	Disagreement in all the cases
Niazi et al. (1981)	—	9/25	—	5/4	No disagreement
Kazy et al. (1982)	165/165	—	—	—	No disagreement
Coleman and Path (1982)	—	12/12	—	0/11	Disagreement in three cases
Simoni et al. (1983)	—	30/32	—	16/14	Mixed XX and XY mitoses in five cases
	—	—	20/20	12/8	No disagreement or maternal cell contamination

In 1975, a study from a Chinese research group from the Anshan Department of Obstetrics and Gynecology (Anshan, 1975) again proposed villi sampling, and a blind transcervical aspiration of the fetal material was employed in that study. Because of the difficulties in tissue culture and chromosome analysis using villi, the aspiration technique was offered only for fetal sex prediction by X chromatin determination. The test was proposed as a possiblility for an intensive population control program. Fetal sexing was directly performed by Barr body evaluation in smears set up immediately after sampling and stained by Papanicolau's method. The sex was predicted in 99 cases out of 100 sampled, and disagreement occurred in six of these. At present, the use of the test for fetal sex selection in China is being avoided because of the foreseen dangerous effect that alterations in the sex ratio might produce in the familial and social composition.

Rhine and associates (1975) reported a sampling procedure to obtain exfoliate trophoblastic cells in the first trimester by endocervical lavage. In the early phase of the work, successful results were obtained in fetal sex prediction using the Y body fluorescence test. In a later phase, the sampled cells were collected for tissue culture and subsequent karyotyping. A male chromosome constitution was diagnosed in one case out of 16 in which suitable mitoses were available for study.

A similar sampling procedure was also used by Goldberg et al. (1980), but a negative evaluation was made on fetal karyotyping using endocervical lavage. These authors were not able to find XY mitoses in cases in which male fetuses were detected by cytogenetic controls after interruption of the pregnancy.

Fetal sex determination on trophoblast cells was done in another investigation reported by Kazy et al. (1982) in which villi samples were obtained in the first trimester of pregnancy by biopsy forceps before inducing abortion. The aim of this work was to evaluate a safe method for obtaining chorionic biopsy specimens for use in measuring enzyme activity in villi in order to detect some metabolic storage disorders. Fetal sex was diagnosed through the combined X and Y chromatin assays by setting up two smears from each villi sample. The acetoorcein staining technique was used to assay X chromatin and acridine staining for Y body visualization. No disagreement was found in this study out of 165 cases investigated.

The possibility of obtaining high efficiency in chorionic villi cultures for first-trimester fetal karyotyping was investigated by Niazi et al. (1981) on samples obtained by transcervical aspiration using a flexible plastic catheter under direct ultrasonic visualization. These authors applied a technique in which the most important step was treatment of the villi with trypsin to remove the covering layers of syncytiotrophoblast and cytotrophoblast, thus promoting the growth of the exposed mesenchymal cells. Moreover, the trypsinization followed by filtration through fine wire gauze also allowed elimination of maternal cell clusters normally adhering to the surface of the villus. In 9 out of the 25 culture specimens the fetal karyotype was diagnosed: five were normal males and four were normal females. On these grounds, the authors concluded that this technique is able to suppress the growth of maternal cells so that one of the major difficulties in using placental villi can be overcome. In spite of the employment of such culture techniques, after carefully selecting villi showing typical morphology under the inverted microscope, heavy maternal cell contamination was found by Simoni et al. (1983) in 32 cultured specimens (see Table 1). The same authors reported that this problem disappeared when Chang medium was used for culture. This hormone-supplemented medium showed a markedly positive effect on the fetal cell growth (Chang et al., 1982; Simoni et al., 1983). After this preliminary observation, the overgrowth of fetal cells using Chang medium was confirmed by comparison of the results obtained culturing villi samples in parallel with RPM I and Chang (Table 2). Recently, a short-term tissue culture method for fetal karyotyping using chorionic villi has been developed by Verlinsky et al. (1984). The method described in Chapter 6 of this Treatise, is very reliable and consistent in obtaining metaphases suitable for chromosome analysis. Even if the use of

Table 2 Comparison of the Cytogenetic Results from First-Trimester Villi in 17 Cases in Which Cultures Were Set Up in Parallel using RPM I and Chang Medium

Karyotype	Number of cases RPM I	Chang
XX	8	9
Mixed XX / XY	4	0
XY	4	8
Totals	16[a]	17

[a]One culture failure.

semisynthetic medium as well as the short-term culture method allowed a maximum success in culturing and in obtaining high efficiency in cytogenetic diagnosis with chorionic villi, the first diagnostic application of chorionic villi sampling for chromosome analysis was made possible through a different approach that proved to be fast, reliable, and efficient (Brambati and Simoni, 1983). This was based on the direct analysis of the fetal spontaneous mitoses present in the villi samples during the first trimester of pregnancy. Cytogenetic results from a first series of 100 diagnostic cases followed by preliminary comments were reported by Simoni et al. (1984).

DIRECT CHROMOSOME ANALYSIS

The presence of dividing cells in trophoblastic tissues has long been a well-known phenomenon, and it is not rare to find pictures of villi showing mitotic figures in old treatise that include chapters on the anatomy and histology of the placenta (Fig.1). Mitoses are frequently observed in the Langhan's cell layer during the first trimester of pregnancy. As reported by Watanabe et al. (1978), mitoses average less than 1% cytotrophoblastic tissue from first trimester samples. Therefore, if we consider that many thousand cells are forming the Langhan's layer in a single placental ramification, we can believe that at least several dozen mitoses are consistently present in each villus. On these grounds, we attempted to adapt to human placental villi the method previously described by Evans et al. (1972) in order to obtain direct chromosome preparations from the membranes of mouse embryos and from the tail tips of newborn mice. The method consists of freeing the spontaneous mitoses of cytotrophoblastic tissue by a short treatment with acetic acid. After sampling, villi are washed once in Hank's saline balanced solution and then transferred to a 35-mm plastic petri dish containing 3 ml of RPM I or medium 199 TC without serum. Colcemid at a final concentration of 0.04 μg/ml is added to the medium, and the sample is left for 1 hr at room temperature. The medium is then removed by a Pasteur pipette and replaced with 3 ml of 1% sodium citrate solution for 10 min. This hypotonic solution is removed, and 3 ml of methanol–acetic acid (3 : 1) fixative is added for 10 min. The first fixative is then replaced with fresh fixative, and the dish is left for 2 hr at –20°C in a deep freezer. The fixative is aspirated with a Pasteur pipette, and 0.5 – 1 ml of aqueous (60%) acetic acid is added to induce cell dissociation. The suspension is then evenly distributed onto the surface of warm (40°–45°C) slides by moving the bent

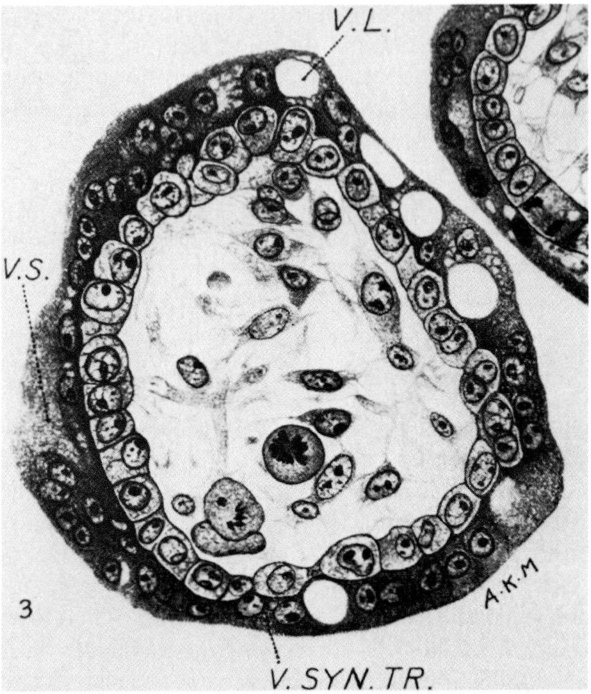

Figure 1 Diagram to illustrate the transverse section of a villus showing spontaneous mitotic figures. This figure, originally from Hamilton and Gladston, was reproduced in *Human Embryology*, p. 71, W. J. Hamilton, J. D. Boyd, and H. W. Mossman, Cambridge, 1957.

tip of a Pasteur pipette symmetrically along the surface of the slide. After air drying the slides overnight in a dry incubator at 40°C, they are stained by routine QFQ-banding technique. Figures 2–4 summarize the successive phases of the procedure until the complete cell dissociation of the villus. The application of the direct chromosome preparations consistently gives a sufficient number of mitoses, and the karyotype may be determined within a few hours after sampling. Moreover, the problem of maternal cell contamination previously encountered with culture seems to be completely ruled out when the direct procedure is used.

As can be seen in Figures 5 and 6, the quality of the metaphases obtainable following the direct preparation is suitable for diagnostic

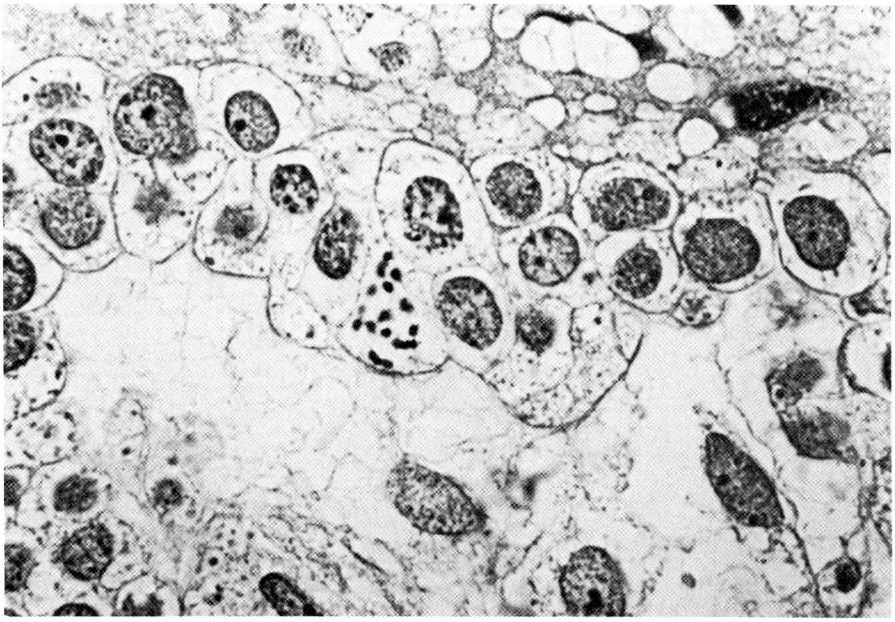

Figure 2 Histological section of a villus after treatment with hypotonic solution showing swollen cells in the cytotrophoblast layer. One of these cells is dividing.

purposes. Short-term incubation (from 12 to 24 hr) of villi in complete culture medium with 5% fetal calf serum in a standard CO_2 incubator at 37°C not only permitted the storage of material but also may have increased the number of mitoses. Colcemid is added during the last hour of incubation, and preparations are obtained following the procedure described above. The storage of incubating villi aliquots has further advantages. In fact, a second attempt to obtain chromosome preparations may be done when the first is not successful, and it is also possible to set up cultures for maintenance of abnormal fetal cells for supplementary investigations. Moreover, a simple incubation of the villi, avoiding the setting up of conventional cultures, may also be useful in applying techniques for which exposure to agents is required. Thus, we were able to obtain RBA-banded mitoses and sister chromatid exchange visualization after bromodeoxyuridine (BUDR) incorporation (Figs. 7 and 8).

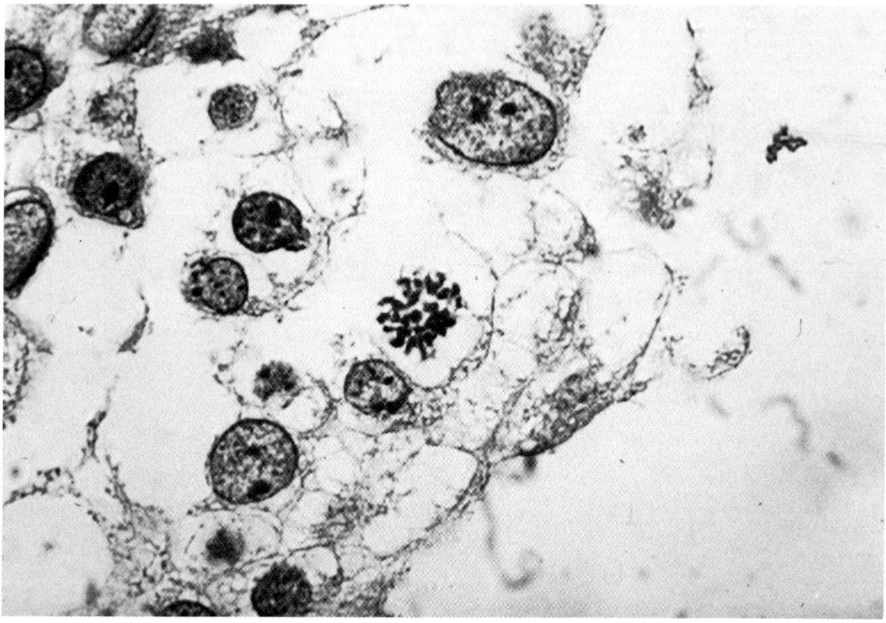

Figure 3 Histological preparation obtained at the moment of the cell dissociation after the addition of aqueous 60% acetic acid solution. Nuclei are being freed from the cytotrophoblast layer. One nucleus is undergoing spontaneous mitosis.

The direct procedure was used in 20 experimental cases in which villi specimens were obtained between 8 and 12 weeks of gestation, and karyotype determination was successful in all of them (Simoni et al., 1983). No chromosomal abnormalities were found, and the chromosome constitution was male in 12 cases and female in 8 cases. Among 582 mitoses obtained by direct preparations from male fetuses, no 46,XX cell was found. This confirmed the reliability of the procedure. We were unable to obtain mitoses using maternal fragments carefully selected under the inverted microscope from several aspirated samples.

DIAGNOSTIC APPLICATION OF THE DIRECT TECHNIQUE

The reliability and efficiency of the direct method being confirmed, it was decided to offer first-trimester chorionic villi sampling (CVS) as an

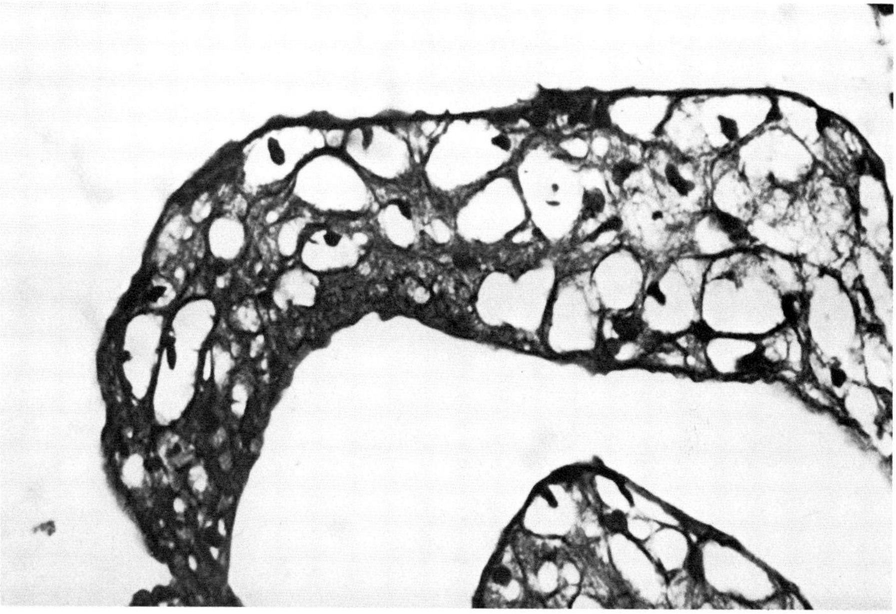

Figure 4 Histological preparation of a villus after a prolonged treatment with acetic acid. Cytotrophoblastic and mesenchymal cells are completely removed, and only residual stroma of the mesenchymal core is preserved.

alternative procedure to second-trimester amniocentesis. From February 1983 to June 1984, 300 pregnancies were investigated at the First Clinic of Obstetrics and Gynecology of Milan University. The results of this experience are shown in Tables 3–5. Direct fetal karyotyping was carried out in 298 cases in which fetal material was obtained at sampling, with five sampling failures and three twin pregnancies. Diagnostic failure occurred in two cases in which an insufficient number of metaphases were found.

Chorionic villus sampling was performed in 269 cases at risk for chromosomal abnormality, in 22 cases for fetal sex determination, in 6 cases at risk for inborn errors of metabolism, and in one case at risk for β-thalassemia. Chorionic villus sampling was used for cytogenic diagnosis in 194 cases with maternal age of 35 years and over, 34 cases with maternal age under 35 years, 26 cases with a previous child showing a chromosomal abnormality, and 15 cases with chromosomal abnormality in one parent. Fetal sex determination was performed in 15 cases at risk for X-linked diseases, in four cases with other genetic risks, and in three

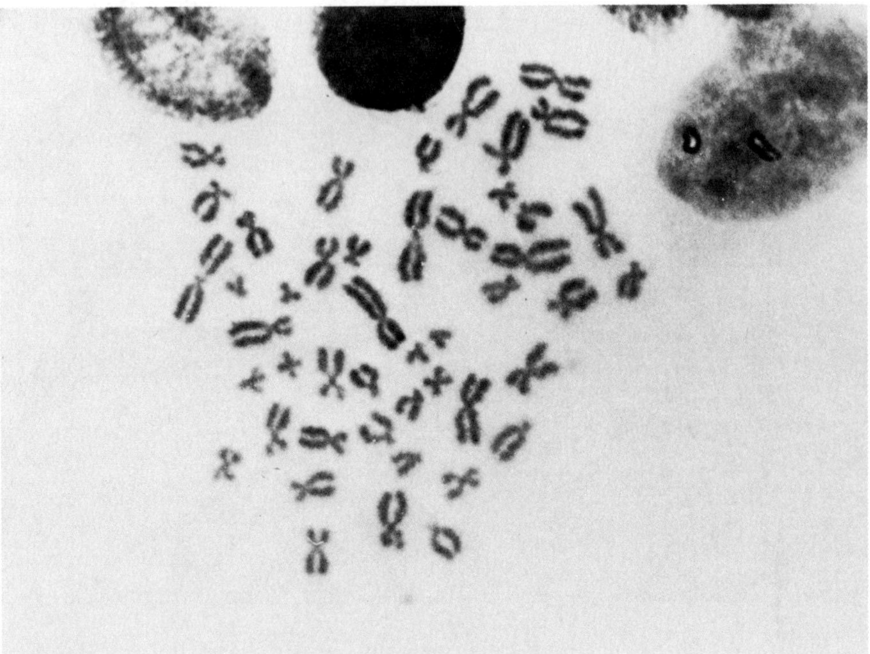

Figure 5 A metaphase obtained by the direct method and stained with Giemsa.

cases as a primary indication after psychiatric evaluation. The six cases at risk for metabolic disorders included GM 1 gangliosidosis, MPS I Hurler syndrome, Niemann-Pick disease, metachromatic leukodystrophy, GM 2 gangliosidosis, and MPS III Sanfilippo syndrome. An abnormal chromosome constitution was found in 24 cases. Of these, 17 were aneuploidies, three were Robertsonian translocations, two were reciprocal balanced translocations, one was a balanced insertion inherited from the father, and one was an inv(X) in a male fetus. Two trisomies were found in female fetuses from pregnancies at risk for X-linked disorders. The cytogenetic controls confirmed the diagnosis in 15 out of 17 cases with abnormal karyotype in which a selective abortion was performed. In two cases showing chromosomal mosaicism, the presence of the abnormal cell line revealed by direct method was not confirmed after interruption of the pregnancy . Both these abnormalities were confined to the chorionic tissue, while a normal chromosome constitution was consistently found in fetal fibroblast cultures obtained

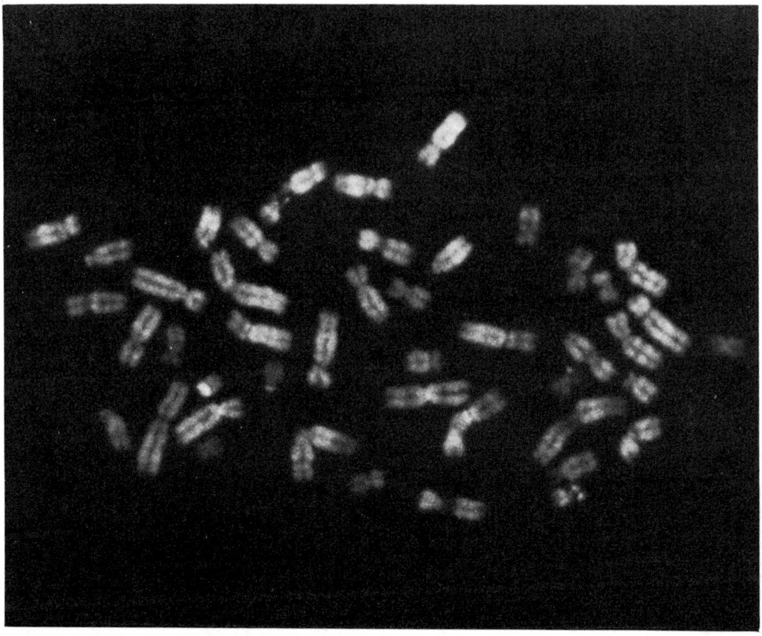

Figure 6 QFQ-banded metaphase spread obtained by direct chromosome analysis of chorionic villi.

from at least two biopsies in each case. The occurrence of these discrepancies between placental cells and fetal fibroblasts emphasizes the need for accurate controls to evaluate the incidence of this phenomenon and its clinical significance.

TECHNICAL AND DIAGNOSTIC PROBLEMS

Some comments arose from the above-mentioned diagnostic experience concerning the advantages and disadvantages of direct chromosomal analysis. We have found that the method is quick and simple for routine application and has a high degree of reliability. Preparations ready for examination can be obtained within a few hours of sampling, and this may be of great consequence in reducing the psychological stress in the woman requesting fetal diagnosis. Thus, the direct chromosomal preparation is of great help in all the cases in which the emotional status of the patient is important. In addition to this first advantage, it should be noted that only

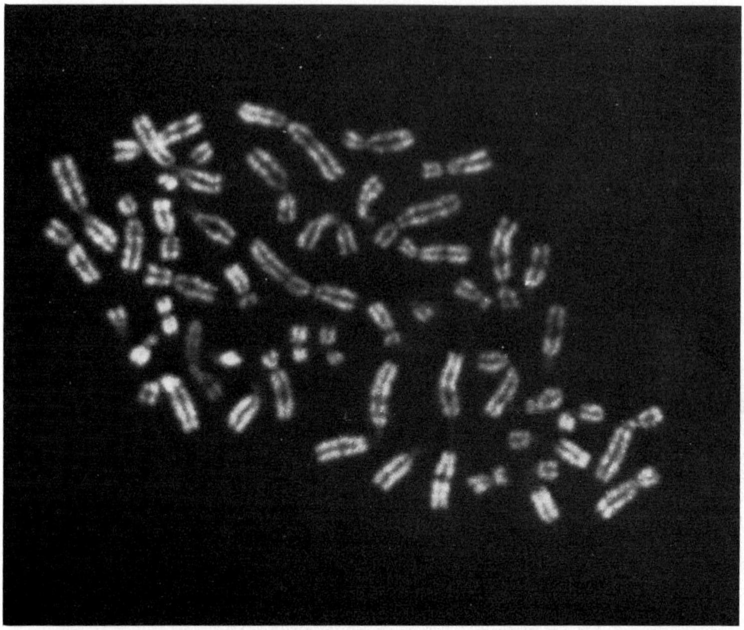

Figure 7 RBA-banded metaphase obtained after 24 hr incubation of the villus at 37°C in 5% CO_2 and 6 hr exposure to BUDR.

two diagnostic failures occurred (0.7%) among 298 samples in which villi were obtained at sampling. The success of chromosomal analysis does not appear to be necessarily correlated with the amount of villi available. In fact, in six cases in which a single villus ramification was aspirated, a sufficient number of metaphases was found in order to determine the fetal karyotype without difficulty. Even if a marked variability is observed in the number of suitable mitoses among different cases, we based the diagnostic result on less than ten mitoses in only four cases. The technique of direct preparation, however, increased the number of metaphases that were distorted and incomplete. We found that these inconveniences are, in part, correlated with the ability to obtain a uniform distribution of cell suspension on the surface of the slide after the acetic acid treatmment. Different operators may have different results using the same cell suspension sample. Therefore, a machine was built for achieving a homogeneous condition in setting up slides (Fig. 9).

After the use of this mechanical distribution of cells was introduced into diagnostic practice, the number of broken mitoses in direct

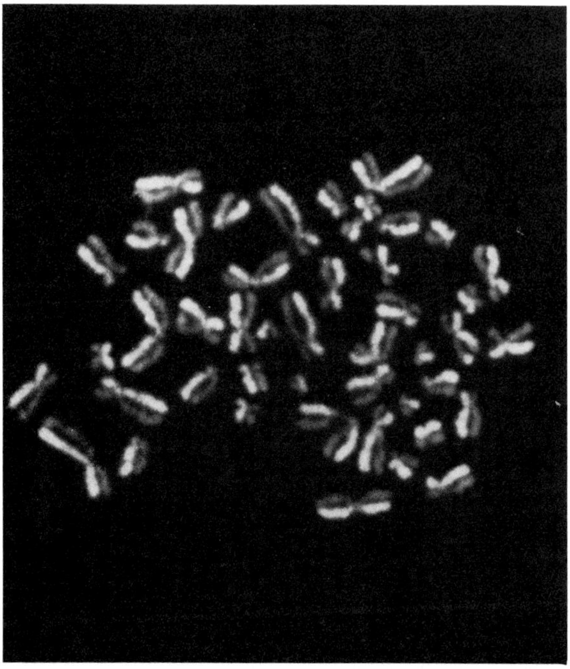

Figure 8 Sister chromatid exchanges visualization after 48 hr incubation of the villus at 37°C in CO_2 with BUDR.

preparation was reduced, if not completely eliminated. A last distinct technical problem of direct procedure is that the quality of banding is not always satisfactory. In fact, routine banding techniques of the chorionic villi cells are not as clear as the banding achieved in cultured amniotic-fluid cells. However, improvement in the banding resolution may be made by minor modifications of the original direct method as well as of the routine banding procedures in order to find the optimal conditions for each laboratory.

In our experience, adequate QFQ banding was best achieved when, at the second fixative change, the villi were placed in a deep freezer (-20°C) for 2 hr before the acetic acid treatment. Gregson and Seabright (1983) reported a modified technique that gave good quality G-banded metaphases using the trypsin banding method. Sachs et al. (1983) proved the usefulness of reverse heat acridine orange (RHA) banding for first-trimester cytogenetic study in a pregnancy at risk for minimal structural chromosome anomalies. The use of RHA banding allowed the

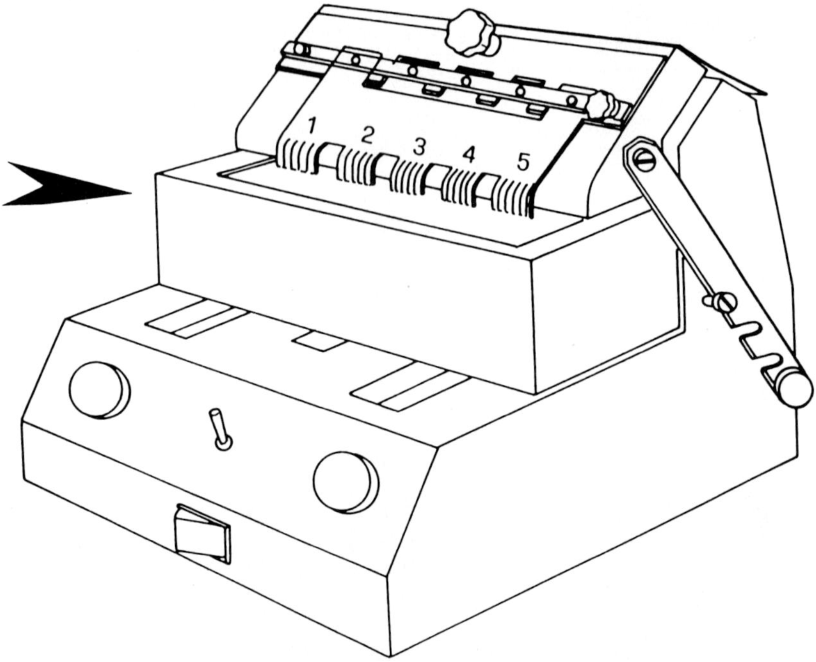

Figure 9 A schematic representation of a machine built in order to have homogeneous distribution of the cell suspension. Five slides may be set up simultaneously. The slow and regular movement of the warm plate (arrow) carrying the slides improves the chromosome spread and reduces the number of incomplete mitoses.

identification of a partial trisomy 17q and of a partial monosomy 9p in the fetal karyotype from a pregnant woman carrier of a double translocation. This is a situation in which excellent quality banding is necessary for diagnosis to be achieved. The major diagnostic problem we encountered was the occurrence of two mosiacs in which the abnormal cell line was strictly confined to trophoblastic tissues. This finding confirmed the possibility of a discrepancy between villi cells and fetal fibroblasts, as reported by Kalousek and Dill (1983). On these grounds, we think that additional second-trimester studies should be offered whenever a mosaic is found in the villus.

At present, even if some technical difficulties are not completely overcome, the direct technique is being successfully applied to diagnostic routine in several laboratories in different countries. In addition to our

Table 3 Total Results by Direct Chromosome Analysis after CVS in 300 Pregnancies[a]

Indication for CVS	No. of cases investigated	Abnormal karyotype (including balanced)	Selective abortion
Chromosomal abnormalities	269	22	14
Fetal sex determination			
Risk of X-linked diseases	15	2	7
Other genetic risks	4	—	—
Other reasons	3	—	2
Enzyme determinations	6[b]	—	1[c]
DNA analysis (β-thalassemia)	1	—	—
Totals	298[d]	24	24

[a] These results are comprehensive of the 100 cases reported by Simoni et al. (1984).
[b] GM 1 gangliosidosis, MPS I Hurler syndrome, Niemann-Pick disease, metachromatic leukodystrophy, GM 2 gangliosidosis Sandhoff disease, MPS III Sanfilippo syndrome.
[c] MPS I diagnosed at 19 weeks on cultured amniocytes.
[d] Sampling failure in five cases; diagnostic failure in two cases; the total includes three twin pregnancies.

Table 4 Cases in Which Fetal Karyotyping Was Primary Indication for CVS

Group at risk	No. of cases investigated	Abnormal karyotype (including balanced)	Type of abnormality
Maternal age ⩾ 35 years	194	11	Tris 21 (4 cases); tris 18 (2 cases); tris 14; tris 16; monosomy X; mos 46,XY/45,X; inv(X) in a male fetus
Maternal age < 35 years	34	—	—
Previous child with chromosomal abnormality	26	2	Tris 13; mos 46, XX/47,XX,+3
Chromosomal abnormality in the parents	15	9	Robertsonian translocations (3 cases); reciprocal balanced translocations (2 cases); balanced ins (18;13)(p11;q13q15);tris 22; t(7q;9q)de novo,+mar[a]; + mar[a]
Totals	269	22	

[a] Two pregnancies from the same woman carrier of a supernumerary small metacentric marker.

Table 5 Cases in Which Fetal Sex Determination Was Primary Indication for CVS

Group at risk	No. of cases investigated	Male	Female	Abnormal karyotype	Type of abnormality
X-linked diseases					
DMD	10[a]	5[b]	4	1	Tris 21 (female)
DMD + HEM A	2[c]	—	2	1	Tris 9 (female)
HEM A	1[d]	1	—	—	
fra (X)(q28)	1	—	1	—	
Testicular feminization (incomplete type McK31308)	1	—	1	—	
Other genetic risks					
Campomelic dysplasia	1	1	—	—	
Congenital hip dislocation (severe form)	1	1	—	—	
Adrenogenital syndrome	2	2	—	—	
Totals	19	10	8	2	

[a] One diagnostic failure.
[b] One pregnancy is continuing in spite of a male fetus diagnosed.
[c] Pregnancies from the same woman.
[d] Second-trimester diagnosis of affected fetus performed at King's College Hospital.

experience, we know that several hundreds of first-trimester diagnoses have already been performed by other centers using direct chromosome procedure. Thus, it is easy to foresee a much greater application of direct cytogenetic analysis in first-trimester prenatal diagnosis in the near future.

ACKNOWLEDGMENTS

We wish to thank Dr. C. Danesino for performing biochemical determinations. We are also grateful to Professor M. Fraccaro for his constructive criticism and help in developing first-trimester chromosome studies. This work was partially supported by a grant from the Associazione Italiana per lo Studio, la Prevenzione e la Terapia delle Malformazioni, Milan, Italy.

REFERENCES

Anshan (1975). Fetal sex prediction by sex chromatin of chorionic villi cells during early pregnancy. *Chin. Med. J.* (Engl) *1*: 117–126.

Brambati, B. and Simoni, G. (1983). Diagnosis of fetal trisomy 21 in first trimester. *Lancet i*:586.

Chang, H.-C., Jones, O. W., and Masui, H. (1982). Human amniotic fluid cells grown in a hormone-supplemented medium: Suitability for prenatal diagnosis. *Proc. Nat. Acad. Sci. USA 79*:4795–4799.

Coleman, D. V. and Path M. R. C. (1982). Endocervical lavage in early pregnancy. *Am. J. Obstet. Gynecol. 142*:118–119.

Evans, E. P., Burtenshaw, M. D., and Fird, C. E. (1972). Chromosomes of mouse embryos and newborn young: Preparations from membranes and tail tips. *Stain Technol. 47*:229–234.

Goldberg, M. F., Chen, A. T. L., Ahn, Y. W., and Reidy, J. A. (1980). First trimester fetal chromosomal diagnosis using endocervical lavage: A negative evaluation. *Am. J. Obstet. Gynecol. 138*:436–440.

Gregson, N. M., and Seabright, M. (1983). Handling chorionic villi for direct chromosome studies. *Lancet ii*:1491.

Hahnemann, N. (1974). Early prenatal diagnosis: A study of biopsy techniques and cell culturing from extraembryonic membranes. *Clin. Genet. 6*:294–306.

Hamilton, W. J., Boyd, J. D., and Mossman, H. W. (1957). *Human Embryology*, p.71. Mossman, Cambridge.

Kalousek, D. K., and Dill, F. J. (1983). Chromosomal mosaicism confined to the placenta in human conceptions. *Science 221*:665–667.

Kazy, Z., Rozovsky, I. S., and Bakharev, V. A. (1982). Chorion biopsy in early prenatal diagnosis of inherited disorders. *Prenat. Diag. 2*:39–45.

Kullander, S., and Sandahl, B. (1973). Fetal chromosome analysis after transcervical placental biopsies during early pregnancy. *Acta Obstet. Gynec. Scand. 52*:355–359.

Niazi, M., Coleman, D. V., and Loeffler, F. E. (1981). Trophoblast sampling in early pregnancy. Culture of rapidly dividing cells from immature placental villi. *Br. J. Obstet. Gynaecol. 88*:1081–1085.

Rhine, S. A., Cain, J. L., Cleary, R. E., Palmer, C. G., and Thompson, T. (1975). Prenatal sex detection with endocervical smears. Successful resulting utilizing Y-body fluorescence. *Am. J. Obstet. Gynecol. 122*:155–160.

Rhine, S. A., Palmer, C. G., and Thompson, J. F. (1977). A simple first trimester alternative to amniocentesis for prenatal diagnosis. *Birth Defects, Orig. Art. Ser. XII 3D*:231–247.

Sachs, E. S., Van Hemel, J. O., Galjaard, H., Niermeijer, M. F., and Jahoda, M. G. J. (1983). First trimester chromosomal analysis of complex structural rearrangements with RHA banding on chorionic villi. *Lancet ii*:1426.

Simoni, G., Brambati, B., Danesino, C., Rossella, F., Terzoli, G. L., Ferrari, M., and Fraccaro, M. (1983). Efficient direct chromosome analysis and enzyme determinations from chorionic villi samples in the first trimester of pregnancy. *Human Genet. 63*:349–357.

Simoni, G., Brambati, B., Danesino, C., Terzoli, G. L., Romitti, L., Rossella, F., and Fraccaro, M. (1984). Diagnostic application of first trimester trophoblast sampling in 100 pregnancies. *Human Genet. 66*:252–259.

Verlinsky, Y., Chu, L., and Pergament, E. (1984). Chromosomal preparations of chorionic villi samples (CVS). *Karyogram 10*:1–3.

Watanabe, M., Ito, T., Yamamoto, M., and Watanabe, G. (1978) Origin of mitotic cells of chorionic villi in direct chromosome analysis. *Human Genet. 44*:191–193.

7

Fetal Karyotyping by Chorionic Tissue Culture

EUGENE PERGAMENT and YURY VERLINSKY
Michael Reese Hospital and Medical Center, Chicago, Illinois

INTRODUCTION

The purpose of this chapter is to describe the role of chorionic cell culture in first-trimester genetic diagnosis. By culturing chorionic villi in vitro, a continuous source of cells reflecting the genotype of the developing fetus is readily available. To accomplish this requires two critical steps. First, any contaminating maternal decidua associated with the villous samples must be carefully stripped away. Second, in order to initiate cell cultures, mesenchymal cells comprising the inner core of the villi layer must be exposed by removal of the covering layer—the syncytiotrophoblast. The development of techniques for the tissue culturing of chorionic villi was reviewed in another chapter. These initial approaches appeared to limit the potential use of chorionic cell culture for first-trimester genetic diagnoses because they were time consuming and because they were at significant risk for microbial contamination due to the number of preparatory steps involved. Recently, the ability to obtain relatively "clean" samples of the chorion combined with the use of physical dispersion and enzymatic treatment has materially simplified the culturing of villous tissue.

This chapter is divided into three sections. The first section outlines in a step-by-step fashion procedures for the short-term and long-term culturing of chorionic villi. The short-term method is specifically designed to provide preparations with the highest possible quality of chromosomal banding. The second section describes the application of chorionic cell culture to first-trimester fetal diagnosis. The results of the karyotypic analyses of 230 pregnancies at significant risk for a broad spectrum of chromosomal disorders are provided in the second section. The third section compares the technical and diagnostic advantages and disadvantages of chorionic cell culture with those associated with direct use of chorionic villi, i.e., without culture.

CHORIONIC CELL CULTURE

The establishment of primary cell culture from chorionic villi is a relatively simple procedure. Villi with large numbers of syncythial buds (50 or more) are selected under a dissecting microscope for direct chromosomal preparations. Villi with reduced or absent syncythial buds are processed for tissue culture. In each case, adherent maternal decidua is meticulously removed by using sterile forceps and needle.

For short-term cell culture, the villi are cut into small pieces by sterile scissors and then placed in 10 ml of trypsin (1:250) for "extended trypsinization" (2 hr or more, e.g., overnight). After centrifugation at 800–1000 rpm for 5–8 minutes, the trypsin is removed. The villi are resuspended with vigorous pipetting in complete media, either Chang's or MEM-Alpha, supplemented with 20% fetal calf serum and antibiotics. The volume of media varies from 0.5 to 5 ml depending on the sample size. The suspended cells are placed on sterile, 22×22 mm coverslips contained within 35-mm petri dishes. The petri dishes are then incubated 24–48 hr in humidified air and 5% CO_2 at 37°C in order for the cells to attach to the coverslip. Approximately 2.5 ml of complete media is then added, and incubation is continued for another 72–120 hr.

Long-term cell cultures can be initiated following "extended trypsinization" by placing approximately 1–2 ml of the cell suspension in a 25-ml tissue culture flask to which 2–3 ml of complete media are added. The flask is then gassed with 10% CO_2 in air and closed tightly. Hereafter, the long-term culturing of villous cells is exactly the same as the standard procedure for culturing fibroblasts or amniocytes.

Harvesting of each coverslip is initiated when a minimum of 4–5 colonies containing 150–200 cells per colony is present. Colcemide (final concentration, 0.04 μg/ml) is added for 2 hr, and incubation is continued in humidified air and 5% CO_2 at 37°C. The media containing Colcemid is then removed from the petri dish and replaced by warmed (37°C) hypotonic solution (0.8% sodium citrate). After 20 min at room temperature, 0.5 ml of methanol–acetic acid (2 : 1) fixative is added directly to the hypotonic solution for approximately 2–5 min. The entire mixture is then removed, and fresh methanol–acetic acid fixative (2 : 1) is placed in the petri dish for several hours (minimum of 1 hr) or overnight.

Spreading of the chromosomes is controlled by exposure to steam. The coverslip is inverted and placed 1 in. above boiling water for 3–5 sec. The degree of chromosomal separation is determined by phase microscopy and, if insufficient, exposure to steam is repeated. After drying in air, the coverslip is mounted (cell side face up!) on a slide. Prior to staining, the slide is placed overnight in a dry incubator at 60°C. The stain consists of Wright's stain diluted in phosphate buffer (1 : 3) to which trypsin–EDTA (0.25 ml per 10 ml of staining solution) has been added. The staining time is usually 2–3 min.

The diagnostic accuracy of chorionic villi and the reliability of the cell culture techniques were evaluated in a series of blighted ovum and incomplete abortions. Villi obtained by catheter aspiration and by suction curettage were cultured in parallel. A total of 16 pregnancies were evaluated. Karyotypic analysis revealed eight specimens with aneuploidy, including trisomies for chromosomes 8 (1 case), 16 (2 cases), 18 (1 case), 21 (1 case), and 22 (2 cases), and 45 X (1 case). There were no apparent instances of maternal contamination detected, although a definitive comparison of chromosomal polymorphisms between the maternal parent and villous specimen was not made.

No significant differences in total hexosaminidase and hexosaminidase A and B activities were present when chorionic cell cultures derived from catheter aspiration and suction curettage were compared.

APPLICATION OF CHORIONIC CELL CULTURE

Chorionic cell cultures, established in the first trimester of pregnancy, were successfully used in diagnosing a spectrum of chromosomal disorders (Table 1). The indication of "advanced maternal age" encompassed the largest number of at-risk parents. Chromosomal analysis in this group indicated that 5.5% of the cultured villi were aneuploid, including 45,X (1 case), trisomy 7 (1 case), trisomy 18 (2 cases), and trisomy 21 (4 cases). Each instance of an abnormal karyotype was confirmed by chromosomal analysis of cultured chorionic and fetal cells established from tissues obtained at the time of elective termination. There was one case of a second affected fetus in 37 parents who had a previous chromosomally abnormal conception. In a 39-year-old woman

Table 1 First-Trimester Fetal Diagnosis Based on Chromosomal Analysis of Chorionic Cell Cultures

	Karyotypes		
Indication	Normal	Abnormal	No Result
Advanced maternal age	145	8	1[a]
Previous chromosomal abnormality	36	1	—
Parental chromosomal rearrangement	6	2	1[b]
X-linked disorder	3	3 (=XY)	—
Chromosomal fragility syndrome	3	—	—
Parental anxiety	1	—	—
Inborn error of metabolism	21	1	—
Total	215	15	2

[a] Bacterial cell contamination present. Chromosomal analysis based on direct preparation only.
[b] Amniocentesis performed. See Table 2 for further details.

whose only previous conception showed triploidy following amniocentesis, cultured chorionic cells exhibited the same polyploid state. This diagnosis was also confirmed at the time of elective termination.

Chromosomal analysis from chorionic cell cultures was successful in seven of eight parents at risk because each carried a structurally altered chromosome (Table 2). In all three instances involving a translocation between chromosomes 14 and 21, the children have been born normal and peripheral blood cultures have confirmed the original diagnosis. In two other translocations, t(11;22) and t(21;22), unbalanced chromosome constitutions were detected in the chorionic cell cultures. Terminations were elected, and the original diagnoses were confirmed in the products of conception. A reciprocal translocation involving chromosomes 1 and 3 present in the paternal parent resulted in a female conceptus with the same complement.

Chromosomal analysis of chorionic cell cultures was not successful in a case involving a paracentric inversion of chromosome 5 carried by the maternal parent. An earlier pregnancy had resulted in a developmentally delayed child with a partial deletion of chromosome 5 due to crossing over within the inversion loop. Unsatisfactory chromosome preparations resulted in this case in part due to the small sample of villi obtained and attempt to complete the chromosomal analysis before the end of the first

Table 2 Karyotypes of Chorionic Cell Cultures from Pregnancies at Risk Because of Structural Chromosomal Rearrangements in the Parents

Type	Parental rearrangement	Chorionic karyotype	Pregnancy outcome
Translocation	46,XY,t(1;3)(q32;p21)	46,XX,t(1;3)(q32;p21)	Continuing
	46,XX,t(11;22)(22q12 – ⟩ 22qter::11qter)	47,XX,tder(22)t(11;22)(q23;q12)	Termination
	45,XX,t(14;21)(p11;q11)[a]	46,XY	Normal
	45,XX,t(14;21)(p11;q11)	45,XX,t(14;21)(p11;q11)	Normal
	45,XX,t(21;22)(p11;q11)	46,XX,t(21;22)(p11;q11)	Termination
	46,XY,t(8;14)(p23;q12)	46,XX,t(8;14)(p23;q12)	Continuing
Inversion	46,XX,inv(5)(p13;q31)	Unsuccessful[b]	Termination
	46,XY,inv(Y)	46,XY,inv(Y)	Continuing

[a] Two cases.
[b] Amniocytes showed 46,XY,del(5)(p13).

trimester. Amniocentesis was performed at 16 weeks gestation, and an unbalanced karyotype was eventually detected.

Fetal sexing for three X-linked disorders (Duchenne muscular dystrophy, hemophilia A, and Wiskott-Aldrich syndrome), was performed on six patients and revealed three XX and three XY sex chromosomal constitutions.

Three pregnancies, at risk for the chromosomal fragility syndromes, Fanconi's anemia and the fragile-X, were successfully monitored by chorionic villi sampling. Previously established methods of analyzing cell cultures (1,2) were applied to chorion cultures. Normal results were confirmed by amniocentesis and at the time of birth.

Polymorphisms of chromosome 9 and the Y chromosome definitively identified that the legal husband had fathered a woman's conception in the case of disputed paternity.

In one set of parents at risk for Tay-Sachs disease, chromosomal analysis of chorionic cell cultures revealed trisomy 16.

Chromosomal mosaicism of the chorion was detected in two cases for which the indication was "advanced maternal age." While the direct preparation in one case revealed a normal chromosomal number in all 25 cells, cell cultures revealed mosaicism for chromosome 21. This diagnosis was confirmed following elective termination in which mosaicism was present in the chorion, amnion, and fetal tissues. In the second case, mosaicism for chromosome 7 was detected in both direct and cell culture preparations and was confirmed following elective termination in chorionic and fetal tissues.

There were two instances of pseudomosaicism: whereas the direct chromosomal preparation revealed a normal chromosomal number, chorionic cell cultures revealed a marker chromosome in one or more colonies harvested in situ. Amniocentesis was performed, and the marker chromosomes were not detected. Both pregnancies were completed with normal outcomes.

Maternal cell contamination was detected in three chorionic cultures with an XY sex chromosome constitution. In two cases, the degree of maternal cell contamination was considered minimal, representing a few 46,XX cells in predominantly 46,XY cultures. In the third case, however, the amount of maternal cell contamination was significant enough that amniocentesis was performed. A normal male with a 46,XY chromosomal complement was delivered.

The overall sex ratio was 111 females to 109 males.

ADVANTAGES AND DISADVANTAGES OF CHORIONIC CELL CULTURE

The purpose of prenatal diagosis is to obtain a sample of cells that precisely reflects the genotype of the developing conceptus. Since the chorion, like the conceptus, is originally derived from the zygote, genetic analysis of the immature placenta should be an accurate assessment of the embryonic or fetal state. The chorion, however, has not been extensively evaluated in this regard. The ability to establish short-term and long-term cell cultures from chorionic villi, in conjunction with the direct use of such tissues, should provide the technical means to support the proposal that heritable disorders, currently diagnosed in the second trimester of pregnancy by amniocentesis, can also be diagnosed in the first trimester. Furthermore, this can be accomplished using conventional methodologies for analyzing chromosomes, enzymatic reactions, or DNA.

The ease with which cell cultures of chorionic tissue can be established was demonstrated at Michael Reese Hospital and Medical Center, Chicago, Illinois. In 16 of 20 samples from blighted ovum or incomplete abortions and in 234 of 236 (99.2%) samples from pregnancies, cell cultures were successfully established and karyotyped. The two diagnostic failures were due to an occurrence of bacterial contamination in one case and the inability to accurately karyotype another case involving an inversion 5 chromosome (See Table 2).

That the chorionic cell culture consistently reflected the genotype of the developing conceptus was demonstrated in the following ways:

1. All aneuploid states detected in the chorion, including two cases of mosaicism, were documented in embryonic and extraembryonic tissues following elective termination.
2. Structural chromosomal rearrangements, originally derived from balanced carrier parents, were detected in chorionic cell cultures. If unbalanced, these structural aberrations were demonstrated to be present in embryonic tissues at termination. If balanced, they were demonstrated to result in normal children following completion of the pregnancy.
3. Pregnancies at risk for an X-linked disorder and then terminated because the fetal sex showed an XY sex chromosome constitution exhibited the same complement in their embryonic tissues. All instances of an XX sex chromosome constitution resulted in the birth of a normal female.

4. Over 100 infants have been born following CVS, and there has been *no* discordance between the phenotype of the newborn and the karyotype based on chorionic cell culture, including sexual designation.
5. The sex ratio closely approximated the expected 1:1 (111 females to 109 males).

The accuracy of the karyotypic analyses for this large number of pregnancies at risk for a variety of chromosomal disorders is a reflection of the efficacy of obtaining chorionic villi, the proficiency in removing any maternal decidua, the ease with which cell cultures can be established in vitro, and as the fact that the chorion consistently represented the fetal genotype.

At present, chromosomal analyses of chorionic villi are best performed by the combined use of direct preparations and cell cultures. Each method had both advantages and disadvantages, but their dual application optimizes the quality of the chromosomal study. On the one hand, chorionic cell culture requires a minimum of 4–7 days of growth before harvesting can be initiated, whereas the results of the direct preparation can be available within hours of sampling. Equipment and media needs for the direct preparation are simple and inexpensive in contrast to the more expensive and technically demanding requirements of cell culture. Microbial and maternal contamination are low-risk factors with direct preparations of villi, but they are potentially significant problems with cell culture.

On the other hand, the morphology of the chromosomes prepared from cell culture is excellent and capable of exhibiting up to 850 bands (see Fig. 1). Direct chromosomal preparations are primarily useful for determining chromosome number, and in certain cases even this may be difficult because of distortion and cell breakage. This significant difference in the quality of the two methods is illustrated in the case of a reciprocal translocation involving chromosomes 1 and 3 (Fig. 2).

Culturing chorionic tissue in vitro has the advantage of providing a continous source of cells for genetic analysis. Moreover, the in vitro system offers relatively greater technical control in the timing of such studies and in diagnosing certain genetic disorders not readily possible with direct preparations. These advantages are illustrated in the following examples. There are disorders whose detection may require the uptake of a radioactive label prior to the initiation of mitosis, e.g., labeling DNA with radioactive thymidine. There are disorders whose

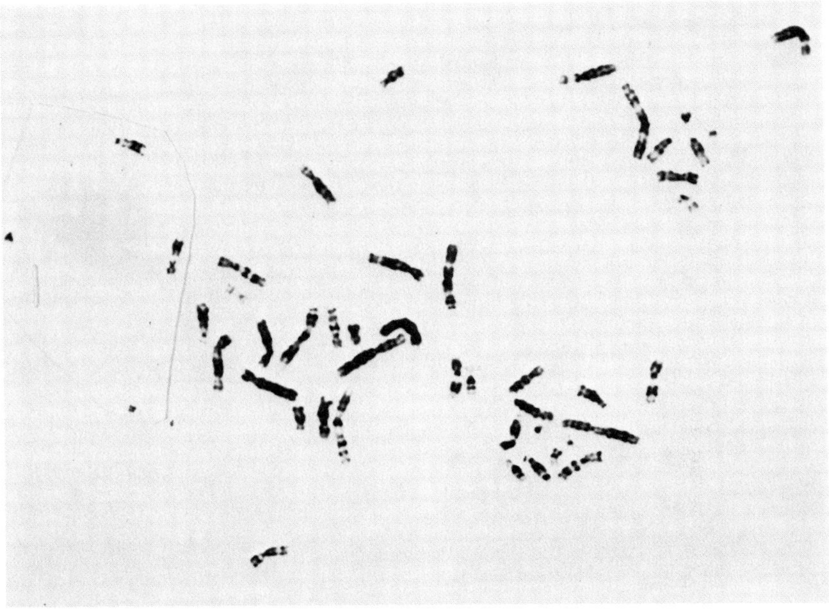

Figure 1 Tissue culture preparation of chorionic villi for chromosomal analysis.

analysis may require two or more consecutive cell divisions, e.g., fragile-X and Fanconi's anemia. Certain enzymes may not be detected on direct analysis of the chorion but can be identified upon cell culture. For example, in the diagnosis of homocystinuria, the enzyme, cystathianine β-synthetase, is not detectable on direct analysis but is active in chorionic cell cultures (M. J. Mahoney, personal communication).

Maternal cell contamination and pseudomosaicism will hinder the accuracy of first-trimester genetic diagnosis. The possibility of maternal cell contamination requires meticulous separation of villi from decidua. Exposure of the original sample to trypsin for extended periods, 2 hr or more, may significantly reduce the ability of maternal cells to attach to the culture surface, while at the same time permitting necessary exposure of the mesenchymal core. The use of small coverslips for primary cultures reduces culture time prior to initiating harvesting and thereby may prevent overgrowth by contaminating maternal cells. With the coverslip method, colonies and not cells are analyzed. Analysis of ten or more mitotic figures should expose maternal cell contamination because cells are selected from different colonies. Similarly, true mosaicism can usually be distinguished

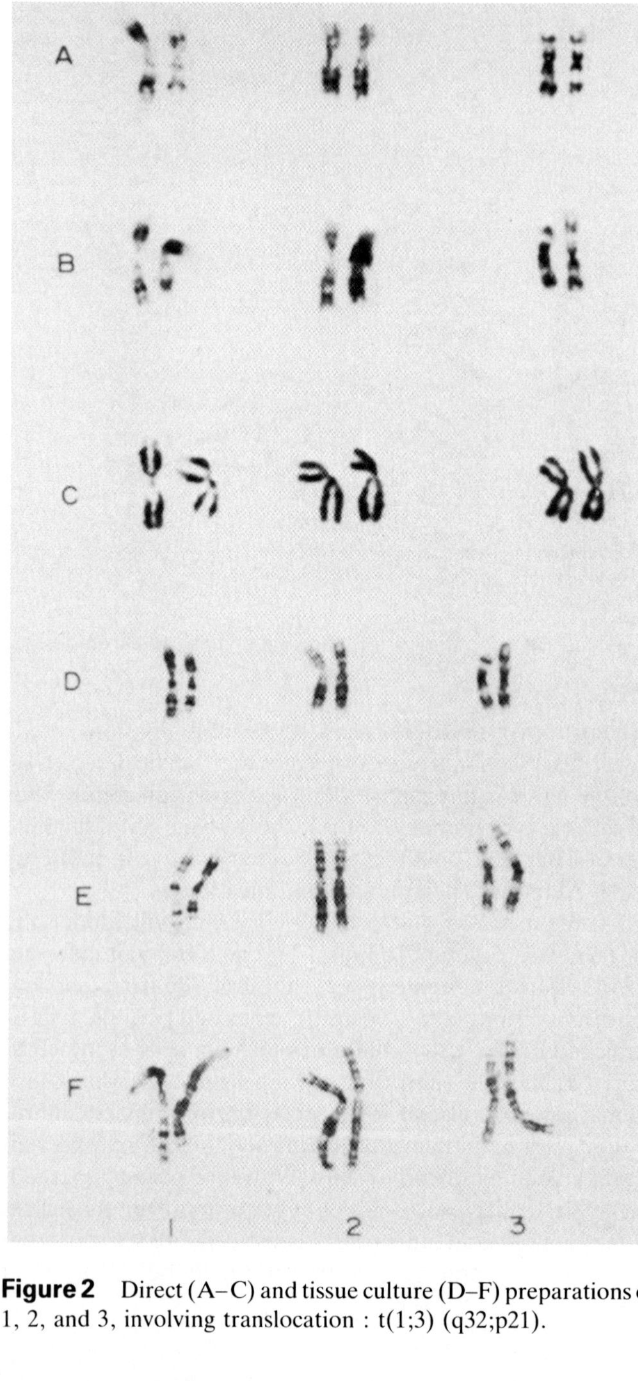

Figure 2 Direct (A–C) and tissue culture (D–F) preparations of chromosomes 1, 2, and 3, involving translocation : t(1;3) (q32;p21).

from pseudomosaicism with this in-situ technique, for the presence of abnormal cells in specific colonies can be readily identified. The chromosomal analysis of primary cultures established on coverslips eliminates the need for trypsinization and seeding onto a second set of plates. Thus, with the in-situ method, the opportunity for increasing the number of cells that do not reflect the genotype of the chorion or fetus is effectively reduced or eliminated.

ACKNOWLEDGMENTS

We wish to thank Ms. Laura Chu for technical support, Ms. Dorothy Halperin for genetic counseling services to patients, and Ms. Rosa Pritchett for constructive criticism and help.

REFERENCES

1. Auerbach, A., Adler, B., and Chaganti S. (1981). Prenatal and postnatal diagnosis and carrier detection of Fanconi anemia by a cytogenetic method. *Pediatrics 67*:128–135.
2. Shapiro, L. R., Wilmot, P. L., Brenholz, P., Leff, A., Martino, M., Harris, G., Mahoney, M. J., and Hobbins, J. C. (1982). Prenatal diagnosis of fragile X chromosome. *Lancet, 1*:99–100.

8

Biochemical Analysis of Chorionic Villi

HANS GALJAARD and WILLEM J. KLEIJER
Erasmus University and University Hospital, Rotterdam, The Netherlands

EARLY DIAGNOSIS AND PREVENTION

At present, more than 3400 conditions in man are known or suspected to be due to a single gene mutation (McKusick, 1983). Their overall incidence among newborns is of the order of 1%, but the incidence of individual genetic diseases may vary considerably among different populations (Table 1).

In a few instances, the occurrence of physical and/or mental handicaps can be prevented by early dietary management or administration of vitamins (cofactors, blood constituents, hormones, or drugs) (for reviews, see Stanbury et al., 1983). Usually, treatment is more effective when started early after birth, and this has been the basis of newborn screening programs in many countries (Bickel et al., 1980).

Unfortunately, for the vast majority of genetic diseases, no treatment is available, and the main emphasis has therefore been on prevention. This is especially important because of the high (recurrence) risks that are involved in the category of diseases with Mendelian inheritance. The main approaches toward prevention are the following:

1. Avoiding environmental factors known to increase the mutation rate
2. Carrier detection prior to reproduction followed by genetic counseling

Table 1 Gene Mutations in Man[a]

Type of mutation	Overall incidence per 1000	Examples	Incidence
Autosomal dominant	0.6–7	Familial hypercholesterolemia	1 : 500
		Huntington's chorea	1 : 5,000
		Osteogenesis imperfecta	1 : 25,000
Autosomal recessive	0.9–2.5	Cystic fibrosis	1 : 2,500
		Phenylketonuria	1 : 12,000
		Mucopolysaccharidoses	1 : 25,000
		Tay-Sachs disease	Varies from < 1 : 100,000 among Caucasians to 1 : 3,000 among Ashkenazy Jews
		Sickle cell anemia	Varies from 1 : 600 among American blacks to < 1 : 100,000 in other populations
		β-Thalassemia	Varies from 1 : 150 in Cyprus to < 1 : 100,000 in other populations
X-linked	0.4–0.7	Duchenne muscular dystrophy	1 : 7,000
		Hemophilia	1 : 10,000
		All others together	1 : 5,000

[a] In 1984 a total of 3500 conditions were known or suspected to be of Mendelian inheritance (McKusick).

3. Early diagnosis of index patients followed by family studies and genetic counseling of couples at risk
4. Prenatal monitoring of pregnancies at risk and selective abortion

The technical possibilities of detecting carriers on a larger scale are as yet limited, but promising results have been obtained with carrier screening for Tay-Sachs disease among Ashkenazy Jews (Kaback, 1977, 1981) and to a lesser extent with screening for hemoglobinopathies (Angastioniotis and Hadjiminas, 1981; WHO, 1981; see also other chapters in this treatise). The great advantage of this approach is that the birth of a first affected child in individual families can be prevented, whereas at a population level, the incidence of a given genetic disease can be significantly reduced. There are, however, a variety of technical, organizational, socio-economic, and cultural–religious factors that determine the ultimate take-up rate and success of a carrier screening program.

Today, the most important approach toward prevention is the early diagnosis of an index patient with a genetic disease followed by genetic counseling of the relatives. Various follow-up studies indicate that 50–90% of couples that have been informed about a high genetic risk refrain from pregnancy (Carter et al., 1971; Emery et al., 1972; Klein and Wyss, 1977). In the case of autosomal-recessive diseases, the diagnosis of an index patient usually is the first signal that both parents are carriers of the same gene mutation. If the diagnosis is established early enough, genetic counseling can at least prevent the birth of subsequent affected children in the same family. In X-linked disorders, it should first be established whether the mother of a patient is a carrier. When this is the case, carrier tests have to be performed on her female relatives, and in this way the birth of further affected males can be prevented. Studies on families with two or more children with Duchenne's progressive muscular dystrophy underline the importance of an early diagnosis and proper genetic counseling (Crisp et al., 1982; O'Brien et al., 1983).

An early diagnosis can often be made on the basis of careful clinical examination. Several genetic diseases, especially in the group of aminoacidopathies and organic acidemias, are characterized by acute neonatal illness. Symptoms, such as vomiting, dehydration, metabolic acidosis, hypertonia or hypotonia, and convulsions, are a reason for further chemical analysis. The same is true during the later development of a child when there are features such as psychomotor retardation, skeletal abnormalities, coarsening facies, visual and/or hearing impairment, hepatosplenomegaly, hypo- or hypertonia, or other neurological manifestations.

More than 100 genetic metabolic diseases, mainly aminoacidopathies and organic acidemias, are associated with characteristic abnormalities of metabolites in urine, blood, and/or other body fluids (Goodman and Markey, 1981; Bremer et al., 1981; Watts, 1984; Stanbury et al., 1983). A variety of qualitative and quantitative abnormalities can now be detected by electrophoresis (mucopolysaccharides and amino acids), thin-layer chromatography (oligosaccharides, oligonucleotides, and amino acids), column chromatography (amino acids) gas chromatography/mass spectrometry (organic acids), and high- performance liquid chromatography (purines and pyrimidines). When such analyses are performed on material from acutely ill neonates or children with developmental problems or other features that might point to a genetic disease, an inborn error of metabolism is found in 4–5% of the cases. Sometimes the diagnosis, management, and genetic counseling can be based on metabolite analysis alone, but if possible the ultimate diagnosis should be based on the demonstration of the responsible (enzyme) protein defect.

In about 10% of the mendelian disorders, the responsible protein defect is known, 210 of which are genetic enzyme deficiencies (McKusick, 1983; Stanbury et al. 1983). When the existence of one of these diseases is suspected, (enzyme) protein analysis can be carried out on organ biopsies, blood (cells), or cultured skin fibroblasts of the patient (for reviews see Galjaard, 1980; Stanbury et al., 1983). The efficiency of diagnostic enzyme studies will depend on the selection of patients by clinical criteria and the results of previous laboratory investigations. The rate of genetic (enzyme) protein defects found is now of the order of 10–20% in the six regional laboratories for metabolic studies in the Netherlands, each of which works in close contact with clinicians in their region of about 1×10^6 people.

When a patient with a possible genetic disease is in a life- threatening condition, it is important to collect urine, blood, and a skin biopsy for the cultivation and storage of fibroblasts. In this way, diagnostic assays can be performed even after the death of the patient. This is essential to permit proper genetic counseling of the parents and other relatives because no accurate information about recurrence risk and preventive measures can be provided without an exact diagnosis. Storage of fibroblasts from the patient and the heterozygous parents is also essential for a prenatal diagnosis in future pregnancies (see the next section).

Table 2 Inborn Errors of Metabolism Which Have Been Diagnosed in Utero

Error	Diagnostic assay
Carbohydrate disorders	
Galactosemia	Galactose-1-phosphate uridyl transferase
Glycogenosis II	α-1,4-Glucosidase
Glycogenosis IV	α-1,4:α-1,4-Glucan-6-glycosyl transferase
Pyruvate carboxylase deficiency	Pyruvate carboxylase
Mucopolysaccharidoses	
Type I (Hurler)	α-L-Iduronidase
Type II (Hunter)[a]	Sulfoiduronide sulfatase
Type III A (Sanfilippo)	Heparan sulfate sulfaminohydrolase
Type III B (Sanfilippo)	α-*N*-Acetyl-*D*-glucosaminidase
Type IV (Morquio)	6-Sulfo-*N*-acetylgalactosaminide sulfatase
Type VI (Maroteaux-Lamy)	4-Sulfo-*N*-acectylgalactosaminide sulfatase
Oligosaccharidoses	
Sialidosis	Lysosomal neuraminidase
Galactosialidosis	β-Galactosidase + lysosomal neuraminidase
Mucolipidosis II ("I-cell-" disease)	Multiple lysosomal deficiency
Mucolipidosis IV	Electronmicroscopy, intralysosomal storage and possibly ganglioside neuraminidase
Fucosidosis	α-Fucosidase
Mannosidosis	α-Mannosidase
Lipidoses	
G_{M1}-Gangliosidosis	β-Galactosidase
G_{M2}-Gangliosidosis Tay-Sachs	Hexosaminidase A
G_{M2}-Gangliosidosis Sandhoff	Hexosaminidase A + B
Niemann-Pick disease	Sphingomyelinase
Gaucher disease	β-Glucosidase/glucocerebrosidase
Krabbe disease	Galactocerebroside-β-galactosidase
Fabry disease[a]	α-Galactosidase
Metachromatic leucodystrophy	Aryl sulfatase A
Wolman disease	Acid lipase
Adrenoleucodystrophy[a]	Cholesterol ester fatty acids
Aminoacidopathies/organic acidemias	
Argininosuccinic aciduria	Argininosuccinase
Citrullinemia	Argininosuccinate synthase
Maple syrup urine disease	Branched-chain α-keto acid decarboxylase
Propionic acidemia	Propionyl CoA carboxylase

Table 2 (Cont.)

Error	Diagnostic assay
Methylmalonic acidemia	
Vitamin B_{12} nonresponsive	Methylmalonyl CoA apomutase
Vitamin B_{12} responsive	Defective cobalamin metabolism
Homocystinuria	Cystathionine β-synthase
Cystinosis	[^{35}S]Cystine chromatography
Isovaleric acidemia	Isovaleryl-CoA dehydrogenase
Glutaric aciduria I	Glutaryl-CoA dehydrogenase
Glutaric aciduria II	Fatty acid oxidation
Nonketotic hyperglycinemia	Glycine: serine ratio in fluid
Tyrosinemia I	Succinyl acetone in fluid
Nucleic acid disorders	
Lesch-Nyhan syndrome[a]	HGPRT assay or [^{3}H]Hypoxanthine autoradiography
Xeroderma pigmentosum	[^{3}H]Thymidine autoradiography after UV radiation
Combined immunodeficiency	Adenosine deaminase
Other genetic disorders	
Sickle cell anemia	Endonuclease restriction site analysis of amniotic fluid cells or chorion
β-Thalassemia	Idem or hemoglobin assay in fetal blood
Menkes syndrome	^{64}Cu incorporation
α_1-Antitrypsin deficiency	Endonuclease restriction site analysis using synthetic oligonucleotides
Congenital adrenal hyperplasia	17-α-Hydroxyprogesterone in amniotic fluid
Congenital nephrosis	α-fetoprotein in amniotic fluid
Acute intermittent porphyria	Uroporphyrinogen-1 synthetase
Cytochrome b_5 reductase deficiency	Cytochrome b_5 reductase
Osteogenesis imperfecta	Proline incorporation in collagen
Hypercholesterolemia[b]	LDH receptor, HMG-CoA reductase
Cystic fibrosis	Intestinal enzymes in amniotic fluid

[a] X-linked inheritance.
[b] Dominant, and all others are autosomal recessive.

In several instances, biochemical assays on cell material from possible carriers permit the demonstration of heterozygosity, but often there is some overlap with control values. At this moment, carrier detection at the individual level is mostly limited to X-linked disorders, such as hemophilia, Duchenne muscular dystrophy, Fabry disease, Lesch-Nyhan syndrome, mucopolysaccharidosis II (Hunter's disease), or Menkes disease. In autosomal-recessive disorders, carrier detection is mainly useful when the prevalence of heterozygotes in a certain population is relatively high. After diagnosing an index patient, siblings and other close relatives can be tested. When people are found to be carriers, they may request further testing of their partners before they consider reproduction.

When couples are found to be at increased risk of having affected offspring, they should be informed about the magnitude of the genetic risk and about the various options to (further) reproduction. As has been mentioned above, a large proportion of couples at high risk are deterred from pregnancy. Yet, this is a difficult decision, especially for couples who do not have a healthy child. When the male is a carrier of a dominant mutation or of the same recessive mutation as his wife, artificial insemination with donor sperm is a possibility in order to have normal offspring. This option is, however, not often chosen, probably because of psychological barriers.

A much more popular alternative for couples at risk is fetal monitoring in early pregnancy with the possibility of selective abortion (for reviews, see Milunsky 1979; Galjaard, 1980, 1982a). In most European countries, the United States, and various other parts of the world, an increasing number of centers for prenatal diagnosis of congenital disorders have developed. During the last decade, hundreds of thousands of pregnancies at risk have been monitored for chromosomal aberrations, genetic metabolic diseases, open neural tube defects, and other fetal malformations. The most common indications are advanced maternal age, previous affected child, and parental carriership. The overall rate of fetal abnormalities detected in the second trimester is 3–5%, depending on the indications used. Prenatal diagnosis is not only a means of preventing the birth of affected children, but also offers a perspective to normal offspring for couples that otherwise would not have dared to have children because of their increased genetic risk.

PRENATAL DIAGNOSIS OF GENETIC METABOLIC DISEASE

Second-Trimester Fetal Diagnosis

Transabdominal amniocentesis at the sixteenth week of pregnancy has become a safe procedure for mother and fetus. In experienced hands, the risk of fetal loss as a result of the puncture can be as low as 0.3%. In our own center, where we perform about 1500 prenatal analyses each year, the amniocentesis, amniotic fluid cell cultivation, and cytogenetic or (micro)biochemical analysis are successful in more than 99% of the cases. In less than 1% repeated amniocentesis 10–14 days later is required, and so far a prenatal diagnosis could be established in all instances.

Some 80 genetic metabolic diseases can be demonstrated by biochemical analysis of cultured amniotic fluid cells (Galjaard, 1980; Patrick, 1984). Practical experience has been acquired with the second-trimester fetal diagnosis of 60 genetic metabolic diseases (Table 2). Since conventional analytical techniques require milligrams of cellular protein, cultivation periods of 2–4 weeks are quite common in order to obtain sufficient numbers of amniotic fluid cells. Ultramicrochemical methods, permitting assays in only dozens, hundreds, or a few thousand cells, have been useful to reduce the cultivation time and hence the waiting period for the couples at risk (Galjaard, 1980, 1982b). By using such sensitive analytical methods, the fetal diagnosis for more than 20 genetic metabolic diseases can be established within 7–14 days after amniocentesis.

For an accurate fetal diagnosis, the analytical results of cultured amniotic fluid cells from the pregnancy at risk must be compared with those of control amniotic fluid cells and of fibroblasts from an index patient and the heterozygous parents. The origin of the cells, conditions of cell cultivation, preparation, and (micro) biochemical analysis must be standardized as much as possible, and a reference enzyme should be measured to test the quality of the sample (Galjaard, 1980).

When the fetus is found to be affected, nearly all parents wish to interrupt their pregnancy. When optimal procedures are used, this can usually be performed between the eighteenth and twentieth week of pregnancy, i.e., before the mother has felt fetal movements. A few aminoacidopathies and organic acidemias can be detected directly after amniocentesis by chromotographic analysis of amniotic fluid supernatant (Jakobs, 1983). Still, termination of a second-trimester pregnancy by instillation of prostaglandins means a psychological stress for many women (for review, see Blumberg, 1984). On the other hand, a recent survey among a few hundred women who underwent termination because of an affected fetus in our own center and who became pregnant again, showed that all of them requested prenatal monitoring again (L. J. Thomassen-Brepols, personal communication).

The proportion of requests for prenatal monitoring because of an increased risk of a genetic metabolic disease is relatively small. In our own series of nearly 10,000 prenatal diagnoses, this was about 500. The percentage of affected fetuses detected in this category is, however, 20% (see Table 3). Most requests were because of an increased risk of one of the mucopolysaccharidoses or sphingolipidoses (Table 3). Similar observations were reported in previous surveys on prenatal diagnoses of genetic metabolic diseases among the main centers in Europe (see Murken et al., 1979) and in the United States (Milunsky, 1979).

Because of the relatively low incidence of most genetic diseases, the highly specialized nature of the microchemical analyses and the necessary availability of proper control cell material, the fetal diagnosis of genetic metabolic diseases should be centralized in one or a few expert center(s). In some instances, collaboration between centers is the most efficient way to deal with requests for prenatal diagnoses of very rare diseases where special substrates or analytical techniques are required.

Table 3 Requests for Prenatal Monitoring in Rotterdam[a]

Total number of pregnancies monitored	9,657
Total number of affected fetuses detected	460 (5%)
Total number of pregnancies at risk for genetic metabolic disease	482

Abnormality	No. of pregnancies monitored	No. of fetal abnormalities
Carbohydrate metabolism	69	12
Mucopolysaccharidoses	149	24
Oligosaccharidoses	20	3
Sphingolipidoses	101	22
Aminoacidopathies/ organic acidemias	65	14
Abnormalities in nucleic acid metabolism	51	8
Other genetic metabolic diseases	27	8
	482	91 (19%)

[a] Data from the Department of Obstetrics (Dr. M. Jahoda and Dr. R. Vosters) and from the Department of Clinical Genetics (Dr. E. S. Sachs and Dr. W. J. Kleijer), University Hospital, Rotterdam.

First-Trimester Fetal Diagnosis

Biochemical Analysis of Normal Chorionic Villi

Direct Assays on Homogenate Kazy et al. (1982) were first to report the results of enzyme assays on homogenates of chorionic tissue obtained by biopsy forceps under control of real-time ultrasound scanning at 6–12 weeks of pregnancy. The activity of six lysomomal enzymes was determined with 4-methylumbelliferyl substrate in 16 specimens obtained in pregnancies prior to termination. Also arylsulfatase A and sphingomyelinase were analyzed. The enzyme activities of normal chorionic villi were in the same range as those of cultured amniotic fluid cells.

Danesino and co-workers also assayed normal activities of a number of lysosomal enzymes and of adenosine deaminase (Simoni et al., 1983), and Kleijer and co-workers established normal values of some 20 enzymes that are involved in genetic metabolic diseases (Table 4). The ranges of activities found in the three studies mentioned are quite similar. Most enzyme activities are lower in chorionic villi than in amniotic fluid cells, which in turn are usually lower than in cultured fibroblasts. Only the activities of α-1, 4-glucosidase and α-fucosidase are higher in chorionic villi. The activities of hexosaminidase A and B, arylsulfatase B, α-mannosidase, and β-glucuronidase are about the same in chorionic villi and cultured amniotic fluid cells.

For diagnostic purposes, analytical data from chorionic tissue will be compared with those of fibroblasts from an index patient and the heterozygous parents. The range of activities in normal fibroblasts is, therefore, given as a comparison in Table 4.

Assays on Cultured Chorionic Cells Quite a number of prenatal tests for genetic metabolic disease are based on the incorporation of radioactive labeled precursors into macromolecules using cultured amniotic fluid cells (for review, see Galjaard, 1980). This is especially the case for inborn errors of amino acid, organic acid, and nucleic acid metabolism. Analogously, we have investigated the feasibility of using cultured chorionic villus cells.

The chorion aspirate is cut into small fragments, which are incubated with 0.25% trypsin in a rotating tube for 20 min at 20°C. Both the villi fragments and the detached cells in suspension can be used for cultivation in Chang medium (Hana, Biological Media). Depending on the type of analysis, a cultivation period of 2–4 weeks is required. When sufficient cells are available, the appropriate labeled precursor can be added to the culture medium, and the assays can be performed according to methods that have been described previously for cultured fibroblasts or amniotic fluid cells (for reviews, see Galjaard, 1980).

The first-trimester fetal diagnosis of some inborn errors of nucleic acid metabolism, such as xeroderma pigmentosum or Lesch-Nyhan syndrome, can be made by autoradiography after incorporation of radiolabeled [^{3}H]thymidine or [^{3}H]hypoxanthine, respectively. Since the analysis of the metabolic defect in these cases is based on grain counts above individual cultured chorionic villous cells, a cultivation period of 12–14 days will be sufficient. Figure 1 shows the relatively weak labeling above the cell nuclei, which represents unscheduled DNA synthesis after ultraviolet radiation in normal cultured chorionic cells. If the fetus was suffering from the autosomal-recessive disease xeroderma pigmentosum, defective DNA repair would be apparent from an absence or reduced

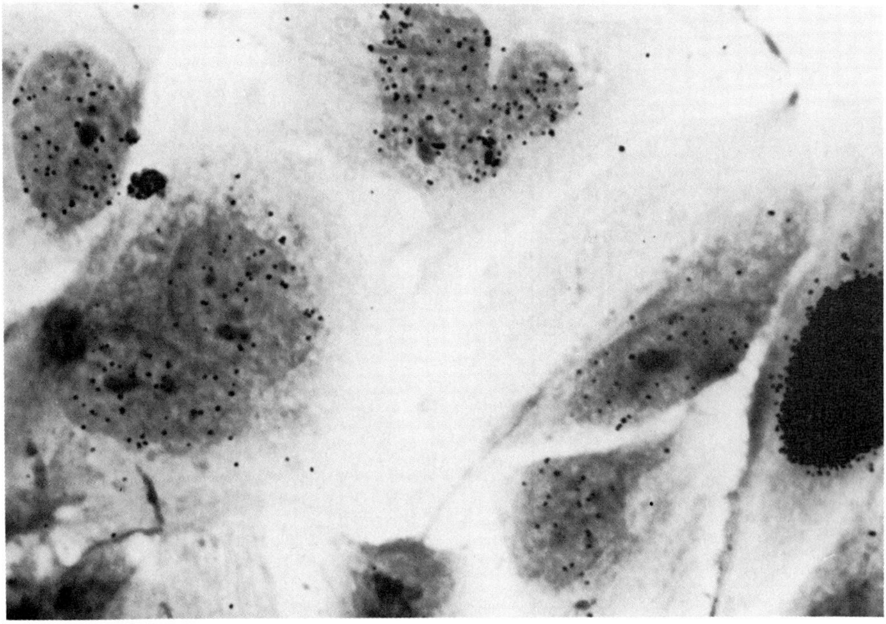

Figure 1 Autoradiography after ultraviolet radiation and [^{3}H]thymidine incorporation into cultured chorionic villous cells (2 weeks after sampling). Heavily labeled cell nucleus indicates DNA synthesis during S phase; weak labeling represents DNA repair that would be absent in the case of xeroderma pigmentosum.

Table 4 Range of Enzyme Activities[a] in Chorionic Villi from Normal Pregnancies

	Chorionic villi			Fibroblast	
	Kazy et al. (1982) range	Danesino (Simoni et al., 1983) range	Kleijer range	Mean	Range
4-Methylumbelliferyl substrate					
β-Hexosaminidase	772–5810		2770–7100	4750	5500–21,000
Hexosaminidase A (%)			57–84%	66%	55–85%
β-Galactosidase	196–739	86–409	142–274	216	450–1,200
α-Galactosidase			15–57	27	45–120
β-Glucosidase	34–179		51–138	101	120–500
α-Fucosidase	76–690		210–503	358	40–180
α-Mannosidase			33–91	56	40–160
α-L-Iduronidase			9–25	12	140–530
β-Glucuronidase	77–354	88–269	31–195	78	40–160
α-Glucosidase			42–106	64	40–160

Arylsulfatase C			250–440	350	5–17
Neuraminidase		8–49			
Chromogenic substrate					
Arylsulfatase A	52–208	40–203	47–139	81	270–970
Arylsulfatase B			170–455	288	350–870
Radiolabeled substrate					
Sphingomyelinase	18–50	40–73	1.9–6.4	4.4	21–45
Cerebroside-β-galactosidase			0.6–1.2	0.9	1.3–3.8
Iduronate sulfatase			65–222	114	30–190
Heparan sulfamidase			1.9–2.3	2.1	1.7–5.5
Adenosine deaminase		2–8			600–1,730
HPRT			50–85	64	77–197
APRT			29–57	44	29–79
Dihydroxyacetone phosphate acyltransferase (Zellweger)			1.8–3.8	2.3	2.1–5.2

[a] Expressed as 10^{-9} moles per hour per milligram except for iduronate sulphatase (10^{-9} moles per 24 hours per milligram) and heparan sulfamidase (percent ^{35}S released per 17 hours per milligram).

amount of [^{3}H]thymidine incorporation, and hence no or fewer grains would be visible. This approach has been successfully used in cultured amniotic fluid cells in pregnancies at risk for xeroderma pigmentosum (Ramsay et al., 1974) and Lesch-Nyhan syndrome (Halley and Heukels-Dully, 1977).

The quantitative analysis of incorporated radioactivity by scintillation counting after isolation of specific cell compounds has a much wider diagnostic scope. In this way, we have analyzed the decarboxylation of [^{14}C]leucine by measuring the $^{14}CO_2$ production according to Wendel et al. (1973) and also the ratio of incorporated [^{14}C]citrulline and [^{3}H]leucine and of [^{14}C]proprionate and [^{3}H]leucine into trichloroacetic acid-precipitated cellular protein (Jacoby et al., 1972; Morrow et al., 1976; for review on methodology, see Galjaard, 1980). The results in Table 5 show that cultured chorionic villus cells give analytical results that are similar to cultured fibroblasts. The large difference between normal and mutant cells indicates the feasibility of first-trimester fetal diagnosis of maple syrup urine disease, citrullinemia methylmalonic acidemia, propionic acidemia, and various other diseases that can be tested in a similar way.

A disadvantage of this approach is the fact that the in vitro cultivation of chorionic villus cells is not always easy and sometimes requires a long time to yield adequate cell numbers. Since the optimal period for chorion sampling is around the ninth week, subsequent cell cultivation should not take longer than 2–3 weeks in order to be able to interrupt the pregnancy by vacuum curettage.

Table 5 Incorporation Studies in Normal Chorionic Cell Cultures[a]

Cells	Maple syrup urine disease ($^{14}CO_2$ production[b])	Citrullinemia $\left(\frac{[^{14}C]\text{citrulline}}{[^3H]\text{leucine}} \times 10^2\right)$	Methylmalonic or propionic acidemia $\left(\frac{[^{14}C]\text{proprionate}}{[^3H]\text{leucine}} \times 10^3\right)$
Chorion cells	1164	77	19
Normal fibroblasts	1322	30	11
Mutant fibroblasts	36	0.9	2.3

[a] Analyses have been carried out after 3 weeks cultivation of chorionic villus cells that were obtained by aspiration in the eighth week of pregnancy.
[b] Activities measured in picomoles per hour per milligram.

Incorporation Studies in Intact Chorionic Villi More or less to our surprise, it also proved possible to perform quantitative incorporation studies with radiolabeled compounds using intact villi directly after chorion sampling. To test the feasibility of a direct diagnosis of maple syrup urine disease (MSUD), chorion tissue fragments of 2–5 mg wet weight were incubated in wells of a microtiter plate with 100 μl substrate containing [^{14}C]leucine. After 4 hr at 20°C, the amount of liberated $^{14}CO_2$ was measured by scintillation counting as well as the amount of [^{14}C]leucine incorporation into trichloroacetic acid-precipitable cellular protein. As is shown in Table 6, the leucine decarboxylation in intact villi directly after sampling was similar to the activity in villi that had been stored for 24 hr in culture medium. Both sets of values were comparable with those of normal cultured fibroblasts. The difference between normal cells and those from a MSUD patient is large enough to permit a reliable diagnosis. Similar results were obtained for the incorporation of [^{14}C]propionate as a measure for diseases such as methylmalonic acidemia or propionic acidemia. The feasibility of incorporation studies using intact chorionic villi was shown by successful first-trimester monitoring for fetal methylmalonic acidemia and by the first diagnosis of fetal citrullinemia (Kleijer et al., 1984c). A. D. Patrick and E. Young (personal communication) have been successful with the first-trimester detection of cystinosis using uptake studies of [^{35}S]cystine into intact chorionic villi (see also Willcox and Patrick, 1974).

First-Trimester Fetal Diagnoses of Genetic Metabolic Disease

At present only few prenatal diagnoses of affected fetuses based on enzyme assays of chorionic tissue have been reported (Gibbs et al., 1984; Grabowski et al., 1984; Kleijer et al., 1984a, b, c; Poenaru et al., 1984; Vimal et al., 1984). From a survey for the *International Symposium on First Trimester Fetal Diagnosis* in Rapallo, October 1984, however, it appears that a total of 106 pregnancies at risk for a genetic metabolic disease had been monitored using chorionic tissue. A total of 27 embryos (25%) were found to be affected and in all these instances the first-trimester diagnosis could be confirmed by biochemical analysis of fetal cells after abortion.

Of the remaining 79 cases where the analytical results were in the heterozygote or control range, confirmatory studies by amniocentesis and biochemical analysis of cultured amniotic fluid cells were reported in 20% of the cases only. In this last group, there were four false negative values, i.e., an enzyme deficiency was found in cultured amniotic fluid

Table 6 Incorporation Studies of Radiolabeled Precursors Using Intact Chorionic Villi

	Test for maple syrup urine disease			Test for methylmalonic or propionic acidemia[b]
	Leucine decarboxylation (dpm released $^{14}CO_2$)[a]	Leucine incorporation in TCA precipitate	Ratio $\times 10^3$	$\left(\frac{[^{14}C]\text{proprionate}}{[^{3}H]\text{leucine}} \times 10^3 \text{ (dpm)}\right)$
Fresh villi (1)	31,300	130,000	242	48–145 (N = 6)
Fresh villi (2)	51,100	183,000	280	
Villi stored in medium for 2 days	44,500	162,000	275	68
Normal fibroblasts	1,900	9,500	200	15–45
Mutant fibroblasts (MSUD and MMA, respectively)	500	18,200	27	1–8

[a]Carbon-14-labeled CO_2 released was measured after 4 hr incubation according to the method of Wendel et al. (1973).
[b]Intact villi were incubated for 17 hr with [^{14}C]propionate and [^{3}H]leucine.

cells (confirmed after termination of the pregnancy), whereas the diagnosis was "unaffected" on the basis of chorion analysis. It is likely that these failures are related to inadequate material in some instances and to insufficient experience with these new diagnostic methods in other cases. Ten babies, predicted normal, had been born and were found healthy, three pregnancies ended with a spontaneous abortion, and the remaining 62 pregnancies predicted normal were continuing.

In our own laboratory, we have so far performed 27 prospective fetal diagnoses for 11 different metabolic disorders. Six fetuses were found to be affected and the diagnosis was confirmed in fetal tissues or fibroblasts obtained after termination in the 9th to 11th week; the diseases involved were Krabbe's disease, the Hunter and Sanfilippo A syndromes, citrullinemia and maple syrup urine disease (see Kleijer et al. 1984a, b, c). In 21 pregnancies at risk normal enzyme activities were shown in the villi, which was confirmed by the analysis of amniotic fluid cells or after birth.

In some pregnancies at risk, the chorionic villus samplings were performed in our own center (Dr. M. Jahoda and Dr. R. Vosters, Department of Obstetrics and Gynecology, University Hospital, Rotterdam) and the tissue was transported to the laboratory in culture medium at room temperature. In other instances, chorionic tissue was referred to us from other countries (France, West Germany, Italy, Spain). Transporting the chorionic tissue in sterile culture medium with antibiotics at room temperature for 1–2 days did not pose any problem. Of course, when samples are sent from tropical countries, prolonged high temperature should be avoided. For DNA analysis, samples could better be frozen (WHO, 1984).

The amount of chorionic tissue needed for biochemical analysis depends on the type of assay. For the diagnosis of hemoglobinopathies using recombinant DNA technology, 10 mg wet weight of chorionic tissue usually yields 2–5 μg DNA, which is just sufficient for analysis (see other chapters in this treatise). About 20 mg wet weight of chorionic tissue provides 10 μg DNA. In the case of direct enzyme assays on cell homogenates, 5–10 mg wet weight is usually sufficient. When 4-methylumbelliferyl substrate and (ultra)microchemical techniques are used, reliable results can be obtained with much smaller amounts of material (for reviews, see Galjaard 1980, 1982). In some assays with natural substrate (such as sphingomyelinase, galactocerebrosidase, and a few enzymes involved in glycosaminoglycan degradation) and especially when the (normal) enzyme activity is low, 10–20 mg of chorionic tissue may be needed. Each first-trimester diagnosis should consist of duplicate or triplicate measurements of the enzyme concerned, a determination of the protein content, and of a reference enzyme, which is especially important after transport in order to test the quality of the sample. The analytical values are then compared with those of mutant fibroblasts from the index patient and cells from the heterozygous parents.

Table 7 illustrates two examples of first-trimester diagnoses based on direct biochemical assays on chorion villous cell homogenate. Embryos affected with Krabbe's disease and with Hunter's syndrome respectively, were detected, and after termination the fetal diagnosis was confirmed in both instances. (Kleijer et al. 1984a, b).

We have, thus far, established two first-trimester diagnoses using incorporation studies of radioactive labeled precursors into intact chorionic villi (see previous section). In a pregnancy at risk for methylmalonic acidemia, chorion sampling was carried out at 10 weeks, and small fragments of chorionic tissue (1–2 mg) were incubated in culture medium containing [^{14}C]propionate and [^{3}H]leucine. After a 17 hr incubation, the amount of incorporated radioactivities into TCA-precipitable protein was measured, and the results showed similar values as in control fibroblasts. The prediction that the fetus would be unaffected was supported by the finding of a normal activity of methylmalonyl-CoA mutase by Dr. B. Fowler (University of Manchester) as well as normal results of amniotic fluid cell assays. A healthy baby was born (Kleijer et al., 1984c).

In a similar way, a fetus affected with citrullinemia was diagnosed at 9 weeks of pregnancy by incubation of intact chorionic villi with [^{14}C]citrulline (Kleijer et al., 1984c). In this case, the fetal diagnosis was confirmed by the demonstration of the metabolic defect in cultured fetal fibroblasts 2 weeks after the interruption. Recently we have also made two first-trimester diagnoses of fetuses affected with maple syrup urine disease by using intact chorionic villi. A. D. Patrick (personal communication) successfully applied the technique of incubating intact villi in the first-trimester monitoring of pregnancies at risk for cystinosis (see also previous section).

In nearly all instances, a fetal diagnosis can probably be established either by direct assays on cell homogenates or by incorporation studies of radioactive precursors using intact villi. In a few instances, biochemical or autoradiographic studies have to be performed after short-term cultivation of chorionic tissue. As a consequence, all advantages of chorionic villus analysis can be maintained, i.e., early sampling, short waiting period, vacuum curettage in case the embryo is affected, and the

Table 7 Examples of First-Trimester Fetal Diagnoses Using Direct Assays on Chorionic Villous Homogenate

	Galactocerebroside β-galactosidase (10^{-9} mol/hr/mg)	Reference enzyme β-galactosidase (10^{-9} mol/hr/mg)	Iduronate sulfate sulfatase (10^{-9} mol/day/mg)
Chorionic villi at risk for Krabbe's disease	0.04	172	—
Control villi	0.54–0.97	95–211	—
Chorionic villi at risk for Hunter's syndrome	—	350	8
Control villi	—	400–550	120–220
Krabbe's disease fibroblasts (index patient)	0.05	443	—
Hunter's syndrome fibroblasts (index patient)			0–3
Control fibroblasts	1.93	400–1000	30–200

possibility for a couple at risk to make their decisions without social pressure.

As in the case of second-trimester fetal diagnosis of genetic metabolic disease, the biochemical analysis of chorionic tissue should be centralized. The annual number of prenatal diagnoses in this category is relatively small and it is, therefore, advantageous if one or a few centers in a country can acquire sufficient experience. Also, for a correct interpretation of the analytical data, the laboratory must have expertise in the investigation of the metabolic pathways involved. It must have access to adequate comparative cell material for index patients and heterozygotes.

Although the first-trimester diagnosis of inborn errors of metabolism is still in its beginning phase, experience has already been gained with diagnostic chorion assays for 32 different genetic metabolic diseases (excluding those analyzed with DNA technology). For each individual disease, only one or a few pregnancies have been monitored; for some others, such as Tay-Sachs disease G_{M1}-gangliosidosis and metachromatic leucodystrophy, series of a dozen or more fetal diagnoses have been established in 8- to 10-week old pregnancies.

Despite the few false negatives, the overall results of diagnostic biochemical chorion analyses are very promising indeed. If the risk of fetal loss will turn out to be low and further evaluation of the biochemical analyses of chorionic tissue prove satisfactory, it is to be expected that amniocentesis in pregnancies at risk for a genetic metabolic disease will gradually be replaced by chorion sampling at 8–10 weeks.

REFERENCES

Angastiniotis, M. A., and Hadjiminas, M. G. (1981). Prevention of thalassemia in Cyprus, *Lancet i*:369–371.

Bickel, H., Guthrie, R., and Hammersen, G. (eds.) (1980). *Neonatal Screening for Inborn Errors of Metabolism*. Springer-Verlag, New York.

Blumberg, B. D. (1984). The emotional implications of prenatal diagnosis. In *Psychological Aspects of Genetic Counseling*, (A.E.M. Emery and I.M. Putten, eds.). Academic Press, New York.

Bremer, H. J., Duran, M., Kamerling, J. P., Przyrembel, H., and Wadman, S. K. (1981). Disturbances of Amino Acid Metabolism: Clinical Chemistry and Diagnosis. Urban and Schwarzenberg, Baltimore.

Carter, L. O., Fraser Roberts, J. A., Evans, K. A., and Bock, A. R. (1971). Genetic clinic: A follow-up. *Lancet i*:281–285.

Crisp, D. E., Ziter, F. A., and Bray, P. F. (1982). Diagnostic delay in Duchenne; muscular dystrophy. J. Am. Med. Assoc. *247*:478–480.

Emery, A. E. H., Watt, M. S. and Clark, E. R.(1972). The effect of genetic counselling in Duchenne muscular dystrophy. *Clin. Genet. 3*:147–150.

Galjaard, H. (1980). *Genetic Metabolic Diseases: Early Diagnosis and Prenatal Analysis*. Elsevier/North Holland, New York.

Galjaard, H. (ed.) (1982a). *The Future of Prenatal Diagnosis*. Churchill Livingstone, Edinburgh.

Galjaard, H. (1982b). Miniaturization of biochemical analysis of cultured amniotic fluid cells. In *Methods in Cell Biology*, Vol. 26, pp. 241–268, S.A. Latt and G. J. Darlington (eds.). Academic Press, New York.

Gibbs D. A., McFadyen, I. R., Crawford, M. d'A., De Muinck-Keizer, E. E., Headhouse-Benson, C. M., Wilson, T. M., and Farrant, P. H. (1984). First-trimester diagnosis of Lesch-Nyhan syndrome. *Lancet 11*:1180–1183.

Goodman, S. I. and Markey, S. P.(1981). *Diagnosis of Organic Acidemias by Gas Chromatography—Mass Spectrometry. In Laboratory and Research Methods in Biology and Medicine*, Vol. 6. Alan R. Liss, New York.

Grabowski, G. A., Kruse, J. R., Goldberg, J. D., Chockkalingam, K., Gordon, R. E., Blakemore, K. J., Mahoney, M. J., and Desnick, R. J. (1984). First-trimester prenatal diagnosis of Tay-Sachs disease. *Am. J. Human Genet. 36*:1369–1379.

Halley, D. and Heukels-Dully, M. J. (1977). Rapid prenatal diagnosis of the Lesch-Nyhan syndrome. *J. Med. Genet. 14*:100–102.

Jacoby, L. B., Littlefield, J. W., Milunsky, A., Shih, V. E., and Wilson, R. S. A. (1972). A microassay for argininosuccinase in cultured cells. *Am. J. Human Genet. 24*321–324.

Jakobs, C. A. J. M.(1983). Contribution to the prenatal diagnosis of inherited metabolic disorders; analysis of metabolites in amniotic fluid. Thesis, State University of Utrecht.

Kaback, M. M. (ed.) (1977). *Tay-Sachs Disease: Screening and Prevention*. Alan R. Liss, New York.

Kaback, M.M.(1981). Heterozygote screening and prenatal diagnosis in Tay-Sachs disease: A world-wide update. In *Lysosomes and Lysosomal Storage Diseases*, (J. W. Callahan and A. J. Lowden, eds.), pp. 331-342. Raven, New York.

Kazy, Z., Rozovsky, I. S., and Bakharev, V. A.(1982). Chorion biopsy in early pregnancy: A method of early prenatal diagnosis for inherited disorders. *Prenat. Diag. 2*:39–45.

Klein, D. and Wyss, D. (1977). Retrospective and follow-up study of approximately 1000 genetic consultations. *J. Genet. Human 25*:47–57.

Kleijer, W. J., van Diggelen, O. P., Janse, H. C., Galjaard, H., Dumez, Y., and Boué, J. (1984a). First-trimester diagnosis of Hunter syndrome on chorionic villi. *Lancet ii*:472.

Kleijer, W. J., Mancini, G. M. S., Jahoda, M. G. J., Vosters, R. P. L., Sachs, E. S., Niermeijer, M. F., and Galjaard, H. (1984b). First-trimester diagnosis of Krabbe's disease by direct enzyme analysis of chorionic villi. *New Engl. J. Med. 311*:1257.

Kleijer, W. J., Thoomes, R., Galjaard, H., Wendel, U., and Fowler, B. (1984).

First-trimester (chorion biopsy) diagnosis of citrullinemia and methylmalonic aciduria. *Lancet ii*:1340.
McKusick, V. A. (1983). *Mendelian Inheritance in Man*, 6th ed. Johns Hopkins University Press, Baltimore.
Milunsky, A. (ed.) (1979). *Genetic Disorders and the Fetus*. Plenum, New York.
Morrow, G., Revsin, B., Mathews, C., and Giles, H. (1976). A simple, rapid method for prenatal detection of defects in propionate metabolism. *Clin. Genet. 10*:218–221.
Murken, J. D., Stengel-Rutkowski, S., and Schwinger, E. (eds.) (1979). Proceedings of the Third European Conference on Prenatal Diagnosis of Genetic Disorders, Enke, Stuttgart.
O'Brien, T. O., Silbert, J. R., and Harper P. S. (1983). Implications of diagnostic delay in Duchenne muscular dystrophy. *Brit. Med. J. 287*:1106–1107.
Patrick, A. D. (1984). Prenatal diagnosis of inherited metabolic disease In Proceedings of the *Eleventh Study Group of the Royal College of Obstetricians and Gynecologists* (C. H. Rodeck and K. H. Nicolaides, eds.), pp. 121–137. Royal College, London.
Poenaru, L., Castelnau, L., Dumez, Y., and Thepot, F. (1984). First-trimester prenatal diagnosis of mucolipidosis II (I-cell disease) by chorionic biopsy. *Am. J. Human Genet. 36*:1379–1385.
Ramsay, C. A., Coltart, T. M., Blunt, S. Pawsey, S. A., and Gianelli, F. (1974). Prenatal diagnosis of xeroderma pigmentosum. *Lancet ii*:1109–1112.
Simoni, G., Brambati, B., Danesino, C., Rossella, F., Terzoli, G. L., Ferrari, M., and Fraccaro, M. (1983). Efficient direct chromosome analyses and enzyme determinations from chorionic villi samples in the first trimester of pregnancy. *Human Genet. 63*:349–357.
Stanbury, J. B., Wyngaarden, J. B., Fredrickson, D. S., Goldstein, J. L., and Brown, M. S. (eds.) (1983). *The Metabolic Basis of Inherited Disease*, 5th ed. McGraw-Hill, New York.
Vimal, C. M., Fensom, A. H., Heaton, D., Ward, R. H. T., Garrod, P., and Penketh, R. J. A. (1984). Prenatal diagnosis of argininosuccinic aciduria by analysis of cultured chorionic villi. *Lancet i*:521–522.
Watts, R. W. E. (1984). Diagnostic and metabolic investigation and treatment of the acutely ill newborn with particular reference to some of the inborn errors of metabolism. In *Screening and Management of Potentially Treatable Genetic Metabolic Disorders* pp. 127–142. (P. F. Benson, ed.), MTP Press, Lancaster.
Wendel, U., Rüdiger, H. W., Passarge, E. and Mikkelsen, M. (1973). Maple syrup urine disease: rapid prenatal diagnosis by enzyme assay. *Humangenetik 19*:127–128.
Willcox, D. and Patrick, A. D. (1974). Biochemical diagnosis of cystinosis using cultured cells. *Arch. Dis. Child. 49*:209–212.
WHO (1981). *Report on the Community Control of Hereditary Anemias,* WHO, Geneva.
WHO (1984). *Report on Perspectives in Fetal Diagnosis of Hereditary Diseases.* WHO, Geneva.

9

First Trimester Fetal Diagnosis of Sickle Cell Anemia by DNA Analysis

MICHEL GOOSSENS
Henri Mondor University Hospital, Créteil, France
and
YVES DUMEZ
University Clinic of Port-Royal, Paris, France

INTRODUCTION

Since 1976, tremendous progress has been made in the development of techniques used in the prenatal diagnosis of hemoglobin disorders. Advances in this field were initially hampered by the fact that these diseases could only be detected by examination of hemoglobin products. The advent of methods for fetal blood sampling has made it possible to carry out several thousand tests by estimation of the relative rates of globin chain synthesis using radiolabeling or analyzing hemoglobin electrophoretic patterns. This study of the products of mutant globin genes has been used extensively over the last 6 years. However, the collection of fetal blood is not without risk to the fetus, although the safety record has improved with experience. More recently, these disorders have been detected by prenatal examination of fetal DNA, which is now performed routinely. Amniocentesis, performed at 16 to 18 weeks of gestation, is a simpler and safer procedure that allows aspiration of fetal nucleated cells floating in the amniotic fluid. The DNA of these cells is analyzed to diagnose the defect at the gene level. However, there are still certain disadvantages: Since the yield of DNA is low, it is often necessary to grow the cells in culture for 2 to 3 weeks in order to obtain sufficient nucleic acid for gene analysis. Amniotic fluid cell sampling cannot be performed until mid-trimester, and mothers at risk have a long wait. Therapeutic abortion is difficult at this late stage of pregnancy.

The need for improved methods of prenatal diagnosis has stimulated research of cellular and molecular techniques and methods of cell sampling. First-trimester fetal tissue sampling was first attempted 10 years ago and was later used for diagnostic purposes in China and the Soviet Union (1,2). More recently, several groups, including our own, developed simple and reliable techniques for trophoblast biopsy in order to perform fetal diagnosis by gene analysis (3–5), chromosome studies (6, 7), or enzymatic assays (8–10).

Between November, 1982 and June 1984, we have used DNA analysis of chorionic villi obtained at 8–11 weeks of gestation as an alternative approach to prenatal diagnosis of sickle cell anemia, a potentially lethal disease resulting from the homozygous expression of a mutant β-globin gene. This very debilitating disorder is one of the most frequently occurring inherited hemoglobinopathies and has its highest incidence in Black Africans and Afro-Americans, although it is also found in Mediterranean countries. Although the clinical severity of the disease is very variable, the availability of prenatal diagnosis is an important development, as there is no specific therapy. In this chapter, we will describe our experience with first-trimester prenatal diagnosis of sickle cell anemia.

PATIENTS

The couples attending our prenatal clinic belong to high-risk populations originating from the French West Indies (Martinique and Guadaloupe) or from north or west Africa. Most of them requested a prenatal test because they have already had a child with sickle cell anemia. Some were identified as carriers following an out-patient visit in early pregnancy. When high-risk couples are seen during genetic counseling sessions, they are informed about the risks and benefits of both amniocentesis and chorionic villus sampling (CVS). Most of them chose to undergo the CVS procedure in order to receive early reassurance or, at worst, to terminate the pregnancy by an earlier and safer therapeutic abortion. Some women had previously had a prenatal diagnosis by fetal blood analysis or amniocentesis, and a few of them had suffered from the psychological trauma of aborting a wanted pregnancy at 22 weeks' of gestation. However, two-thirds of the women at risk attending our center are still detected too late for first-trimester prenatal testing.

ACQUISITON OF CHORIONIC VILLI: THE BIOPSY FORCEPS METHOD

Several methodological approaches are in use for diagnostic purposes in chorionic villi sampling. To date the majority of CVS have been performed by a transcervical aspiration technique with a flexible catheter under ultrasound guidance (10,11). A different technique has been developed and is used in our centre. This technique consists of sampling the chorionic villi by means of a rigid biopsy forceps guided by ultrasound (5). By the end of June 1984, our experience with this technique consisted of about 85 prenatal diagnoses performed for hemoglobinopathies, metabolic diseases, and fetal sex determinations. We will briefly outline the main features of this CVS procedure.

The biopsies are performed as an out-patient procedure, without anesthesia or premedication. At the first visit, the patient is informed about the benefits of the procedure and its potential danger. The patient undergoes an initial evaluation that consists of an ultrasound examination to determine the gestational age (crown–rump length), the uterine position, and the implantation site and to assess fetal viability. A real-time ultrasound scanner with a 3.5 MHz transducer is used to guide the biopsy forceps, which is highly echogenic. After cleaning the external genitalia and vagina with an antiseptic solution, the cervix is visualized by a speculum and grasped with a Pozzi tenaculum. The biopsy forceps (Storz, 2 mm in cross section) is then introduced transcervically under ultrasound guidance and directed toward the chorionic plate. When the tip of the forceps has reached the appropriate position, a biopsy specimen is taken, and the forceps is slowly withdrawn (Figs. 1 and 2). The villi are then placed in a sterile saline solution and are microscopically examined under low-power. They are stripped of any maternal decidua present and are sent to the laboratory. Biopsy specimens obtains in this way usually consist of pieces of undamaged villi with no or little maternal contamination, in contrast with the minced and often contaminated chorionic villi obtained by suction.

Owing to the rigidity of the biopsy forceps, it may be more difficult to obtain a sample when the placenta is anteriorly located in an anteverted uterus or, on the contrary, when it is posterior in a retroverted uterus. Nevertheless, these problems can be dealt with by moving the tenaculum or by taking the sample with a full bladder. Once the biopsy has been taken, the pregnancy is again monitored by ultrasound. The patient

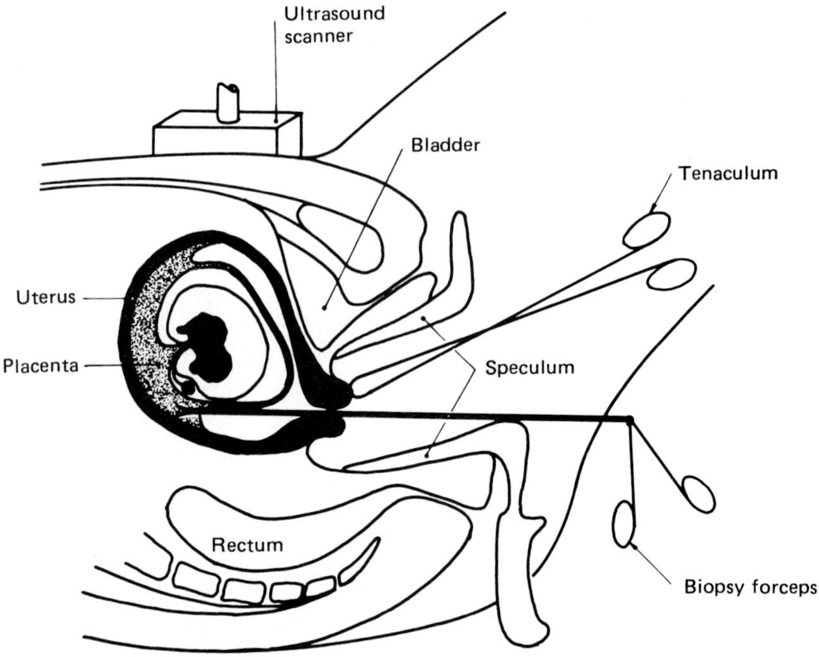

(a)

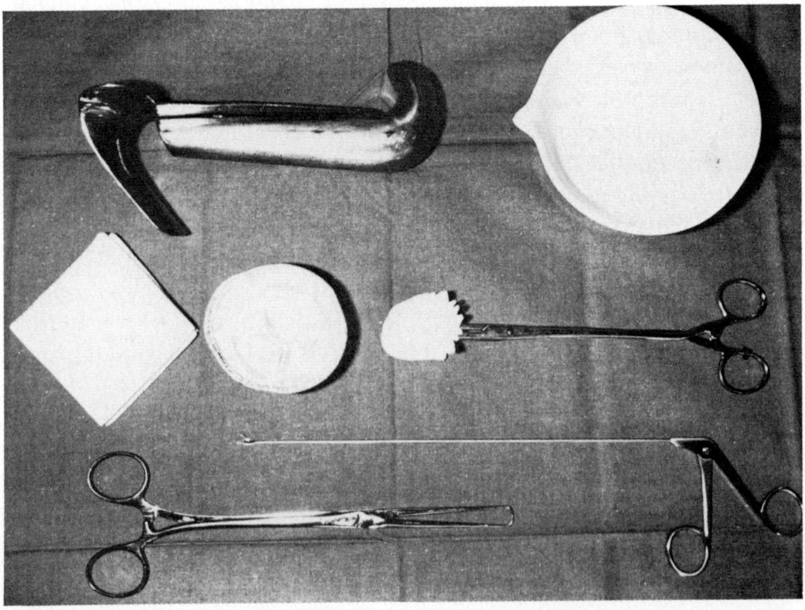

(b)

Figure 1 (a) First-trimester chorionic villus sampling using a biopsy forceps introduced under ultrasound guidance. (b) Instruments used for chorionic villus sampling.

leaves the clinic with written instructions for the follow-up studies. An ultrasonic control is made 15 days later.

Initially, fetal tissue sampling was performed early, at 7–8 weeks, of gestation. It was subsequently decided to perform the sampling around the tenth to eleventh week, when spontaneous abortion is known to be less common, and the procedure is easier and safer. No sampling failure has occurred so far, and this biopsy technique always gives sufficient chorionic tissue for all diagnositc purposes.

DNA ANALYSIS OF THE SICKLE CELL DEFECT

Over the last few years, new advances in recombinant DNA technology have made it feasible to examine genes directly and have defined the basic defect causing hemoglobinopathies and several other genetic diseases. Restriction nuclease analysis has become a major tool in gene analysis and is now being used routinely for prenatal diagnosis. Since the DNA defect is present in every cell, amniotic fluid cells or trophoblastic tissues can serve as a source of fetal DNA to carry out a prenatal test. After purification, the DNA is cut with the appropriate enzyme and the resulting fragments are electrophoresed in agarose. This separates them according to their size. The fragments are then rendered single stranded by alkali treatment and are transferred to a membrane by a process called Southern blotting. The membrane is then soaked in a solution containing ^{32}p-radiolabeled single strands of the gene probe. Once the molecular hybridization of complementary sequences is completed, the membrane is washed to remove unhybridized radioactivity. The size of the fragments containing the gene to be studied is determined by analysis of the position of autoradiographic bands on X-ray films.

Diagnosis of the Sickle Cell Mutation by Linkage

Initially, an indirect approach by linkage analysis was used to diagnose the sickle mutation (12,13). This defect is frequently associated with another mutation which eliminates a *Hpa* I restriction site located on the 3′ side (downstream) of the β-globin gene. As a result, the gene is contained in a fragment of different length, either 7.6 or 13.0 kilobases long. This is the first time that a restriction fragment length (RFLP) polymorphism, which can be detected in the DNA of any nucleated cell, has been used to document the inheritence of the sickle cell gene in mid-trimester amniocytes. However, this approach requires family

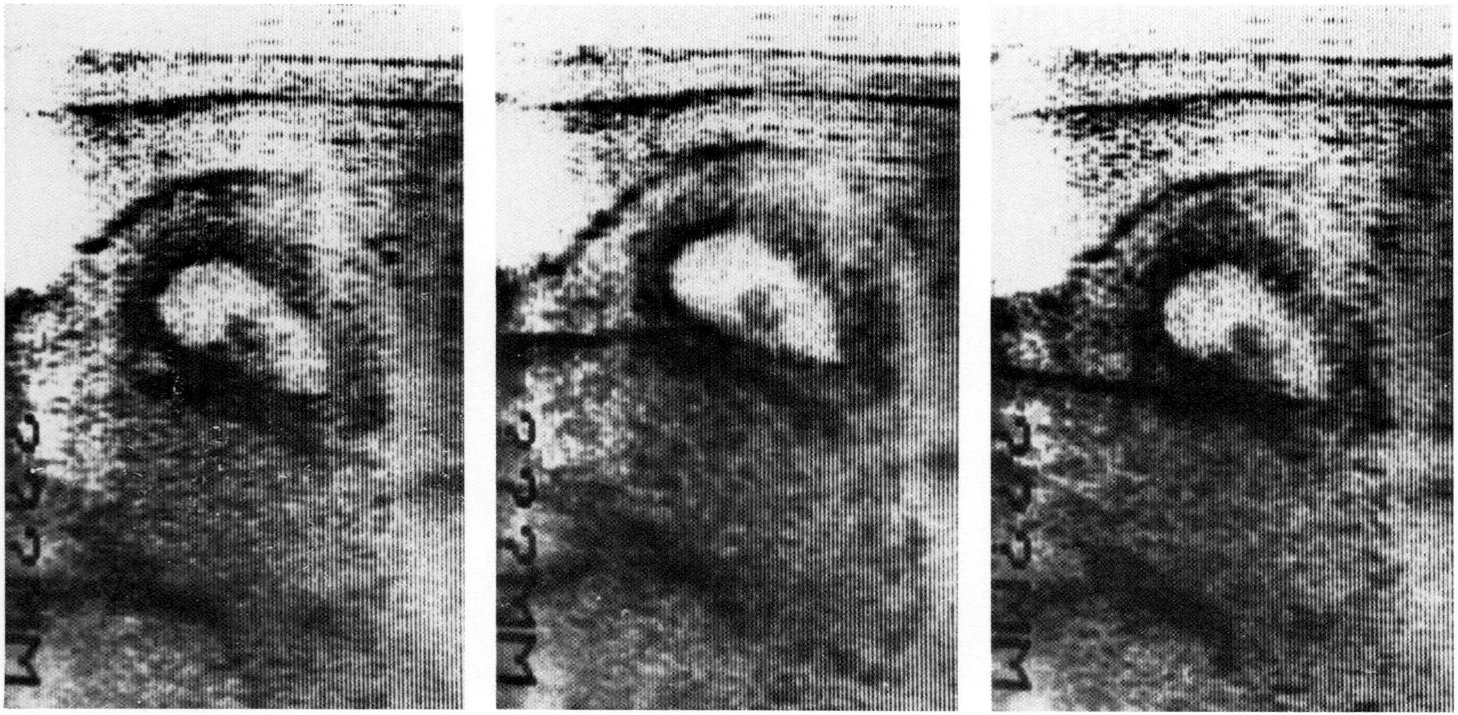

(a) (b) (c)

Figure 2 Ultrasonic scans showing the introduction of the biopsy forceps (a). Uterus before introduction (b) appearance of the echogenic biopsy forceps. (c) Biopsy forceps in position.

studies to establish the linkage arrangement and has been superseded by a direct assay.

The Direct Detection of the Sickle Globin Mutation

The gene mutation changes a glutamic residue, coded by the triplet GAG, for a valine residue, coded by the triplet GTG, at position 6 in the β-globin chain of hemoglobin (see Fig. 3). This A–T nucleotide change alters the sequence of a region normally recognized and cleaved by several restriction endonucleases. The enzyme *Mst* II (or its isoschizomers *Cvn* I, *Aoc* I, or *Sau* I) cleaves DNA at the sequence CCTNAGG (N = any of the four bases), which occurs in the normal β-globin gene in the region corresponding to amino acids 5, 6, and 7 (Pro-Glu-Glu: CCT-GAG-GAG). This cleavage generates multiple DNA fragments, one of them which is 1200 base pairs (bp) in length and can be visualized with a radiolabeled 5′ β-globin gene probe. The β-globin gene containing the sickle cell mutation has the sequence CCTGTGG and so is not

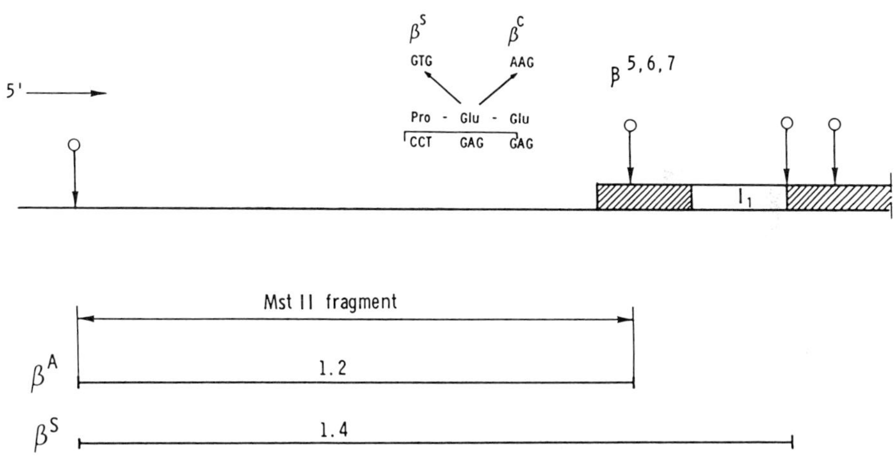

Figure 3 *Mst* II restriction map of human β-globin gene. Arrows indicate the *Mst* II sites in the 5′ flanking (line) and coding (hatched boxes) regions of the normal (β^A) gene. Using the ^{32}p-labeled 1.2-kb *Mst* II fragment indicated in the diagram as probe, the 1.2-kb fragment is seen in normal DNA, and the 1.4-kb fragment in sickle DNA. I1 denotes the first (5′) intervening sequence. At the top of the figure is a nucleotide sequence of β^A gene for codons 5, 6, and 7 where the *Mst* II cleavage sequence (CCTNAGG, where N = G) is underlined. The A→T substitution in the β^S gene alters this cleavage sequence, whereas the G→A substitution in the β^C gene does not.

cleaved at this site by *Mst* II. A restriction fragment of a different length (1400 bp) is therefore generated (Fig. 4). This allows identification of the chromosome bearing the β^s gene and assessment of the fetus genotype if fetal DNA is used in the assay (14–16).

In pregnancies at risk of hemoglobin SC disease, the linkage approach must be used since the enzyme *Mst* II will not distinguish the β^C from β^A gene. The *Hpa* I enzyme can be used in conjunction with *Mst* II, since the 13-kb *Hpa* I pattern is linked to the β^C gene in over 95% of cases (17).

Methods

The preparation of DNA, digestion with the specific restriction endonuclease, and blot hybridization are carried out as decribed (5,18)

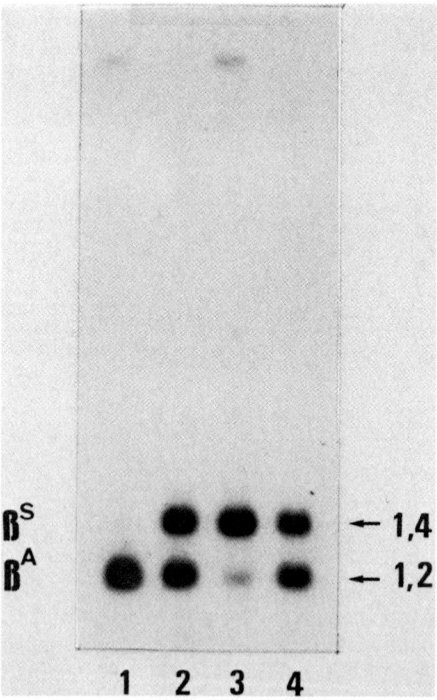

Figure 4 Autoradiogram of a filter with *Mst* II-digested DNA. Four DNA samples isolated from chorionic villus biopsy specimen are shown. 1, AA genotype; 2 and 4, AS genotype; and 3, SS genotype. Note the faint band in the β^A position in sample 3, due to slight maternal contamination of the sample. Sizes (kb) of the β^A and β^S *Mst* II fragments are indicated.

Several commercial preparations of the specific restriction endonuclease are now available (*Mst* II, New England Biolabs or *Sau* I, Boerhinger Manheim). We routinely use 1.2% agarose gels to fractionate DNA samples (5–10 μg) that have been digested with the restriction enzyme *Sau* I. After transfer, the filters are hybridized with a 5′-β-globin gene probe. This probe is the 1.2-kb *Mst* II fragment extending from the β-globin gene codon 6 *Mst* II site in a 5′ direction to the next *Mst* II site in the flanking region (Fig. 3). This genomic fragment has been subcloned in pBR328. The gel-purified 1.2-kb insert is labeled with [α-^{32}p]dCTP and dTTP by nick- translation (19). Specific activities $>5 \times 10^8$ cpm/μg are routinely obtained. Figure 4 shows the typical result of such a restriction enzyme mapping of trophoblast DNA.

DNA analysis of chorionic villi is much easier than that of uncultured amniotic fluid cells. The amount of DNA obtained is always sufficient (10–50 μg), even from small pieces of chorionic tissue, and if necessary, the DNA analysis can be repeated. Misdiagnosis due to maternal contamination can be excluded by careful visual selection of only characteristic chorionic villi for analysis. Since the pattern in the homozygous fetus differs from that in both parents (see Fig. 4), additional confirmation is built into the DNA method in many cases. Because of the high sensitivity of the gene analysis procedure, results are usually obtained within 6 to 10 days after sampling. The laboratory procedures involve many critical steps and require expensive reagents, but several samples can be handled simultaneously without extra work, which reduces the cost of the test. At the moment, these procedures can only be performed close to a research laboratory. The availability of an efficient nonradioactive labeling technique for the gene probe could drastically change the magnitude of these technical problems.

Results and Conclusions

We have attempted prenatal diagnosis of sickle cell anemia in 33 fetuses at risk by analysis of trophoblastic DNA. The results obtained and the outcomes of the pregnancies are described in Table 1. Ten infants have been born, and the diagnoses have been confirmed at birth by cord blood analysis. When the result of the prenatal test led to termination of pregnancy, fetal material was retrieved and the diagnosis confirmed by DNA analysis in every homozygous fetus.

Three cases of fetal loss have been observed at the beginning of our experience. One of these three losses can be attributed to a chromosomal aberration (triploidy). Pathological evaluation was not possible in the

Table 1 Outcomes of First-Trimester Diagnostic Pregnancies (Dec. 1982 to June 1984)[a,b]

Cases (N)	Fetal genotype	No. of termination	Intrauterine[b] fetal death	Continuing pregnancies	Deliveries
22	AA,AS or AC	—	3	9	10
11	SS[c]	10	—	—	1

[a]Fetal DNA was extracted from chorionic villi samples obtained by ultrasound guided biopsy and analyzed by Southern blotting after digestion with the restriction enzyme *Mst* II (or its isoschizomers). Linkage analysis was used for β^c gene detection (*Hpa* I polymorphism).
[b]Respectively, 3 weeks, 15 days, and 1 month after sampling.
[c]One SS woman decided to continue the pregnancy.

two other cases. The risk of fetal loss in the total number of first-trimester diagnoses performed with this sampling technique in our center appears to be 7%. (In addition to sickle cell anemia, 51 pregnancies at risk for a metabolic or an X-linked disease have been investigated.)

The introduction of chorionic villi analysis in the eighth to tenth week of pregnancy is an important breakthrough in prenatal monitoring. Because it reduces the waiting period, allows the couple to maintain privacy about the pregnancy, and permits earlier and safer therapeutic abortion, CVS is now almost always chosen by couples at risk for hemoglobinopathies when CVS is proposed during genetic counseling in our center. The main problem remains the evaluation of the true obstetric risk, since the rate of spontaneous abortion at this early stage of pregnancy may be as high as 5%. Significant risk figures can only be defined after large numbers of cases have been collected by international cooperation. Many single-gene disorders, such as sickle cell anemia, may be directly detectable by DNA restriction analysis or may be diagnosed by the study of restriction endonuclease site polymorphisms, provided that a cloned DNA sequence close to the affected gene is available. When linkage analysis is necessary, the advantage of chorionic biopsy is that more than 20 μg of DNA can be obtained, facilitating the detection of mutant genes when several enzymes are required to achieve the diagnosis. It is likely that this new approach could, in the near future, replace amniotic fluid cells analysis in many instances. If this is the case, the population at risk will have to be educated to consult their physician early in pregnancy.

ACKNOWLEDGMENTS

This work was supported by grants from the Institut National de la Santé et de la Recherche Médicale (INSERM) and the Ministère de l'Industrie et de la Recherche (82E 1140 and DGRST-PVD 8 IL 0528). We are indebted to J. Rosa and R. Henrion for their support and encouragement, to P. Duquesnoy and C. Chabret for excellent technical assistance, and to A.M. Dulac for her help in preparing the manuscipt.

REFERENCES

1. Anshan, Department of Obstetrics and Gynaecology (1975). Fetal sex prediction by sex chromatin of chorionic villi cells during early pregnancy. *Chin. Med. J. (Engl.), 1*:117–126.
2. Kazy, Z., Rokovsky, I, and Bakharev, V. A. (1982). Chorion biopsy in early pregnancy: A method of early prenatal diagnosis for inherited disorders. *Prenatal Diag. 2*:34–45.
3. Old, J. M., Ward, R. J., Karagozlu, F., Petrou, M., Modell, B., and Weatherall, D. J. (1982). First-trimester fetal diagnosis for haemoglobinopathies: Three cases. *Lancet ii*:1414–1417.
4. Gosden, J. R., Mitchell, A. R., Gosden, C. M., Rodeck, C. J., and Morsman, J. M. (1982). Direct vision chorion biopsy and chromosome-specific DNA probes for determination of fetal sex in first-trimester prenatal diagnosis. *Lancet ii*:1416–1419.
5. Goossens, M., Dumez, Y., Kaplan, L., Lupker, M., Chabret, C., Henrion, R., and Rosa, J. (1983). Prenatal diagnosis of sickle cell anemia in the first trimester of pregnancy. *N. Engl. J. Med. 309*:831–833.
6. Brambati, B., and Simoni G. (1983). Diagnosis of fetal trisomy 21 in first trimester. *Lancet i*:546.
7. Gustavi, B. (1983). First trimester chromosomal analysis of chorionic villi obtained by direct vision technique. *Lancet ii*:507–508.
8. Pergament, E., Ginsberg, N., Verlinsky, Y., Cadkin, A., Chu, L., and Trinka, L. (1983). Prenatal Tay-Sachs diagnosis by chorionic villi sampling. *Lancet ii*:286.
9. Poenaru, L., Castelnau, L., Dumez, Y., and Thepot F. (1984). First trimester prenatal diagnosis of mucolipidosis II (I-cell disease) by chorionic biopsy. *Am. J. Hum. Genetics 36*:1379–1385
10. Simoni, G., Grambati, B., Danesino, C., Rossella, F., Terzoli, G. L., Ferrari, M., and Fraccaro, M. (1983). Efficient direct chromosome analyses and enzyme determinations from chorionic villi samples in the first trimester of pregnancy. *Human Genet. 63*:349–357.

11. Ward, R. H. T., Modell, B., Petrou, M., Karagozlu, F., and Douratsos, E. (1983). Method of sampling chorionic villi in first trimester of pregnancy under guidance of real time ultrasound. *Br. Med. J. 286*:1542–1544.
12. Kan, Y. W., and Dozy, A. M. (1978). Polymorphism of DNA sequence adjacent to human β-globin structural gene: Relationship to sickle mutation. *Proc. Natl. Acad. Sci. USA, 75*:5631–5635.
13. Kan Y. W., and Dozy, A. M. (1978). Antenatal diagnosis of sickle cell anemia by DNA. Analysis of amniotic-fluid cells. *Lancet 2*:910–912.
14. Geever, R. F., Wilson, L. B., Nallaseth, F. S., Milner, P. F., Bittner, M., and Wilson, J. T. (1981). Direct identification of sickle cell anemia by blot hybridization. *Proc. Natl. Acad. Sci. USA 78*:5081–5085.
15. Orkin, S. H., Little, P. F. R., Kazazian, H. H., Jr., and Boehm, C. D. (1982). Improved detection of the sickle mutation by DNA analysis: Application to prenatal diagnosis. *N. Engl. J. Med. 307*:32–36.
16. Chang, J. C., and Kan, Y. W. (1982). A sensitive new prenatal test for sickle cell anemia. *N. Engl. J. Med 307*:30–32.
17. Kan Y. W., and Dozy, A. M. (1980). Evolution of the hemoglobin S and C genes in world populations. *Science 209*:388–391.
18. Goossens, M. G., and Kan, Y. W. (1981). DNA analysis in the diagnosis of hemoglobin disorders. *Methods in Enzymology* Vol. 76, pp. 805–817. Academic Press, New York.
19. Durnam, D. M. and Palmiter, R. D. (1983). A practical approach for quantitating specific mRNAs by solution hybridization. *Anal. Biochem. 131*:385–393.

10

Restriction Fragment Length Polymorphisms: Diagnosis of Hemoglobinopathies and Other Gene Defects

JOHN M. OLD
John Radcliffe Hospital, Oxford, England

INTRODUCTION

The hemoglobinopathies are the first group of genetic disorders to be studied comprehensively by the techniques of molecular biology and recombinant DNA technology. Restriction endonuclease analysis and DNA sequencing of cloned DNA has revealed a wide variety of molecular defects, ranging from large DNA deletions, such as those responsible for α-thalassemia (1), to single nucleotide substitutions or deletions, which have been found in the majority of the β-thalassemias (2). However, polymorphisms of DNA sequence are not restricted to the differences between normal and abnormal DNA. Analysis of normal DNA sequences by restriction endonuclease analysis and DNA sequencing has shown that small differences in the DNA sequences between individuals are very common, both in coding and noncoding regions of the genome. Fifteen DNA polymorphisms have now been found in the normal β-globin gene cluster, and these have recently been reviewed by Orkin et al. (2).

Restriction endonucleases are enzymes that cut DNA by recognizing and cleaving a specific sequence. Every few hundred nucleotides or so along each chromosome a polymorphic single nucleotide change can be found that either abolishes a restriction enzyme recognition site or creates a new one. Such polymorphisms result in different-sized restriction fragments after digestion of DNA. These fragments can be used as markers to distinguish chromosomes carrying normal or abnormal genes. Closely linked restriction fragment length polymorphisms (RFLPs) have now been found for many single gene disorders other than β-thalassemia, for example, phenylketonuria (3), hemophilia B (4), antithrombin III deficiency (5), growth hormone deficiency (6), Huntington's chorea (7), and Duchenne muscular dystrophy (8). Unlike classic expressed markers, RFLPs can be found in regions of the genome that do not code for any particular protein. Therefore, RFLPs can be used that are located in closely linked anonymous DNA regions, as in the case of Huntington's chorea and Duchenne muscular dystrophy, in which neither the primary gene defect nor its precise chromosomal location is known.

The new technique of chorionic villus sampling has enabled fetal DNA to be obtained in large quantities in the first trimester of pregnancy (9). Chorionic villus DNA has been shown to be suitable for prenatal diagnosis of β-thalassemia (10) and sickle cell anemia (11), and provided that chorionic villus sampling procedure will eventually be found not to be associated with a significant risk to the fetus, it will be used for the prenatal diagnosis of many other genetic diseases in the future.

PREPARATION OF CHORIONIC VILLI DNA

Deoxyribonucleic acid may be easily prepared from chorionic villi samples by the standard method of proteinase K digestion and phenol extraction (12), modified slighly to take into account the nature and size of the villus sample. If transportation of the sample is necessary, the DNA is best protected by either freezing the sample or by placing it in a buffer containing 8 *M* urea that denatures any DNases.

Methods

To prepare DNA from a frozen sample, it is first thawed and gently homogenized in a total of 0.5 ml of buffer [150 m*M* NaC1/25 m*M* ethylonediaminetetraacetic acid (EDTA)] using a standard 0.5 ml microtissue grinder (Wheaton Scientific). Proteinase K (25 μg) and Sodium dodecyl sulfate (SDS) (to a final concentration of 0.1%) are added to the homogenate in an Eppendorf tube, and the mixture is incubated at 37°C. After approximately a 3-hr incubation, the mixture becomes clear upon complete digestion of the cellular protein, and the DNA may be isolated by phenol extraction. The mixture is extracted twice with an equal volume of phenol–chloroform to remove the proteinase K and twice with an equal volume of chloroform–isoamyl alcohol to remove the traces of phenol. The DNA is then precipitated by the addition of 2 volumes of ethanol plus one-tenth volume of 4 *M* NaC1 and collected by centrifugation.

For transportation of a chorionic villus sample at room temperature, it can be placed in 0.5 ml of buffer containing 8 *M* urea, 0.3 *M* NaC1, 10 m*M* Tris, 10 m*M* EDTA, and 2% SDS (J.R. Gosden, personal communication). Upon receipt, the sample is homogenized as described above and then the mixture is extracted twice with chloroform–octan-2-o1 (24 : 1) to remove the urea. The DNA can then be precipitated by ethanol, redissolved, and digested with proteinase K as described above.

DNA Purification

In my experience, I have found it necessary to purify the DNA further in order to ensure the routine complete digestion of the DNA sample so that even the smallest DNA yields (less than 5 μg) can be digested with confidence. The DNA is purified by precipitation with spermine at a final concentration of 3 m*M* at which most other non-DNA components, such as RNA, stay in solution (13). The DNA precipitate is collected by centrifugation and redissolved (slowly) in a small volume of 0.5 *M* NaC1 by vigorous mixing of the solution for several minutes. The DNA is recovered by the addition of 2 volumes of ethanol, and the precipitate is dried before finally being dissolved in 25–50 μ1 of distilled water. One-tenth of the final DNA solution is sacrificed to measure the DNA concentration in a UV spectrophotometer.

DNA Yields

The above method has been used reliably to prepare DNA from over 40 chorionic villi samples in a pilot program for first-trimester diagnosis of the hemoglobinopathies at Oxford. The DNA yields have varied from 100 μg to 2.5 μg depending on the size of the villus sample. The average yield from the 40 samples was found to be 40 μg, which is a very reasonable amount of DNA for restriction endonuclease analysis—enough for eight digestions.

RESTRICTION ENDONUCLEASE ANALYSIS

Gene deletions and polymorphic restriction endonuclease sites are detected by the technique of restriction endonuclease analysis (often termed gene mapping). Deoxyribonucleic acid prepared from either peripheral blood or chorionic villi (usually 5 μg) is digested with 10–20 units of each restriction enzyme under the conditions recommended by the manufacturers. However, with some restriction enzymes, partial digestions often occur with DNA prepared from peripheral blood containing heparin, resulting in larger fragments than expected and making a diagnosis impossible. Spermine precipitation of large amounts of DNA can be difficult, and, therefore, another method is used to overcome the inhibitory effect of contaminating materials. Spermidine (14), when added to the restriction enzyme buffer at concentrations ranging from 0.5 to 5 m*M* usually relieves this inhibition and permits complete digestion.

Digested DNA consists of many differently sized fragments that can be separated according to size by electrophoresis in an agarose gel (12). The fragments are then made single stranded by soaking the gel in alkali before being transferred out of the gel onto the surface of a nitrocellulose filter by the method of Southern blotting (15). The filter bound DNA is then hybridized to a single-stranded ^{32}P-labeled DNA probe. The filter is washed to remove the unhybridized probe and subjected to autoradiography. By this method, the one or two fragments that are complementary to the probe appear as bands on the developed X-ray film. By comparing the position of these bands with those of known molecular weight marker DNA fragments, the size of the fragments can be determined.

The probes used are usually either genomic DNA fragments subcloned into plasmids from cloned DNA sequences or complementary DNA (cDNA) made from mRNA with reverse transcriptase and cloned into plasmids. Genomic DNA probes are usually part of the whole gene containing both coding and noncoding sequences, whereas cDNA probes normally contain the whole coding sequence of the gene. Therefore, cDNA probes generally hybridize to a larger region of DNA and thus to more fragments than cloned genomic DNA probes. This can be very useful when searching for new RFLPs. However, for prenatal diagnosis, the presence of many bands on the autoradiograph can interfere with the interpretation of the result, and, therefore, very small genomic fragments often have to be used.

PRENATAL DIAGNOSIS

Prenatal diagnosis of any genetic disorder by restriction enzyme analysis can be performed by (a) the determination of the presence or absence of normal DNA fragments in fetal DNA (if the disorder is caused by a gene deletion); (b) the detection of abnormal fragments that result from the molecular basis of the genetic disorder; and (c) the establishment of linkage to restriction fragment length polymorphisms by a family study.

Diagnosis by Direct Analysis

If a particular genetic disorder is caused by a gene deletion that removes only part of the DNA in the region under study or by a mutation that affects a useful restriction enzyme site, the disorder can be detected directly by the presence of a characteristic abnormal fragment. A normal individual will have two normal restriction fragments, a heterozygote will have one normal and one abnormal fragment, and a homozygote will have only abnormal fragments. Therefore, after the identification of this type of defect in both husband and wife, a diagnosis can be carried out on their first pregnancy. Examples of such hemoglobinopathies are the severe type of α-thalassemia, several types of β-thalassemia, sickle cell anemia, and hemoglobin Lepore.

α-Thalassemia

There are three common types of gene deletions that, in their homozygous state, result in infants with hemoglobin Bart's hydrops fetalis syndrome. These deletions produce characteristic abnormal restriction fragments from the α-globin gene cluster, which enable these types of α-thalassemia to be distinguished. Therefore, the detection of these abnormal fragments in chorionic villus DNA, together with the absence of any normal α-globin gene fragments, will indicate a Bart's hydrops fetalis.

One of the three deletions is found in patients of southeast Asian origin, and the other two have been found in patients from the Mediterranean area. All three deletions can be analyzed by digestion of DNA with the restriction enzyme *Bgl* II and hybridization with a ζ-gene probe. Figure 1 shows the restriction fragments observed from normal DNA: a 7.4-kb fragment containing the $\alpha 1$ gene; a 12.6-kb fragment containing the $\alpha 2$ gene and the $\psi\zeta$ gene; and a fragment containing the ζ gene that is variable in size because it also contains a hypervariable region (16). The southeast Asian deletion ($--^{SEA}$) starts immediately 3′ to the $\psi\zeta$ gene and extends beyond both α genes. The deletion occurs on a chromosome that contains the 10.5-kb ζ gene fragment. The abnormal $\psi\zeta$ gene fragment is usually also 10.5-kb (17), although this fragment can

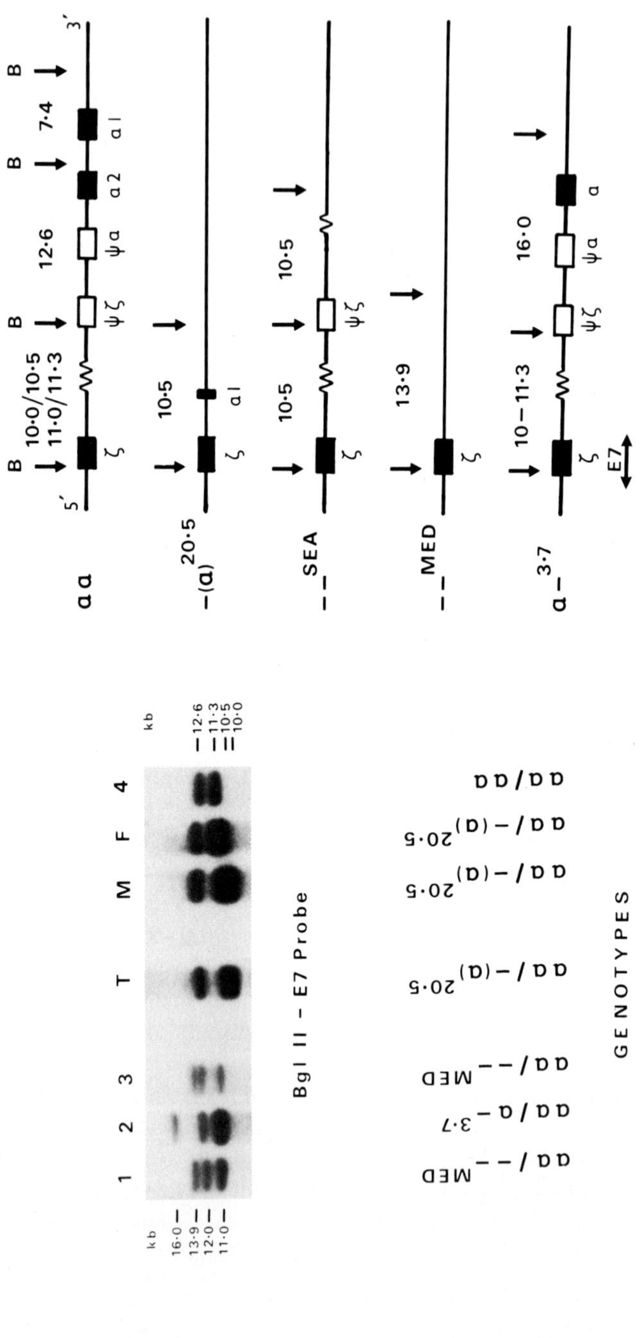
1 2 3 T M F 4
kb
16·0
13·9
12·0
11·0
kb
12·6
11·3
10·5
10·0
Bgl II - E7 Probe
αα/− −MED
αα/α−3·7
αα/− −MED
αα/−(α)20·5
αα/−(α)20·5
αα/−(α)20·5
αα/αα
GENOTYPES
αα
B B B B
10·0/10·5
11·0/11·3
12·6
7·4
5′ 3′
ζ ψζ ψα α2 α1
−(α)20·5
10·5
ζ α1
− −SEA
10·5 10·5
ζ ψζ
− −MED
13·9
ζ
α−3·7
10−11·3
16·0
ζ ψζ ψα α
E7

vary slightly, possibly because the 3′ end contains another hypervariable region. Detection of a single 10.5-kb band in fetal DNA, together with the absence of a 12.6-kb band and any detectable α gene fragments would indicate a fetus homozygous for the southeast Asian deletion.

The band patterns observed in DNA from patients heterozygous for the two Mediterranean deletions are shown in Figure 1. The more common deletion, designated $--^{MED}$, starts on the 5′ side of the $\psi\zeta$ gene and extends beyond both α genes (18). This deletion creates a characteristic abnormal ζ gene fragment of 13.9-kb instead of the normal 10.0 to 11.3-kb variable fragment and also results in the loss of the 12.6-kb and 7.4-kb fragments. Therefore, the homozygous state for this type of deletion produces a single band at 13.9-kb. The less common type, designated $-(\alpha)^{20.5}$, is a 20.5-kb deletion that starts on the 3′ side of ζ gene and ends inside the $\alpha 1$ gene, removing the whole of the $\psi\zeta$ and $\alpha 2$ genes and the 5′ end of the $\alpha 1$ gene (19). This deletion creates an abnormal 10.5-kb fragment that hybridizes to both ζ and α gene probes (in contrast to the $--^{SEA}$ deletion).

Figure 1 shows a first-trimester diagnosis for a couple in which both mother and father were carriers for the $-(\alpha)^{20.5}$ gene. The chorionic villi DNA from the fetus showed three bands: 12.6, 10.5, and 10.0-kb, indicating that the fetus was heterozygous for the α-thalassemia defect (inheriting the normal ζ gene fragments from the mother because of the presence of the 10.0-kb band, and therefore inheriting the $-(\alpha)^{20.5}$ defect from the father).

Figure 1 Autoradiograph showing the result of a first-trimester diagnosis for α^0-thalassemia together with a physical map of the normal α-globin gene cluster ($\alpha\alpha$) and the common α-thalassemia genes that generate abnormal ζ gene fragments. DNAs from the father (F), mother (M), chorionic villi sample (T), α-thalassemia heterozygote for the single α gene deletion type α-$^{3.7}$ (2), α-thalassemia heterozygote for the two α-gene deletion type $--^{MED}$ (1) and (3), and finally normal DNA (4) were digested with *Bgl* II (B), blotted, and hybridized to a ζ-gene probe (plasmid E7, containing an *Eco–Bam* fragment, a gift from Dr. N. Proudfoot). The sizes of the observed fragments are shown, together with the determined genotypes for each DNA sample. Because the autoradiograph was overexposed, the abnormal 10.5-kb band from the $-(\alpha)^{20.5}$ deletion gene has merged with either a neighboring 10.0-kb (M) or an 11.0-kb fragment (F). In the map, transcribed genes are shaded, the pseudogenes are unshaded, and the location of hypervariable regions are represented by a zig-zag symbol. The $\psi\zeta$ gene also contains two small variable regions that account for the $\psi\zeta$ gene fragment in (1) to be smaller than the usual 12.6-kb.

Sickle Cell Anemia

The β^S-gene is a single base substitution of A to T in codon 6 of the β-globin gene. This base substitution abolishes three different restriction enzyme recognition sites in the normal β gene. The first to be identified was the enzyme *Mnl* I, then *Dde* I, and finally *Mst* II. The first two enzymes both produce very small normal and abnormal β-globin gene fragments, and although prenatal diagnosis of sickle cell anemia with *Dde* I was shown to be possible (20), the small fragments generated were found to blot and hybridize very inefficiently. This resulted in a very limited use of the direct method in preference to the established indirect method of linkage of the β^S gene to a polymorphic *Hpa* I site as described in the section on diagnosis by linkage analysis. However, the third enzyme to be found, *Mst* II, generates much larger fragments that blot and hybridize normally (21,22), and this method is now used by most centers for the prenatal diagnosis of sickle cell anemia.

The principle of the method of restriction enzyme analysis with *Mst* II is shown in Figure 2. *Mst* II normally cuts 5′ to the β-globin gene and at

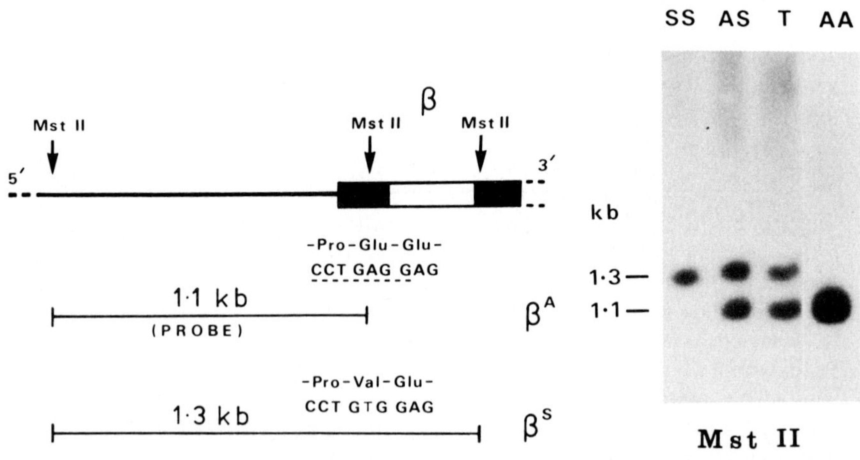

Figure 2 Autoradiograph showing the result of a first-trimester diagnosis of sickle cell anemia, together with a physical map of the β^A and β^S globin genes. DNAs from a normal patient (AA), a patient with sickle cell trait (AS), a patient with sickle cell anemia (SS) were digested with *Mst* II as controls to the digestion of a chorionic villi biopsy (T) from a couple at risk for sickle cell anemia. The DNAs were hybridized to a 1.1-kb *Mst* II fragment prepared from a β-globin gene probe. The map includes the recognition sequence of *Mst* II (CCTGAGG, underlined) located at the site of the β^S lesion.

the GAG codon to generate a 1.1-kb fragment and at a third site 200 base pairs 3′ to codon 6 to generate a 0.2-kb fragment that is not usually detected. The sickle cell mutation destroys the middle recognition site, and a 1.3-kb fragment is generated that is the sum of the two normal ones. Figure 2 also shows a first-trimester diagnosis on chorionic villi DNA together with various DNA samples to act as controls. Both the 1.1-kb and the 1.3-kb bands were observed in the fetal DNA sample, showing that the fetus was heterozygous for sickle cell anemia.

β-Thalassemia

β-Thalassemia is caused by at least 30 different mutations (2). One of these is a 619 base pair deletion in the β-globin gene that is detectable directly by restriction enzyme mapping. The remainder are either single nucleotide changes or very small deletions or insertions that result in (a) the creation of a nonsense codon that terminates mRNA translation, (b) the interference with the splicing mechanism of newly transcribed mRNA, (c) a frameshift mutation that affects the normal functioning of mRNA, or (d) the reduction in function of the promotor regions that are important for mRNA transcription.

At present, 5 of the 30 types of β-thalassemia gene are associated with an alteration of a restriction enzyme site and therefore can be detected directly by gene mapping (2). Unfortunately none of these types of β-thalassemia have been found to be particularly common, and therefore most cases of β-thalassemia have to be diagnosed by linked DNA polymorphisms or by hybridization with oligonucleotide probes (as described later). One of these five types has been shown to be caused by a frameshift deletion in codon 6 of the β-globin gene and results in the loss of the same *Mst* II site that is altered in the β^S gene (23). This type β^o-thalassemia, originally described in patients from Calabria in Italy, has now been observed in a British family with a homozygous β^o-thalassemic child. Figure 3 shows the restriction fragment pattern obtained by digestion with *Mst* II, together with the family pedigree and haplotype data.

The β-thalassemia gene resulting from a 619 base pair deletion (24) has only been found in β^o-thalassemia patients from India and Pakistan. However, it appears to be quite common, as it accounts for 18% of the β-thalassemic chromosomes of the Asian Indian immigrant population in the United Kingdom (25). The Indian deletion β^o-gene is directly detectable by digestion of DNA with the enzymes *Bgl* II or *Pst* I, both of which cut on either side of the β-globin gene. For example, the deletion results in a characteristic 4.6-kb *Bgl* II fragment instead of the normal

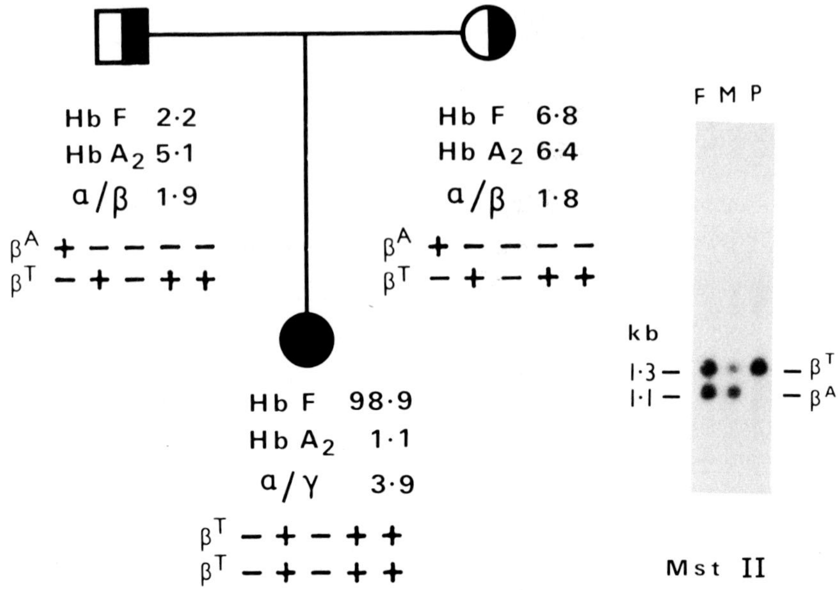

Figure 3 Family pedigree showing hematological data and the chromosomal haplotypes for a British family with β-thalassemia, together with an autoradiograph showing the result of an *Mst* II analysis. DNAs from the father (F), mother (M), and patient with homozygous β-thalassemia (P) were digested with *Mst* II and hybridized to the 1.1-kb *Mst* II β fragment. The haplotypes shown are derived from linkage analysis of the first five polymorphic sites 5′ to the β-globin as illustrated in Figure 7.

5.2-kb globin gene-containing fragment. An example of a first-trimester diagnosis that involved the detection of the β^o deletion gene is shown in Figure 4. In this case, the father carried the β^o-deletion gene, while the mother carried a nondeletion type of β-thalassemia that could be identified by an *Ava* II polymorphism following linkage analysis (see Figure nine). Analysis of chorionic villus DNA with both *Bgl* II and *Pst* I showed only the normal β-globin restriction fragments, showing that the fetus had inherited the normal chromosome from the father and not the β-thalassemia deletion gene. To complete the diagnosis, the fetal DNA was also digested with *Ava* II as described later.

One other type of β^o-thalassemia deletion gene has been reported, a 10-kb DNA deletion found in a Dutch family (26). However, in this case, the β^o-thalassemia gene was associated with significantly increased γ-globin chain production and is therefore similar to the $(\delta\beta)^o$-

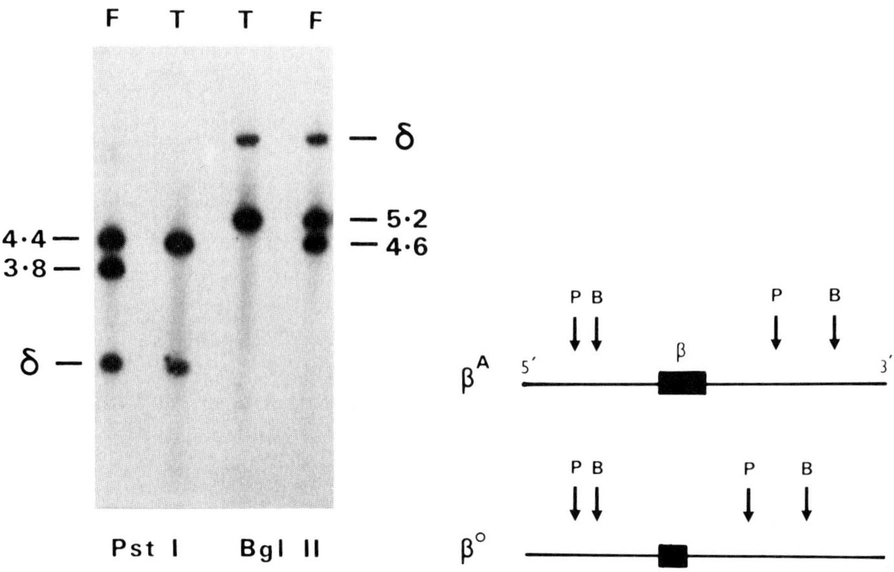

Figure 4 Autoradiograph showing the result of a first-trimester diagnosis of the deletion type of β°-thalassemia, together with a physical map of the normal β-globin gene and the 0.6-kb deletion β°-thalassemia gene. DNAs from the father (F) and the chorionic villi biopsy (T) were digested with *Bgl* II (B) or *Pst* I (P) and hybridized to a β-globin gene probe. Cross-hybridizing δ fragments are indicated (δ).

thalassemia disorders (27) in that the raised level of Hb F results in a more moderate clinical condition than β-thalassaemia in homozygotes, and prenatal diagnosis is not usually required.

Hemoglobin Lepore

Hemoglobin Lepore is produced from a $\delta\beta$ hybrid gene that results from an unequal crossing-over between the δ and β genes at meiosis. The hybrid gene is transcribed very inefficiently, which results in the homozygous condition for Hb Lepore with a clinical picture very similar to homozygous β-thalassemia. Therefore, although the homozygous condition is very rare, it is a suitable candidate for prenatal diagnosis. The Hb Lepore gene is associated with the deletion of 7-kb of DNA extending between the δ and β genes and can be detected directly with the enzyme *Xba* I (28). *Xba* I cuts on the 5′ side of the δ-globin gene and on the 3′ side of the β-globin gene to produce a 10.8-kb fragment from normal DNA and a characteristic fragment of 3.8-kb from the Hb Lepore gene. Figure 5 shows a first-trimester diagnosis for a couple (a first cousin marriage) at risk for Hp Lepore. Only the 10.8-kb band was observed, indicating the fetus had inherited both normal chromosomes.

Oligonucleotide Probes

A new approach has recently been developed that can detect genetic disorders resulting from single base changes. This approach is based on the differential hybridization of a pair of short oligonucleotide probes to blots of digested DNA (29). The first genetic disorders to be analyzed by oligonucleotide probes were sickle cell anemia (30) and the common Mediterranean β^+-thalassemia (31). As most of the β-thalassemia mutations have now been identified to be single base changes, this method could be used for the direct detection and diagnosis of the majority of cases of β-thalassemia.

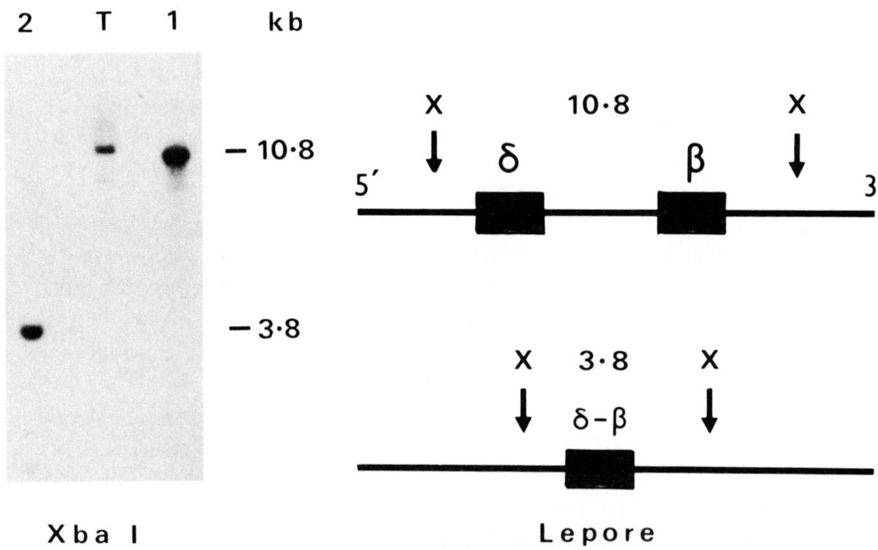

Figure 5 Autoradiograph showing the result of a first-trimester diagnosis for hemoglobin Lepore togehter with a physical map of the normal δ and β genes and the Hb Lepore gene. DNAs from a normal individual (1), chorionic villus sample (T), and a Hb Lepore homozygote (2) were digested with *Xba* 1 (X) and hybridized to a β-globin gene probe.

Although extremely useful in theory, the technique is more difficult than restriction enzyme mapping and has not yet proved to be as sensitive and reliable for prenatal diagnosis. The technique is no quicker than restriction enzyme analysis, and, in most populations, there are several common different β-thalassemia mutations. Therefore, the use of oligonucleotide probes in these populations would require the synthesis of a battery of probes and the study of the parental DNA before prenatal diagnosis to identify which pair of pairs (if the mutant genes are different) of probes to use. Although oligonucleotide probes have proved very useful for assigning β-thalassemia mutations to haplotypes in population surveys (32), very few centers involved in prenatal diagnosis are using oligonucleotide probes as a first line approach. Oligonucleotide probes are perhaps most useful for population in which one β-thalassemia mutation is the predominant type, such as Cyprus (33) and Sardinia (34), and recently it was reported that all cases of prenatal diagnosis of β-thalassemia in Sardinia are now being carried out by the direct detection of the β-39 nonsense mutation by using oligonucleotide probes on fetal DNA from amniotic cluid cells or chorionic villi (35).

Diagnosis by Linkage Analysis

Within the β-globin gene cluster there are at least 14 polymorphic restriction endonuclease recognition sites (2). The polymorphic sites are due to natural variations in the DNA sequence (usually single nucleotide changes) that lead to the presence (+) or absence (−) of the recognition site. Different sizes of DNA fragments are obtained after digestion, and these restriction fragment length polymorphisms (RFLPs) are inherited in a simple mendelian manner and can be used as markers for chromosomes carrying normal or abnormal genes.

For the purpose of prenatal diagnosis, the polymorphic sites must be close enought to the locus of the mutant gene so that the chance of recombination between the polymorphic site and the mutant gene is very small. This occurs if the polymorphic sites are located in or around the mutant gene, as in the case of the β-globin gene cluster DNA polymorphisms and β-thalassemia. The frequency of meiotic crossing-over has been calculated to be 1 per 10^8 base pairs per meiosis. Therefore, the probability of a cross over between a gene and a linked polymorphic site 20 kb distant from it (as in the case of most of the β-globin DNA polymorphisms) is of the order of 1 in 5000 (36), although regions of DNA with a much higher than average frequency of recombination exist in the genome, and the presence of one of these hot spots for recombination would increase the probability of a cross over.

Allele-Linked Restriction Fragment Length Polymorphisms

The frequencies of most of the β gene DNA polymorphisms have now been studied in different ethnic groups and in different types of chromosomes bearing mutant β-globin genes (2). Apart from a few polymorphisms that occur only in American Blacks (such as *Taq 1* and *Hinf* I) (2), there is generally very little difference between the frequency of the presence (+) of a polymorphic site in normal and β-thalassemic chromosomes. However, several examples of linkage disequilibrium between the presence of a polymorphic site and a mutant β-globin gene have been found, the most important being the difference between an *Hpa* 1 polymorphism and the β^S gene in West Africans (37) and a *Bam* H1 polymorphism with β^o-thalassemia in Sardinians (38).

Digestion of DNA with *Hpa* 1 for the majority of normal chromosomes generates either a 7.6-kb fragment or, much less frequently, a 13-kb fragment. However, chromosomes carrying the β^S gene in patients of West African origin were found to generate only the 13-kb band. Therefore, the *Hpa* 1 polymorphism can be used for prenatal diagnosis of sickle cell anemia in cases where both parents are heterozygous for the *Hpa* 1 polymorphism. Such a first-trimester diagnosis for sickle cell anemia has been reported (10). However, in other populations, the β^S gene has been found linked to the more common 7.6-kb fragment. Therefore, prenatal diagnosis of sickle cell anemia has to be carried out by using *Mst* II, as previously described, since this enzyme can be used to detect sickle cell genes from all racial groups.

The *Bam* H1 polymorphism is illustrated in Figure 6. *Bam* H1 digestion of normal DNA generates either 8.3-kb (+) or 22-kb (−) β-globin gene fragments. In Sardinians, the β^o-thalassemia gene, which accounts for the majority of β-thalassemia in the island population, is found only on the 8.3-kb fragment. Therefore, identification of a 22-kb fragment in fetal DNA indicates the presence of a normal chromosome. Figure 6 shows the digestion patterns of a Sardinian β^o-thalassemia homozygote and his parents, illustrating the linkage of the thalassemia gene to the 8.3-kb fragment (+). This linkage disequilibrium has been used for prenatal diagnosis in Sardinia using amniotic fluid DNA (31). The Sardinian β^o-thalassemia has also been found to be always associated with a (+) *Ava* II DNA polymorphism in the β-globin gene (34). Therefore, the presence of an *Ava* II (−) polymorphism can also be used

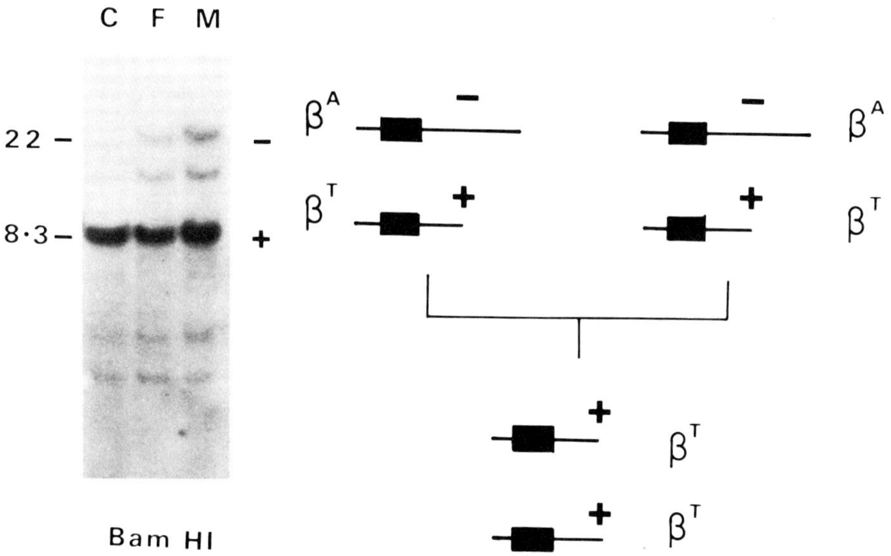

Figure 6 Linkage analysis of the *Bam* H1 polymorphic site in a Sardinian family with a homozygous β^{o}-thalassemic child. DNAs from the father (F), mother (M), and child (C) were digested with *Bam* H1 and hybridized to a β-globin gene probe. The polymorphic 22-kb and 8.3-kb β fragments are indicated (−) and (+), respectively. The unlabeled bands are cross-hybridizing δ gene fragments. The diagram shows the linkage of the 8.3-kb RFLP (+) and the 22-kb RFLP (−) to the normal (β^{A}) and thalassemic (β^{T}) chromosomes.

to identify a normal chromosome in Sardinians, although in practice a family study would normally be done to establish the linkage.

Linkage Analysis

Because most of the polymorphic restriction sites in the β-globin gene cluster occur on both normal and β-thalassemic chromosomes, it is necessary to establish linkage between a particular RFLP and the mutant gene by a family study. This is easily carried out if the couple at risk have a normal or homozygous β-thalassemic child. However, if the couple requiring prenatal diagnosis have only children with β-thalassemia trait or it is their first pregnancy, the parents of the couple or lateral relatives may be used to establish linkage in most cases. At present, most laboratories involved in prenatal diagnosis study seven RFLPs to

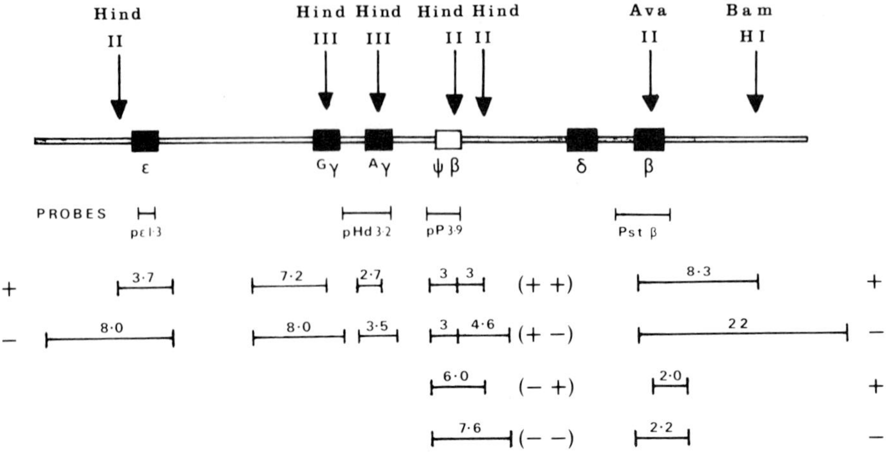

Figure 7 The location of seven RFLP sites in the β-globin gene cluster together with the sizes of the polymorphic fragments generated by the digestion of DNA and hybridization to the appropriate ^{32}P-labeled probe as previously described (39).

establish linkage in each case. These seven RFLPs are illustrated in Figure 7. The combination of the results for the presence (+) or absence (−) of each polymorphic site along the chormosomes can be worked out from the family study. The combination, called a haplotype, is determined for the normal and β-thalassemia chromosomes of each When the haplotypes are different from each other, it is possible for prenatal diagnosis by restriction enzyme analysis to be carried out.

An example of a family study is shown in Figure 3. The five polymorphic restriction sites 5′ to the β-globin gene (see Figure 7) were analyzed in each family member (father, mother, and homozygous β-thalassemic child), and the haplotypes were determined. The normal chromosome in both parents had the haplotype +−−−−, and the β-thalassemia chromosome had haplotype −+−++. In this case, the normal β chromosome can be distinguished from the abnormal β-thalassemia chromosome at four out of the five sites. In most cases, it is possible to use more than one polymorphic site for a diagnosis, and, usually, enough DNA is obtained from a chorionic villi sample so that all the informative polymorphic sites can be studied to give the best possible chance for a successful diagnosis.

Feasibility

The feasibility of first-trimester diagnosis by RFLP analysis for a couple at risk is determined by the haplotypes of their normal and β-thalassemia chromosomes. The four possible outcomes are shown in Figure 8. A diagnosis is possible when the haplotypes are different in each parent. The diagnosis may be performed by analysis of one polymorphic site, or it may require a different polymorphic site for the differentiation of the two chromosomes in each parent (Fig. 8b). Occassionally, especially with the Asian Indians, one β-thalassemia gene can be identified directly and the other by linkage analysis. An example of such a two enzyme diagnosis is illustrated in Figure 9, in which the linkage of an *Ava* II polymorphism was used to identify the β-thalassemia gene inherited from the mother, and *Pst* I, the β^{o}-deletion gene from the father. The fetus was found to have inherited the normal gene from the father (data are shown in Fig. 4) and the β-thalassemia gene from the mother. In a recent study of the Cypriot and Asian Indian populations of the United Kingdom (39), 35% of the Cypriot families at risk for β-thalassemia and 76% of the Asian Indian families could have a diagnosis by one or two enzymes. This, latter figure compares well with the results of a study in the United States of a group of couples of mixed nationality at risk for β-thalassemia (Italian, Greek, Asian Indian, and Chinese) in which a diagnosis was possible in 80% (40). The low result for the Cypriot population results from the fact that the Cypriot β^{+}-thalassemia gene occurs on the most frequent haplotype found on normal chromosomes, making it impossible to differentiate the normal and β-thalassemia chromosomes in many individuals.

The third possible outcome of a feasibility study is shown in Figure 8c, in which the normal chromosome can be distinguished from the β-thalassemia chromosome in only one parent. In these cases, there is a 50% chance of obtaining a successful diagnosis by RFLP analysis. Prenatal diagnosis would give the result of either a normal or heterozygous fetus if the β-thalassemic chromosome were found to be absent, or a result of either a heterozygote or homozygote for β-thalassemia if it were found to be present. The former result, statistically obtained in 50% of the diagnosis, would be considered a successful result as no further action would be necessary. If the latter result were obtained, further analysis by fetal blood sampling would be necessary to determine if the fetus was a β-thalassemia homozygote. Nineteen percent of the Asian families and 45% of the Cypriot families studied fell into this category.

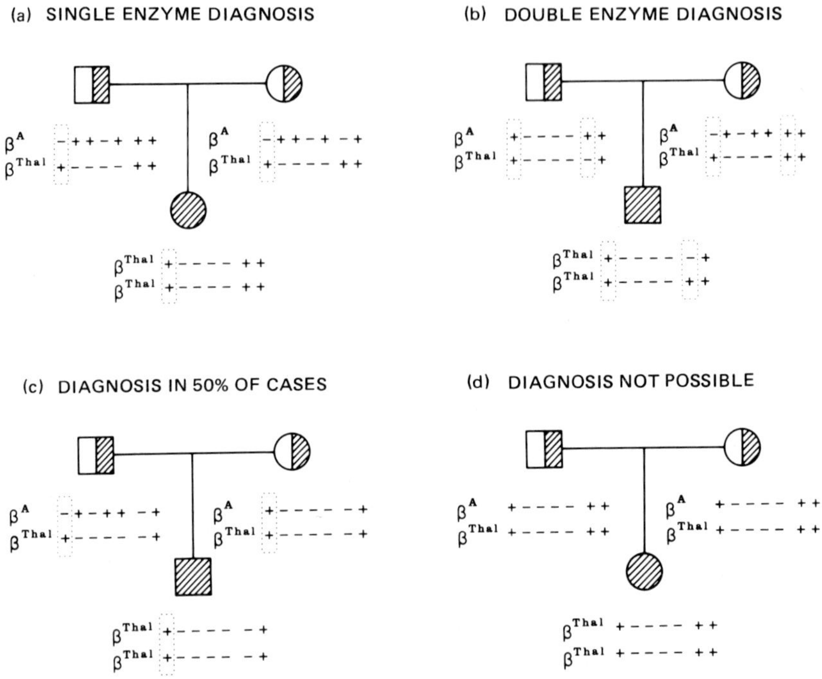

Figure 8 Analysis of four families illustrating the different possibilities for prenatal diagnosis. (a) Illustration of a family in which a diagnosis is possible using one enzyme. The informative sites are either *Hind* II-ε, *Hind* III-γ, or *Hind* II-$\psi\beta$. For example, analysis of the *Hind* II-ε site would give the polymorphism pattern of $(-/-)$ for a normal fetus, $(+/-)$ for a β-thalassemia heterozygote, and $(+/+)$ for a β-thalassemia homozygote. (b) Illustration of a family in which a diagnosis is possible using a combination of two enzymes. The informative sites are either the *Hind* II-ε, *Hind* II-γ, or *Hind* II-$\psi\beta$ for the first enzyme and *Ava* II-β for the second. Analyzing the *Hind* II-ε and *Ava* II-β sites respectively, a result of $(+/-)$, $(+/+)$ would indicate a normal fetus, results of $(+/+)$, $(+/+)$, or $(-/+)$ would indicate a β-thalassemia heterozygote, and a result of $(+/+)$, $(-/+)$ would indicate a β-thalassemia homozygote. (c) Illustration of a family in which there is only a 50% chance of a successful diagnosis using DNA polymorphisms. The informative sites are either *Hind* II-ε, *Hind* III-γ, or *Hind* II-$\psi\beta$. For example, analysis of the *Hind* II-ε site would give either $(+/-)$ indicating a normal fetus of a β-thalassemia heterozygote (successful diagnosis) or $(+/+)$ indicating either a β-thalassemia heterozygote or homozygote (requiring further analysis by fetal blood sampling). (d) Illustration of a family in which diagnosis is not possible using DNA polymorphisms as there are no informative sites.

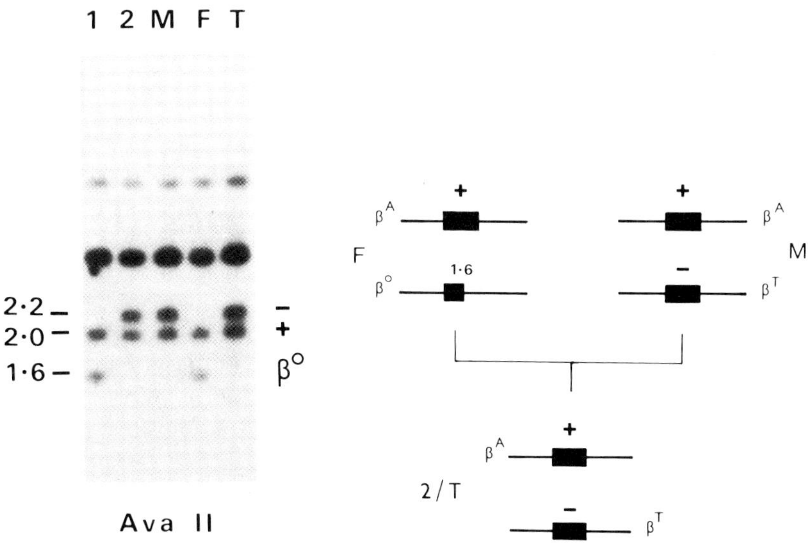

Figure 9 An example of a first-trimester diagnosis in which two different restriction enzyme digestions were required. The father was heterozygous for the Indian β^o-deletion gene, and the result of a diagnosis with both *Bgl* II and *Pst* I is shown in Figure 4. Digestion of DNA from the father (F), the mother (M) and two children (1 and 2) heterozygous for β-thalassemia with *Ava* II showed that the mother was (+/−), the father's DNA showed the 1.6-kb abnormal fragment characteristic of the β^o deletion gene (25) and a (+) for the normal chromosome (β^A). The DNA pattern from child 2 was +/−, with no abnormal 1.6-kb band. Therefore, child 2 had inherited the normal chromosome (+) from the father and the β-thalassemia chromosome (−) from the mother, thus establishing the linkage shown in the diagram. The chorionic villus sample (T) showed an *Ava* II pattern of (+/−), indicating that the fetus had inherited the β-thalassemia gene of the mother and a normal β-globin gene from the father.

Finally, the fourth possible outcome is shown in Figure 8d. In this case the two chromosomes cannot be dintinguished in either parent, and no diagnosis by RFLP analysis is possible. In 5% of the Asian families and 20% of the Cypriots, RFLPs could not be used for prenatal diagnosis. Because of the nonrandom association of the β-globin RFLPs (41), analysis of the other known polymorphisms in the β-globin gene cluster is unlikely to be of any use for couples in this category. Therefore, at present, the only method of prenatal diagnosis by DNA analysis for these couples is the oligonucleotide approach, although new, more useful polymorphic restriction sites may be discovered in the future.

Problems

Although prenatal diagnosis by RFLP analysis has proved very successful, there are certain problems associated with the method. The main limitation of the method is the need to establish a linkage of an abnormal β chromosome to a particular RFLP, and this requires a family study. If an affected or normal child is not available, it is often very difficult to obtain blood samples from grandparents or lateral relatives. In a small number of cases, even a complete study of the family pedigree may not establish linkage (for example, if both grandparents are heterozygous for β-thalassemia).

Having established linkage of polymorphic restriction sites, it is still possible to arrive at an incorrect diagnosis even though the particular RFLP's in fetal DNA have been correctly determined. One source of error is the slight risk of meiotic recombination between the polymorphic restriction site and the β-thalassemia mutation. A second source of error is nonpaternity. If the true paternal chromosome carried a β-thalassemia gene and had the same haplotype as the husband's normal chromosome, it would pass undetected and could lead to a serious misdiagnosis. Finally, there is the possibility that the wrong linkage was established in the family study. This could arise, for example, if the linkage analysis was achieved using fetal DNA obtained from an aborted fetus following an incorrect diagnosis of a β-thalassemia homozygote by fetal blood sampling.

One problem in using chorionic villi for prenatal diagnosis is that the chorionic tissue must be free of contaminating maternal cells. The chorionic villi after sampling can be easily identified by microscopic examination and separated from the maternal decidua by gentle dissection. Provided that the villi are not cultured before the preparation DNA, it seems that maternal contamination is not a problem for diagnosis by restriction endonuclease analysis. In the three first reported cases of first-trimester diagnosis for hemoglobinopathies, one of the diagnoses, a homozygote, showed no evidence of any faint maternal normal fragments present in the chorionic villi DNA sample (10). Studies on two chorionic villi DNA samples with a specific DNA probe for the X chromosome have also demonstrated the complete absence of any maternal contamination (42). A statistical analysis of a much larger series of first-trimester diagnoses should finally show that maternal contamination is not a problem.

OTHER GENETIC DEFECTS

For the purpose of prenatal diagnosis, genetic disorders can be grouped into those in which the mutant gene has been identified and cloned and those in which the mutant gene is unknown. Once the gene has been cloned, the cloned DNA can be used to identify polymorphic restriction sites and to examine the molecular basis of the inherited disorder.

Gene-specific probes have now been isolated for many genetic disorders: for example, coagulation factors IX and VIII, for hemophilia and Christmas disease, phenylalanine hydroxylase for phenylketonuria, antithrombin III for antithrombin III deficiency, α_1-antitrypsin for α_1-antitrypsin deficiency, and a collagen α_1 (1)-like gene for inherited disorders of connective tissue. Many of these disorders will probably be very heterogeneous for their molecular defects as shown by the thalassemia syndromes. Already both complete gene deletions and nondeletional type of defects have been reported for the disorders of antithrombin III deficiency (5) and Christmas disease (hemophilia B) (43). Those conditions that result from gene deletions will be amenable to prenatal diagnosis by direct analysis of fetal DNA; the remainder will have to be approached by linkage analysis with RFLPs, at least until their molecular defects have been characterized. It might then be possible to use direct methods of diagnosis in a few cases, as in the example of α_1-antitrypsin deficiency, which is caused by a point mutation and has been detected by the use of oligonucleotide probes (44). However, because of the heterogeneity and the fact that many genetic disorders have a high frequency of new mutations, the linkage of genetic disorders to RFLPs will be the major approach for diagnosis. At present, RFLPs associated with the probes for hemophilia B (4), antithrombin III deficiency (5), and phenylketonuria (3) have been discovered and shown to be useful for carrier detection and prenatal diagnosis if required.

Genetic disorders in which the mutant gene is unknown include Huntington's chorea, Duchenne muscular dystrophy, and cystic fibrosis. For these disorders, many research groups are currently using random DNA probes to define RFLPs that are scattered throughout the genome and to construct a detailed human genetic linkage map. By carrying out detailed family studies, specific RFLPs can be related to particular genetic disorders, and the mutant genes can be localized. This approach has resulted in the Huntington's chorea gene being closely linked to a RFLP on chromosome 4 (7) and to the finding of one RFLP on either side of the locus of the Duchenne muscular dystrophy (*DMD*) gene on the X chromosome (8). All three RFLPs each have an 85% linkage to the mutant gene locus, which is not sufficient for their use for prenatal diagnosis on their own. However, in the case of muscular dystrophy, if the two flanking RFLPs are analyzed together, the chance of recombination separating both RFLPs from the *DMD* locus is much smaller, only 2%, which is probably adequate for prenatal diagnosis in families heterozygous for both RFLPs. Unfortunately, only a small proportion of families have been found to be heterozygous for both RFLPs, and, therefore, more informative RFLPs closer to the DNA locus are being sought.

FUTURE PROSPECTS

In the near future, prenatal diagnosis of many genetic disorders other than the hemoglobinopathies will be possible by RFLP analysis. A pilot program of first-trimester diagnosis in the hemoglobinopathies using chorionic villi for 34 cases at Oxford has been reported to be very successful (45). Therefore, if the method of chorionic villus sampling is found to have an acceptable risk to the fetus, it will become used more widely for the prenatal diagnosis of the hemoglobinopathies and other genetic disorders.

The technology of RFLP analysis will also undergo changes in the future. At present, the method is lengthy, expensive in materials, and requires the handling of radioisotopes. The methodology will probably be simplified so that small DNA samples can be handled, thus reducing costs and eliminating the use of radioisotopes. Already a number of nonradioactive labeling methods have been developed (46,47), and it will nto be long before these can be applied routinely to the detection of single copy genes in genomic DNA. These methods will enable large batches of labeled probes to be prepared and stored for long periods without deterioration, eliminating the need to make a fresh ^{32}P-labeled probe for each diagnosis. These improvements should enable the technique of RFLP analysis to be performed in laboratories other than the few specialized research laboratories.

ACKNOWLEDGMENTS

I wish to thank Mr. H. Ward, Dr. B. Modell, and Mr. C. Rodeck for supplying the cases used for the illustrations of RFLP analysis, Miss A. Fitches and Miss C. Heath for their technical assistance, Mr. R. Nicholls for his unpublished data on the $-(\alpha)^{20.5}$ deletion depicted in Figure 1, and Dr. J.S. Wainscoat for the autoradiograph shown in Figure 6.

REFERENCES

1. Higgs, D. R. and Weatherall, D. J. (1983). α-Thalassemia. In *Current Topics in Hematology*, (S. Piomelli and S. Yachnin, eds), Vol. 4, pp 37–97. Alan R. Liss, New York.
2. Orkin, S. H., Antonarakis, S. E. and Kazazian, H. H. (1983). Polymorphism and molecular pathology of the human beta-globin gene. *Prog. Hematol. 13*:49–73.
3. Woo, S. L. C., Lidsky, A. S., Guttler, F., Chandra, T. and Robson, K. J. H. (1983). Cloned human phenylalanine hydroxylase gene allows prenatal diagnosis and carrier detection of classical phenylketonuria. *Nature (London) 306*:151–155.
4. Gianelli, F., Anson, D. S., Choo, K. H., Rees, D. H. G., Winship, P. R., Ferrari, N., Rizza, C. R. and Brownlee, G. G. (1984). Characterisation and use of an intragenic polymorphic marker for detection of carriers of haemophilia B (factor IX deficiency). *Lancet i*:239–241.
5. Prochownik, E. V., Antonarakis, S., Bauer, K. A., Rosenberg, R. D., Fearon, E. R. and Orkin, S. H. (1983). Molecular heterogeneity of inherited antithrombin III deficiency. *New Engl. J. Med. 308*:1549–1552.
6. Phillips, J. A. Parks, J. S., Hjelle, B. L., Herd, J. L., Plotnick, H. L. P., Migeon, C. J., and Seeberg, P. H. (1982). Genetic analysis of familial isolated growth hormone deficiency Type 1. *J. Clin. Invest. 70*:489–495.
7. Gusella, J. F., Wexler, N. S., Conneally, P. M., Naylor, S. L., Anderson, M. A., Tanzi, R. E., Watkins, P. C., Ottina, K., Wallace, M. R., Sakaguchi, A. Y., Young, A. B., Shoulson, I., Bonilla, E. and Martin, J. B. (1983). A polymorphic DNA marker genetically linked to Huntington's chorea. *Nature (London) 309*:234–238.
8. Davies, K. E., Pearson, P. L., Harper, P. S., Murray, J. M., Obrien, T., Sarfazi, M., and Williamson, R. (1983). Linkage analysis of two cloned DNA sequences flanking the Duchenne muscular dystrophy locus on the short arm of human X chromosome. *Nucl. Acids Res. 11*:2303–2310.
9. Williamson, R., Eskdale, J., Coleman, D. V., Niazi, M., Loeffler, F. E. and Modell, B. (1981). Direct gene analysis of chorionic villi; a possible technique for the first trimester diagnosis of hemoglobinopathies. *Lancet ii*:1125–1127.
10. Old, J. M., Ward, R. H. T., Petrou, M., Karagozlu, F., Modell, B., and Weatherall, D. J. (1982). First trimester diagnosis for haemoglobinopathies: A report of 3 cases. *Lancet ii*:1413–1416.
11. Goossens, M., Dumez, Y., Kaplan, L., Lupker, M., Chabret, C., Henrion, R., and Rosa, J. (1983). Prenatal diagnosis of sickle-cell anemia in the first trimester of pregnancy. *New Engl. J. Med. 309*:381–833.
12. Old, J. M. and Higgs, D. R. (1983). Gene analysis. In *The Thalassaemias: Methods in Haematology*. Churchill Livingstone, Edinburgh.
13. Hoopes, B. C. and McClure, W. R. (1981). Studies on the selectivity of DNA precipitation by spermine. *Nucl. Acids Res. 9*:5493–5504.

14. Bouche, J. P. (1981). The effect of spermidine on endonuclease inhibition by agarose contaminants. *Anal. Biochem. 115*:42–45.
15. Southern, E. M. (1975). Detection of specific sequences among DNA fragments separated by gel electrophoresis. *J. Mol. Biol. 98*:503–517.
16. Higgs, D. R., Goodbourn, S. E. Y., Wainscoat, J. S., Clegg, J. B., and Weatherall, D. J. (1981). Highly variable regions of DNA flank the human α-globin genes. *Nucl. Acids Res. 9*:4213–4223.
17. Pressley, L., Higgs, D. R., Clegg, J. B., and Weatherall, D. J. (1980). Gene deletions in α-thalassaemia prove that the 5′ ζ locus is functional. *Proc. Natl. Acad. Sci. USA 77*:3586–3589.
18. Sophocleous, T., Higgs, D. R., Aldridge, B., Trent, R. J., Pressley, L., Clegg, J. B. and Weatherall, D. J. (1981). The molecular basis for the haemoglobin Bart's hydrops fetalis syndrome in Cyprus. *Br. J. Haemat. 47*:153–156.
19. Orkin, S. H. and Michelson, A. (1980). A partial deletion of the α-globin structural gene in human α-thalassaemia. *Nature (London) 286*:538–540.
20. Chang, J. C. and Kan, Y. W. (1981). Prenatal diagnosis of sickle cell anaemia by direct analysis of the sickle mutation. *Lancet ii*:1127–1128.
21. Chang, J. C. and Kan, Y. W. (1982). A sensitive new prenatal test for sickle cell anemia. *New Engl. J. Med. 307*:30–32.
22. Orkin, S. H., Little, P. F. R., Kazazian, H. H., and Boehm, C. D. (1982). Improved detection of the sickle mutation by DNA analysis. *New Engl. J. Med. 307*:32–36.
23. Chang, J. C., Alberti, A., and Kan, Y. W. (1983). A β-thalassaemia lesion abolishes the same *Mst* II site as the sickle mutation. *Nucl. Acids Res. 11*:7789–7794.
24. Spritz, R. A. and Orkin, S. H. (1982). Duplication followed by deletion accounts for the structure of an Indian deletion β^0 thalassaemia gene. *Nucl. Acids Res. 10*:8025–8029.
25. Thein, S. L., Old, J. M., Wainscoat, J. S., Modell, B., Petrou, M., and Weatherall, D. J. (1984). Population and genetic studies suggest a single origin for the Indian deletion β^0 thalassaemia. *Br. J. Haemat. 57*:271–278.
26. Gilman, J. G., Huisman, T. H. J., and Abels, J. (1984). Dutch β^0-thalassemia: A 10 kilobase DNA deletion associated with significant γ-chain production. *Br. J. Haemat. 56*:339–348.
27. Weatherall, D. J. and Clegg, J. B. (1981). *The Thalassaemia Syndromes*, 3rd ed. Blackwell Scientific Publ. Oxford.
28. Flavell, R. A., Kooter, J. H., DeBoer, E., Little, P. F. R., and Williamson, R. (1978). Analysis of the $\beta-\delta$ globin gene loci in normal and Hb Lepore DNA: Direct determination of gene linkage and intergene distance. *Cell 15*:25–41.
29. Wallace, R. B., Schold, M., Johnson, M. J., Dembek, P., and Hakura, K. (1981). Oligonucleotide directed mutagensis of the human β-globin gene: A general method for producing specific point mutations in cloned DNA. *Nucl. Acids Res. 9*:3647–3656.

30. Conner, B. J., Reyes, A. A., Morin, C., Itakura, K., Teplitz, R. L., and Wallace, R. B. (1983). Detection of sickle β^S-globin allele by hybridization with synthetic oligonucleotides. *Proc. Natl. Acad. Sci. USA, 80*:278–282.
31. Orkin, S. H., Markham, A. F., and Kazazian H. H. (1983). Direct detection of the common Mediterranean β thalassemia gene with synthetic DNA probes. An alternative approach for prenatal diagnosis. *J. Clin Invest 71*:775–779.
32. Kazazian, H. H., Orkin, S. H., Markham, A. F., Chapman, C. R. Youssoufian, H., and Waber, P. G. (1984). Quantification of the close association between DNA haplotypes and specific β-thalassaemia mutations in Mediterraneans. *Nature (London) 310*:152–154.
33. Wainscoat, J. s., Old, J. M., Weatherall, D. J., and Orkin, S. H. (1983). The molecular basis for the clinical diversity of β-thalassaemia in Cypriots. *Lancet i*:1235–1237.
34. Wainscoat, J. S., Bell, I., Old, J. M., Weatherall, D. J., Furbetta, M., Galanello, R., and Cao, A. (1983). Globin gene mapping studies in Sardinian patients homozygous for β^o-thalassaemia. *Mol. Biol. Med. 1*:1–10.
35. Rosatelli, C., Falchi, A. M., Tuveri, T., Scalas, M. T., Di Tucci, A., Monni, G., and Cao, A. (1985). Prenatal diagnosis of β-thalassaemia with the synthetic–oligomer technique. *Lancet i*:241–243.
36. Kurnit, D. M. and Hoeh, H. (1979). Prenatal diagnosis of human gene variation. *Ann. Rev. Genet. 13*:235.
37. Kan, Y. W. and Dozy, A. M. (1978). Polymorphism of DNA sequence adjacent to human β-globin structural gene: Relation to sickle mutation. *Proc. Natl. Acad. Sci. USA 75*: 5631–5635.
38. Kan, Y. W., Lee, K. Y., Furbetta, M., Angius, A. and Cao, A. (1980). Polymorphism of DNA sequences in the beta globin gene region. Application to prenatal diagnosis of β^o thalassaemia in Sardinia. *New Engl. J. Med. 302*:185–188.
39. Old, J., Petrou, M., Modell, B. and Weatherall, D. J. (1984). Feasibility of antenatal diagnosis of β-thalassaemia by DNA polymorphisms in Asian Indian and Cypriot populations. *Br. J. Haemat. 57*:255–263.
40. Boehm, C. D., Antonarakis, S. E., Phillips, J. A., III, Setten, G., and Kazazian, H. H. (1983). Prenatal diagnosis using DNA polymorphisms: Report on 95 pregnancies at risk for sickle cell disease or β thalassemia. *New Engl. J. Med. 308*:1054–1058.
41. Antonarakis, S. E., Boehm, C. D., Giardina, P. J. V., and Kazazian, H. H. (1982). Non-random association of polymorphic restriction sites in the β globin gene cluster. *Proc. Nat. Acad. Sci. USA 79*:137–141.
42. Elles, R. G., Williamson, R., Niazi, M., Coleman, D. V., and Horwell, D. (1983). Absence of maternal contamination of chorionic villi used for fetal-gene analysis. *New Engl. J. Med. 308*:1433–1435.
43. Gianelli, Choo, K. H., Rees, D. J. G., Boyd, Y., Rizza, C. R., Brownlee, G. G. (1982). Gene deletions in patients with haemophilia B and anti-factor 1X antibodies. *Nature (London) 303*:181–182.

44. Kidd, J. V., Wallace, B., Itakura, K., and Woo, S. L. C. (1983). α_1-Antitrypsin deficiency detection by direct analysis of the mutation in the gene. *Nature (London) 304*:230–234.
45. Old, J. M., Weatherall, D. J., Ward, R. H. T., Petrou, M., Modell, B., Rodeck, C. H., Warren, R., and Morsman, J. M. (1985). First trimester diagnosis of the hemoglobin disorders. *Ann. N.Y. Acad. Sci* (in press).
46. Leary, J. J., Brigati, D. J., and Ward, D. C. (1983). Rapid and sensitive colorimetric method for visualizing biotin-labeled DNA on nitrocellulose: Bio-blots. *Proc. Natl. Acad. Sci. USA 80*:4045–4049.
47. Renz, M. and Kurz, C. (1984). A colorimetric method for DNA hybridization. *Nucl. Acids Res. 12*:3435–3444.

11

First Trimester Diagnosis of Thalassemias by DNA Analysis in the Mediterranean Area

MAURIZIO FERRARI and SILVANA TEDESCHI
Istituti Clinici di Perfezionamento, Milan, Italy

MAURIZIO SAMPIETRO and GEMINO FIORELLI
Third Institute of Clinical Medicine, University of Milan, Milan, Italy

ANNA SERRA, GIUSEPPE SAGLIO, and CLARA CAMASCHELLA
Institute of Internal Medicine, University of Turin, Turin, Italy

INTRODUCTION

Thalassemia has the highest frequency of any genetic disease in the world. β-Thalassemia is probably the most common of the several thalassemia syndromes. This defect, which is clinically silent in heterozygous subjects, causes a severe chronic transfusion-dependent anemia in homozygous patients. Prevention programs for this disease, based on medical and educational approaches, have been started in several countries (Modell and Berdoukas, 1984). At present, prenatal diagnosis based on globin chains synthesis studies with fetal blood obtained by fetoscopy is an important part of these programs. The first prenatal diagnoses by this method were made at the end of 1974 (Kan et al., 1975), and since then the demand for the procedure has risen.

In the last 9 years, several centers for prenatal diagnosis of thalassemia have been organized in the areas with higher incidence of thalassemia: Athens, Cyprus, Israel, and Italy (Cagliari, Ferrara, Milan, Palermo, Rome, and Turin). Recently, Alter (1984) summarized the world experience, evaluating the figures for more than 5000 cases on the obstetric and hematological problems connected with the procedure. Prenatal diagnosis made in the second trimester of pregnancy also involves medical and psychological problems. For these reasons, in recent years, the work of several investigators has been aimed at earlier prenatal diagnosis of thalassemia in the first trimester of pregnancy.

First-trimester prenatal diagnosis of β-thalassemia has became a feasible procedure because of the recently developed techniques of chorionic villi sampling and DNA analysis. With chorionic villi sampling, one can obtain tissue of fetal origin during the first trimester of pregnancy (Simoni et al., 1983). This technique has been widely used for chromosomal analysis and biochemical assays (Simoni et al., 1984). The amount of fetal material obtained by this procedure is sufficient for DNA extraction for molecular analysis (Williamson et al., 1981).

Thalassemia is one of the most thoroughly studied genetic diseases at the molecular level, and a large number of molecular defects have been characterized. Several of these defects can be detected for prenatal diagnostic purposes by direct or indirect analysis (Orkin and Kazazian, 1984). In both types of analyses, DNA is digested with endonucleases, and electrophoretically separated fragments are hybridized with specific ^{32}P-labeled probes. The direct methods recognize large deletions of globin genes and point mutations affecting restriction sites (Orkin et al., 1978). Recently, small synthetic probes (oligomers) that are complementary to normal and thalassemic sequences have been developed (Wallace et al., 1981). These probes make it possible to detect thalassemia defects due to point mutations directly. Indirect methods employ DNA restriction fragment length polymorphism (RFLP) linked to β-thalassemia defects as genetic "markers" for these mutations (Kazazian et al., 1980). In this way, the segregation of the abnormal gene in a family can be known even when the defect cannot be detected by direct analysis.

The molecular analysis of DNA extracted from chorionic villi has three main advantages over the common techniques of fetal blood sampling and globin chain synthesis study: (a) the procedure is performed during the first trimester of pregnancy; (b) the diagnosis is independent of phenotypic variations; and (c) the sampling procedure is less invasive than fetoscopy. If chorionic villi sampling proves to be safe for the fetus in a larger study, this approach will probably be widely introduced for populations in which thalassemia is a major problem.

MOLECULAR DEFECTS THAT CAUSE β-THALASSEMIA IN THE MEDITERRANEAN POPULATION

The molecular study of β-thalassemia in the Mediterranean area has demonstrated a wide heterogeneity of this defect. Most types of β-thalassemia in this area are caused by point mutations or few nucleotide deletions that alter, in different ways, the expression of the β gene to interfere with transcription, RNA processing, or RNA translation.

The molecular defects can be classified as follows:

1. *Transcription mutants*: The mutation C→G in position −87 in the 5′ flanking region of the β gene alters a promoter unit for transcription, probably interfering with the recognition site for RNA polymerasis (Orkin et al., 1982; Treisman et al., 1983). This mutation, which appears to be rare in the Mediterranean area, gives rise to a β^+-thalassemia.
2. *Mutants affecting mRNA processing*: Native mRNA undergoes a number of modifications in the nucleus, the most important of which is the "splicing" of sequences corresponding to the introns of the gene. The splicing of introns requires the presence of two invariant dinucleotides, GT and AG, at the two extremities of the intron. At least four different types of mutations may interfere with splicing in Mediterranean β-thalassemia: (a) mutation G→A in position 1 in the first (*IVS-1*) (Orkin et al., 1982) or second intron (*IVS-2*) (Baird et al., 1981). Normal splicing sites are not functional, and other sites, which are not used physiologically (cryptic sites), are employed. In both cases, the thalassemia has a β° phenotype. (b) When the mutation takes place in the consensus sequence of the dinucleotide GT (mutation T→C in position 6 in *IVS-1*) (Orkin et al., 1982), the activity of the normal site is reduced, and cryptic sites are partially used. This defect causes a β^+-thalassemia. (c) The mutation G→A in position 110 in the *IVS-1* gives rise to the common type of β^+-thalassemia seen in the Mediterranean area (Spritz et al., 1981). In this case, a new splicing site that arises in the first intron is used preferentially to the normal AG site. (d) The mutation C→G in position 745 in the *IVS-2* creates a new GT site (Orkin et al., 1982). As a result of double splicing, an abnormal exon is created. The phenotype of this defect is a β^+-thalassemia.
3. *Mutants affecting mRNA translation*: The most common type in the Mediterranean area is the defect that causes the β^o-thalassemia that is common in Sardinia. A mutation C→T in the second exon (codon 39) gives rise to a codon TAG that causes premature termination of translation (Moschonas et al., 1982; Orkin and Goff, 1981; Trecartin et al., 1981). Two other types of

β°-thalassemia are caused by frameshift mutations in the first exon [deletion of a nucleotide in codon 6 (Kazazian et al., 1983), deletion of two nucleotides in codon 8 (Orkin and Goff, 1981)].

Among all the mutations recognized in the Mediterranean area, direct detection is possible for only four, in which the mutations affect known restriction sites. These defects are mutation G → A in position 1 in the *IVS-2* detected by *Hph* I (Baird et al., 1981); mutation C → G in position 745 in the *IVS-2* detected by *Rsa* I (Orkin et al., 1982); mutation C → G in position −87 detected by *Avr* II (Orkin et al., 1982); and the frameshift deletion in codon 6 detected by *Mst* II (Chang et al. 1983). However, these defects are rare in the Mediterranean area. The direct detection of other mutations is feasible only with specific synthetic oligomers complementary to single mutations (Wallace et al., 1981).

DNA POLYMORPHISMS IN THE β-GLOBIN GENE CLUSTER

Deoxyribonucleic acid polymorphisms can be defined as those neutral variations in base sequences that are observed with given frequency in a population. They provide a powerful tool for the identification of gene mutations by genetic linkage analysis. The first polymorphism in the β-globin gene cluster was recognized by the enzyme *Hpa* I, by Kan and Dozy (1978). This polymorphism made possible the identification of the gene carrying the sickle mutation in individuals from western Africa. The first polymorphic site to be employed for detection of a β-thalassemic gene was the *Bam* HI site, located 3′ to the β gene, which in Sardinians has been employed to identify the common β° mutation (Kan et al., 1980). Subsequently, a large number of other polymorphic restriction sites were identified in the β-globin gene cluster (Jeffreys, 1979; Orkin and Goff, 1981; Orkin et al., 1982, 1983a; Semenza et al., 1984; Old and Wainscoat, 1983; Kan et al., 1980; Antonarakis et al., 1982).

At present, 17 different polymorphic sites have been identified in a region spanning about 60 kb around the β-globin gene. Each polymorphic site may be present (+) or absent (−) on a chromosome. The combination of different sites on a chromosome is called a haplotype. Only a few haplotypes among the theoretically possible combinations are usually observed in a population because of the linkage disequilibrium between different polymorphic sites. Haplotypes represent the structural background on which the thalassemia mutations have been established, and their frequencies vary in different ethnic groups. In the Mediterranean area, Orkin et al. (1982) found nine different haplotypes linked to at least eight β gene mutations.

Determination of haplotypes can be used to identify the type and incidence of β-thalassemia defects in a population. To obtain more information about the geographical distribution of thalassemia defects in Italy, we have determined the haplotypes for 101 thalassemia major patients at the pediatric clinics in Turin and Milan. These patients are heterogeneous in their geographical origins, since in the industrialized areas of Turin and Milan (northwest of Italy), there is major internal

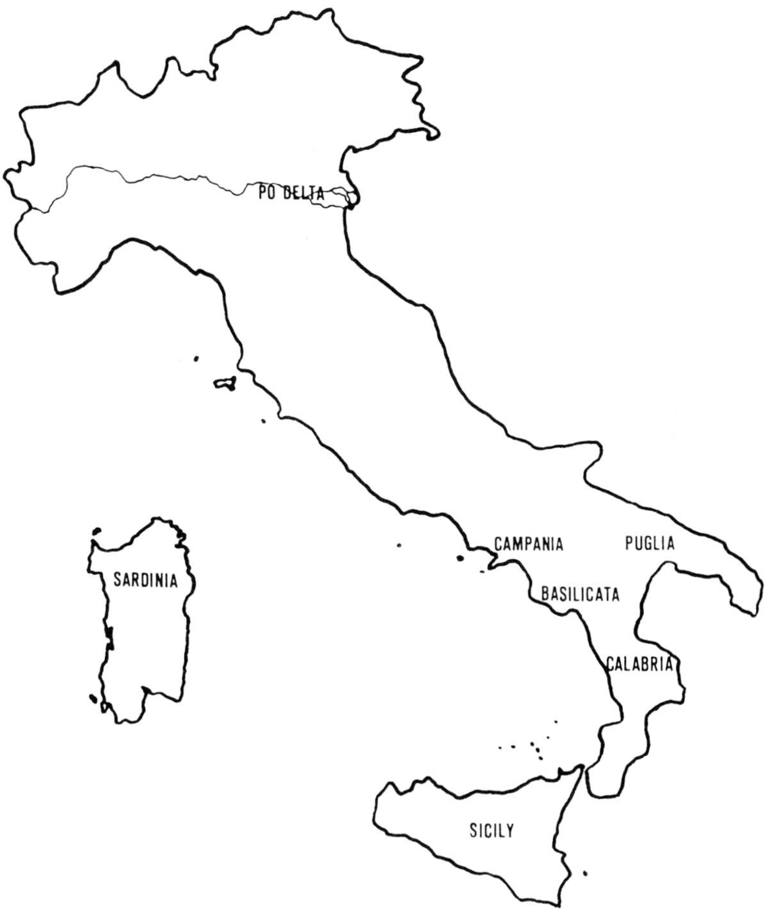

Figure 1 Regions of Italy involved in the haplotype study.

migration from other regions of Italy (Fig. 1). We have studied only few cases from Sardinia at this stage of the study, as it is already known that a single type of mutation (Wainscoat et al., 1983) is prevalent in the island. Four endonucleases, to establish the patterns of seven polymorphic sites, were used. The endonucleases employed were *Hinc* II, *Hind* III, *Ava* II, and *Bam* HI (Fig. 2). In Tables 1 and 2, the incidence and geographical distributions of haplotypes for 202 chromosomes are reported. In accordance with the findings of Orkin et al. (1982), the most frequent haplotypes were the I (41.6%), II (26.7%), and VI (11.9%). The defects linked to these haplotypes (Kazazian et al., 1984) are the common β^+-thalassemia (mutation G→A in position 110 in the *IVS-1*), the common β^o-thalassemia (mutation C→T in the second exon codon 39), and the mild β^+-thalassemia (substitution T→C in position 6 in the *IVS-1*). Haplotype VI deserves special attention, as it has been shown to be linked to a "mild" β^+-thalassemia (Tamagnini et al., 1983, Troungos et al., 1983). Subjects homozygous for this haplotype always have a clinical picture of thalassemia intermedia, while double heterozygotes for this defect and for β^o or β^+-thalassemia may have typical pictures of

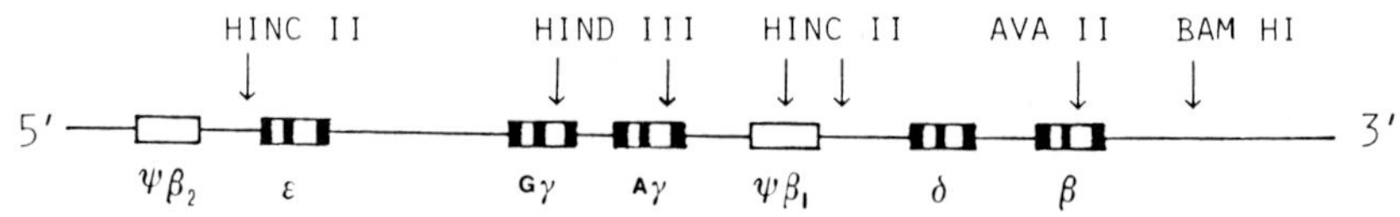

HAPLOTYPE	HINC II	HIND III	HIND III	HINC II	HINC II	AVA II	BAM HI
I	+	−	−	−	−	+	+
II	−	+	+	−	+	+	+
III	−	+	−	+	+	+	−
IV	−	+	−	+	+	−	+
V	+	−	−	−	−	+	−
VI	−	+	+	−	−	−	+
VII	+	−	−	−	−	−	+
VIII	−	+	−	+	−	+	−
IX	−	+	−	+	+	+	+

Figure 2 Polymorphic restriction sites in the β-globin gene cluster. The arrows show the polymorphic site. The presence of a site is indicated by + and the absence by −. The common Mediterranean haplotypes are shown.

Table 1 Haplotype Distribution in 202 β-Thalassemic Chromosomes

Haplotype	No.	Percentage
I	84	41.6
II	54	26.7
III	3	1.5
IV	—	—
V	11	5.4
VI	24	11.9
VII	9	4.5
VIII	—	—
IX	15	7.4
A	2	1.0

Table 2 Geographic Distribution and Haplotypes of 202 β-Thalassemic Chromosomes

	Haplotypes							
Regions	I	II	III	V	VI	VII	IX	A
Basilicata	6	3	1	—	1	—	—	—
Calabria	23	9	—	6	6	5	3	—
Campania	6	—	—	1	—	—	—	—
Po Delta	16	10	—	—	—	—	7	—
Puglia	17	17	2	3	10	3	1	2
Sardinia	—	4	—	—	—	—	—	—
Sicily	16	11	—	1	7	1	4	—

transfusion-dependent thalassemia major. This fact must be taken into account in genetic counseling of subjects at risk for this type of defect.

We have never observed haplotypes IV and VIII, linked to rare mutations, in our group of patients. We have observed an unusual haplotype, identified in Tables 1 and 2 by "A," with a pattern $- - - - + + +$. This haplotype, which we found in a subject from southern Italy, has been previously reported in Africans (Antonarakis et al., 1984).

As for the geographical distribution of haplotypes, we observed great heterogeneity, with the possible exception of the area of the Po Delta, where only three haplotypes (I, II, and IX) have been found. Since haplotypes II and IX are linked to the same mutation, in this region only two β-thalassemic mutations should be present, as suggested in the paper recently published by Pirastu et al. (1984).

In conclusion, our data confirm the great heterogeneity of thalassemia in Italy. Nevertheless, the haplotype study suggests that three defects account for more than 80% of thalassemic genes. Unfortunately, direct detection of these defects by endonucleases is not possible. Their identification, at present, should be carried out either by haplotype study of the family or by means of specific synthetic oligomers complementary to the mutation.

FEASIBILITY OF PRENATAL DIAGNOSIS IN THE MEDITERRANEAN AREA

Prenatal diagnosis of thalassemia, as mentioned before, can be carried out by two different approaches: (a) study of polymorphisms by restriction endonucleases, as markers of a normal or thalassemic gene in a family, or (b) direct identification of the mutation affecting the restriction site with endonucleases or synthetic oligomers complementary to the mutation. The first approach is at present more widely used. It may be difficult because polymorphism study must be carried out on couples at risk and their previous offspring (normal or affected). If there are no offspring, the study must be extended to other relatives, and, in some cases, it may still not be possible to identify a linkage between polymorphisms and a thalassemia mutation. Direct detection of β-thalassemic defects affecting a restriction site is possible in only few cases because there are only four mutations in this type, and they occur rarely in the Mediterranean area.

Recent developments of molecular techniques have provided an alternative tool for the direct detection of β-thalassemias caused by point mutation. It is possible to synthesize short fragments of DNA (oligomers) that, under appropriate experimental conditions, can hybridize to their complementary sequences but not to sequences bearing a mutation (Wallace et al., 1981). Several oligomers have been already employed for prenatal diagnosis of sickle cell anemia and β-thalassemia (Pirastu et al., 1983; Conner et al., 1983; Orkin et al., 1983b). Apart from the technical problems of this method, the use of oligomers is obviously more advantageous for populations (such as Sardinians) that carry a predominant single type of thalassemia (Wainscoat et al., 1983). In other areas in which there are several thalassemia defects, it is necessary to carry out the analysis with more oligomers or, alternatively, to choose the appropriate oligomer after previous haplotype study.

From the practical point of view, the introduction in a given population of first-trimester diagnosis of thalassemia by analysis of DNA from chorionic villi has to be preceded by an evaluation of its feasibility. In fact, in different populations, the number of couples at risk who could benefit from RFLP analysis is variable, depending on the number of defects, their haplotypes, and the haplotypes that are present in the normal population.

Preliminary data on the feasibility of prenatal diagnosis by RFLP studies were evaluated in the Italian population from the haplotypes of 12 families (with an affected child) living in northern Italy but originating from different regions of Italy. In 8 of the 12 couples (66.6%), prenatal diagnosis was completely feasible. In other words, the allele carrying the β-thalassemic gene was always detectable (Table 3). In 4 of the 12 couples (33.3%), prenatal diagnosis had a feasibility of 50%. In other words, only one allele carrying the β-thalassemic gene was detectable (Table 3). In these four couples, prenatal diagnosis was not completely feasible because one parent was homozygous for haplotype I.

Since haplotype I is the most frequent in Italy, both in the normal and thalassemic allele (Orkin, et al., 1983), we think that subjects homozygous for haplotype I may be the major problem in prenatal diagnosis by haplotype study. An oligomer complementary to the most

Table 3 Feasibility of Prenatal Diagnosis by Haplotype Study in 12 Families at Risk for β-Thalassemia

Family	Haplotypes			Feasibility (%)
	Mother	Father	Patient	
1	I/IV	I/V	I/I	100
2	I/IX	I/IX	I/I	100
3	I/II	I/II	II/II	100
4	I/VII	II/VII	I/II	100
5	II/V	II/V	II/II	100
6	I/I	II/IX	I/IX	50
7	II/V	II/IX	II/II	100
8	I/I	I/V	I/I	50
9	I/III	I/VII	I/I	100
10	I/I	II/IX	I/II	50
11	I/II	I/I	I/II	50
12	I/II	II/IX	II/II	100

frequent mutation of haplotype I (Orkin et al., 1982) could solve this problem for these couples. Complementary oligomers will also be necessary for those couples at risk who do not have a homozygous (normal or affected) child and for whom an extended family study is not helpful. In the Italian population, the simultaneous use of three oligomers corresponding to the more frequent defects could cover more than 80% of prenatal diagnosis.

In any case, as the demand for first-trimester prenatal diagnosis increases, even for first pregnancies, the choice of oligomers could be suggested by a haplotype study prior to the pregnancy.

APPENDIX

Restriction endonuclease analysis in subjects with Cooley's anemia and in 12 couples of their parents was performed as described by J. M. Old et al. (1983). Human DNA obtained by phenol–chloroform extraction was digested with restriction endonucleases under the conditions recommended by manufacturers. The resulting DNA fragments were separated by size electrophoresis in an agarose gel and transferred to a nitro-cellulose filter. Filters were then hybridized with ^{32}P-labeled probes and autoradiographed on X-ray films.

ACKNOWLEDGMENTS

The Authors are indebted to Professor G. Masera and Professor V. Carnelli, Pediatric Clinic, University of Milan, and to Professor W. Gabutti, Pediatric Clinic, University of Turin, for encouraging this study. We gratefully acknowledge the useful suggestions and help by J. S. Wainscoat, MRC Molecular Haematology Unit, Oxford. We are particularly grateful to the patients and their parents for their helpful collaboration.

This study was partially supported by grants from Regione Piemonte, Ricerca Finalizzata n. 36, 1982. S.T. is supported by a grant from "Associazione Italiana per lo Studio delle Malformazioni," "Associazione Lombarda per il Bambino Emopatico," and "Comitato De Marchi per la Lotta contro la Talassemia".

REFERENCES

1. Alter, B. P. (1984). Antenatal diagnosis of thalassemia: A review. *Ann. N. Y. Acad. Sci.* (in press).

2. Antonarakis, S. E., Boehm, C. D., Giardina, P. J. V., and Kazazian, H. H. Jr. (1982). Nonrandom association of polymorphic restriction sites in the β-globin gene cluster. *Proc. Natl. Acad. Sci. (USA) 79*:137–141.
3. Antonarakis, S. E., Boehm, C. D., Sergeant, G. R., Theisen, C. E., Dover, G. J., and Kazazian, H. H., Jr. (1984). Origin of the β^S-globin gene in Blacks: The contribution of recurrent mutation or gene conversion or both. *Proc. Natl. Acad. Sci. (USA) 81*:853–856.
4. Baird, M., Driscoll, C., Schreiner, H., Sciarratta, G. V., Sansone, G., Niazi, G., Ramirez, F., and Bank, A. (1981). A nucleotide change at a splice junction in the human β-globin gene is associated with β^o-thalassemia. *Proc. Natl. Acad. Sci. (USA) 78*:4218–4221.
5. Chang, J. C., Alberti, A., and Kan, Y. W. (1983). A β-thalassemia lesion abolishes the same *Mst* II site as the sickle mutation. *Nucl. Acids Res. 11*:7789–7794.
6. Conner, B. J., Reyes, A. A., Morin, C., Itakura, K., Teplitz, R. L., and Wallace, R. B. (1983). Deletion of sickle β^S-globin allele by hybridization with synthetic oligonucleotides. *Proc. Natl. Acad. Sci. (USA) 80*:278–282.
7. Jeffreys A. J. (1979). DNA sequence variants in the $^G\gamma$-, $^A\gamma$-, and β-globin genes of man. *Cell 18*:1–10.
8. Kan, Y. W. and Dozy, A. M. (1978). Polymorphism of DNA sequence adjacent to the human β-globin structural gene: Relationship to sickle mutation. *Proc. Natl. Acad. Sci. (USA) 75*:5631–5635.
9. Kan, Y. W., Golbus, M. S., Klein, P., and Dozy, A. M. (1975). Successful application of prenatal diagnosis in a pregnancy at risk for homozygous β-thalassemia. *N. Engl. J. Med. 292*:1096–1099.
10. Kan, Y. W., Lee, K. Y., Furbetta M., Angius, A., and Cao, A. (1980). Polymorphism of DNA sequence in the β-globin region: Application to prenatal diagnosis of β^o-thalassemia in Sardinia. *N. Engl. J. Med. 302*:185–188.
11. Kazazian, H. H. Jr., Phillips, J. A. III, Boehm, C. D., Vic, T. A., Mahoney, M. J., and Ritchey, A. K. (1980). Prenatal diagnosis of β-thalassemias by amniocentesis: Linkage analysis using multiple polymorphic restriction endonuclease sites. *Blood 56*:926–930.
12. Kazazian, H. H. Jr., Orkin, S. H., Boehm, C. D., Sexto, J. P., and Antonarakis, S. E. (1983). β-Thalassemia due to deletion of the nucleotide which is substituted in sickle cell anemia. *Am. J. Human Genet. 35*:1028–1033.
13. Kazazian, H. H. Jr., Orkin, S. H., Markham, A. F., Chapman, C. R., Youssoufian, H., and Waber, P. G. (1984). Quantification of the close association between DNA haplotypes and specific β-thalassemia mutations in Mediterraneans. *Nature (London) 310*:152–154.
14. Modell, B. and Berdoukas, V. (1984). *The Clinical Approach to Thalassemia*, pp. 354–378. Grune and Stratton, New York.
15. Moschonas, N., de Boer, E., Grosveld, F. G., Dahl, H. H. M., Shewmaker,

C. K., and Flavell, R. A. (1982). Structure and expression of a cloned β-thalassemia globin gene. *Nucl. Acids Res. 9*:4391–4401.
16. Old, J. M. and Wainscoat, J. S. (1983). A new DNA polymorphism in the β-globin gene cluster can be used for antenatal diagnosis of β-thalassemia. *Br. J. Haematol. 53*:337–341.
17. Orkin, S. H. and Kazazian, H. H., Jr. (1984). The mutation and polymorphisms of the human β-globin gene and its surrounding DNA. *Ann. Rev. Genet. 18*:131–171.
18. Orkin, S. H. and Goff, S. C. (1981). Nonsense and frameshift mutations in β-thalassemia detected in cloned β-globin genes. *J. Biol. Chem. 256*:9782–9784.
19. Orkin, S. H., Alter, B. P., Altay, C., Mahoney, M. J., Lazarus, H., Hobbins, J. C., and Nathan, D. G. (1978). Application of endonuclease mapping to the analysis and prenatal diagnosis of thalassemias caused by globin gene deletion. *N. Engl. J. Med. 299*:166–172.
20. Orkin, S. H., Kazazian, H. H., Antonarakis, S. E., Goff, S. C., Boehm, C. D., Sexton, J. P., Waber, P. G., and Giardina, P. J. V. (1982). Linkage of β-thalassemia mutations and β-globin gene polymorphisms with DNA polymorphisms in the human β-gene cluster. *Nature (London) 296*:627–631.
21. Orkin, S. H., Antonarakis, S. E., and Kazazian, H. H. Jr. (1983a). Polymorphism and molecular pathology of the human β-globin gene. *Prog. Hematol. 13*:49–73.
22. Orkin, S. H., Markham, A. F., and Kazazian, H. H. Jr. (1983b). Direct detection of the common Mediterranean β-thalassemic gene with synthetic DNA probes. An alternative approach for prenatal diagnosis. *J. Clin. Invest. 71*:775–779.
23. Pirastu, M., Kan, Y. W., Cao, A., Conner, B. J., Teplitz, R. L., and Wallace, R. B. (1983). Prenatal diagnosis of β-thalassemia: Detection of a single mutation DNA. *N. Engl. J. Med. 309*:284–287.
24. Pirastu, M., Del Senno, L. Conconi, F., Vullo, C., and Kan, Y. W. (1984). Ferrara β^o-thalassemia caused by the β^{39} nonsense mutation. *Nature (London) 307*:76.
25. Semenza, G. L., Malladi, P., Poncz, M., Delgrosso K., Schwartz, E., and Surrey, S. (1984). Detection of a novel DNA polymorphism in the β-globin cluster and evidence for site-specific recombination. *Ped. Res. 18*:225A.
26. Simoni, G., Brambati, B., Danesino, C. Rossella, F. Terzoli, G. L., Ferrari, M., and Fraccaro, M. (1983). Efficient direct chromosome analysis and enzyme determinations from chorionic villi samples in the first trimester of pregnancy. *Human Genet. 63*:349–357.
27. Simoni, G., Brambati, B. Danesino, C., Terzoli, G. L., Romitti, L., Rossella, F., and Fraccaro, M. (1984). Diagnostic application of first trimester trophoblast sampling in 100 pregnancies. *Human Genet. 66*:252–259.
28. Spritz, R. A., Jagadeeswaran, P., Choudary, P. V., Biro, P. A., Elder, J. T.,

de Riel, J. K., Manley, J. L., Gefter, M. L., Forget, B. G., and Weissman, S. M. (1981). Base substitution in a intervening sequence of a β^+-thalassemic human globin gene. *Proc. Natl. Acad. Sci. (USA) 78*:2455–2459.

29. Tamagnini, G. P., Lopes, M. C., Castanheira, M. E., Wainscoat, J. S., and Wood, W. G., (1983). β^+-Thalassemia-Portuguese type: Clinical, hematological, and molecular studies of a newly defined form of β-thalassemia. *Br. J. Haematol. 54*:189–200.
30. Trecartin, R. F., Leibhaber, S. A., Chang, J. C., Lee, Y. W., and Kan, Y. W. (1981). β^o-Thalassemia in Sardinia is caused by a nonsense mutation. *J. Clin. Invest. 68*:1012–1017.
31. Treisman, R., Orkin, S. H., and Maniatis, T. (1983). Specific transcription and RNA splicing defects in five cloned β-thalassemia genes. *Nature (London) 302*:591–596.
32. Troungos, C. Sortino, G., Cacciola, R., Lombardo, T., Cacciola, E., and Labie, D. (1983). Haplotype-VI associated mild β^+-thalassemia in Sicily: Mediterranean type? *Lancet ii*:509–510.
33. Wainscoat, J. S., Bell. I., Old, J. M., Weatherall, D. J., Furbetta, M., Galanello, R., and Cao, A. (1983). Globin gene mapping studies in Sardinian patients homozygous for β^o-thalassemia. *Mol. Biol. Med. 1*:1–10.
34. Wallace, R. B., Schold, M., Johnson, M. J., Dembek, P., and Itakura, K. (1981). Oligonucleotide directed mutagenesis of the human β-globin gene: A general method for producing specific point mutations in cloned DNA. *Nucleic Acids Res. 9*:3467–3656.
35. Williamson, R., Eskdale, J., Coleman, D. V., Niazi, M., Loeffler, F. E., and Modell, B. M. (1981). Direct gene analysis of chorionic villi: A possible technique for first trimester antenatal diagnosis of hemoglobinopathies. *Lancet ii*:1125–1127.

12

Risk Assessment for Teratogenesis due to Chorionic Villus Sampling

SERGIO FABRO and ANTHONY R. SCIALLI
Columbia Hospital for Women, Georgetown University, Washington, D.C.

INTRODUCTION

Teratology, from a strict etymological point of view, is the science concerned with the study of birth defects as permanent structural abnormalities. This term is too restrictive for the evaluation of the potential hazards of chorionic villus sampling (CVS), and the term poor pregnancy outcome is preferred. Any attempt to evaluate a possible relationship between CVS and poor pregnancy outcome must be able to identify and exclude the background occurrence of poor pregnancy outcome (see the chapters by Dr. Warburton and by Dr. Simpson in this treatise).

Poor pregnancy outcome is a collective term encompassing all types of reproductive abnormalities and/or failure. It is a significant event in the human reproductive process. About 3% of newborns present serious congenital malformations, 8–10% are premature, and 4% are small for gestational age. We have to add to these poor pregnancy outcomes the rate of spontaneous abortion (15–20%), stillbirths (1%), and neonatal deaths (1%). Furthermore, defects that appear later in life (e.g., learning disabilities and behavioral abnormalities) should also be added to the list. Basic knowledge about the various aspects of human reproduction is incomplete, particularly as it relates to mechanisms by which alterations of the normal reproductive process are brought about. A number of mechanisms have been proposed. For example, it is thought that some abnormalities are due to single gene actions (e.g., achondroplasia or phenylketonuria), to individual environmental exposures (e.g., rubella or aminopterin), or to the interaction of multiple environmental factors and/or genes (e.g., dislocated hip or cleft palate). The last may account for the majority of congenital abnormalities (Shepard, 1983).

In recent times, there has been growing concern that both the physical and chemical environment may play an important role in affecting intrauterine development and may be responsible for a significant number of poor pregnancy outcomes. Although this belief is not supported by scientific evidence, every type of exposure or procedure must be questioned for its possible deleterious effect on human pregnancy and on reproduction in general. The procedures used for prenatal recognition of structural and biochemical abnormalities in the human conceptus have not been excluded from this scrutiny. With regard to CVS, attention has been directed at three sources of possible adverse pregnancy effects: the ultrasound examination used to guide placement of the cannula, the physical effects related to cannula placement and chorion removal, and the introduction of infectious agents.

ULTRASOUND

Ultrasound is a mechanical energy form in which small particles in a medium are made to oscillate. This energy form is similar to audible sound except that the frequencies of oscillation used are above the limits of human hearing. The amount of energy reaching a given tissue depends on the intensity of the sound energy directed at the tissue, the attenuation of the energy as it traverses intervening tissues, and the time over which the sound exposure occurs. Adverse biological effects of ultrasound have appeared in the literature since the 1920s. Many of these reports concern a variety of ultrasound frequencies, intensities, and doses in a number of different species and in vitro systems and are not applicable to the use of diagnostic ultrasound in humans (National Council on Radiation Protection and Measurements, 1983; WHO, 1982; Stewart and Stratmeyer, 1982). Much of the early work on the potential hazards of medical ultrasound was performed in the fruit fly, *Drosophila melanogaster*. A possible mechanism for ultrasound effects on developing flies was suggested by the observation that the blastoderm cells of insonated *Drosophila* eggs move rapidly in the sound field (Selman and Counce, 1953). It is generally believed, however, that ultrasound damage to larvae, pupae, and adult flies occurs as a result of cavitation (violent contraction) of gas bubbles that are a part of the animal's respiratory system (National Council on Radiation Protection and Measurements, 1983; WHO, 1982).

Chromosomal effects of ultrasound energy have been studied in a number of species as well as in human cells in vitro. Insonation of peripheral human blood for 1 hr does not result in an increase in chromosomal abnormalities in blood cells in spite of ultrasound energy sufficient to raise the temperature of the medium 2.5°C (Buckton and Baker, 1972). Cultured human lymphocytes, however, show an increase in sister chromatid exchanges (SCE) after prolonged exposure to real-time ultrasound similar to that used in diagnostic obstetrics (Liebeskind et al., 1979; Haupt et al., 1981). Pregnant mice treated with ultrasound do not show an increase in SCE either in maternal marrow cells or in fetal tissues (Au et al., 1982). Similarly, no increase in SCE are noted also after Doppler ultrasound exposure in hamster ovary cells (Wegner et al., 1980). Of greatest reassurance to those concerned with CVS is the finding that when first-trimester human embryos are exposed to prolonged insonation prior to elective abortion, there is no increase in chromosomal abnormalities compared to control abortuses (Ikeuchi et al., 1973).

The possibility that ultrasound induces nonchromosomal abnoralities has been investigated in a number of mammals. Most of the studies have been performed in rodents. Consistent effects have not been noted; however, one study found an association between ultrasound exposure and reduced birth weight (Pizzarello et al., 1978). The American Institute on Ultrasound in Medicine considered the available mammalian data in 1982 and concluded that there are no independently confirmed significant biological effects in mammals of ultrasound in the low megahertz frequency range when intensities are below 100 mW/cm^2. In addition, at higher intensities with exposure times of less than 500 sec, biological effects have not been established as long as the product of the intensity and exposure time (including time off for pulsed ultrasound) is less than 50 $joules/cm^2$ (National Council on Radiation Protection and Measurements, 1983).

Epidemiological studies of human populations exposed to ultrasound have not established any adverse effect of insonation. Some of these studies have not been controlled (Hellman et al., 1970), but controlled studies have also concluded that adverse reproductive effects of ultrasound cannot be demonstrated (Scheidt et al., 1978; Stark et al., 1984).

MECHANICAL INJURY

The introduction of a foreign object into the conceptus raises the possibility of direct mechanical injury that may have adverse effects on development. Any discussion of such effects must consider the potential for injury related to an older technique of mechanically invading the conceptus, i.e., amniocentesis, in order to place into perspective the relative risks of these prenatal diagnostic techniques.

Major injuries attributed to amniocentesis include ileocutaneous fistula, gangrene of the arm, placental separation, and umbilical cord occlusion secondary to hematoma formation (Rickwood, 1977; Lamb, 1975). Such consequences of amniocentesis are uncommon, however. Of greater concern is whether amniocentesis results in an increased risk of pregnancy loss. Two large collaborative studies found no increased loss in pregnancies subjected to amniocentesis (NICHD National Registry for Amniocentesis Study Group, 1976; Simpson et al., 1976), while a third study reported a 1.0–1.5% increased risk of pregnancy loss after the procedure (United Kingdom Medical Research Council Working Party of Amniocentesis, 1978). This last study, however, used controls that differed in important parameters (such as age) from subjects. It is generally accepted now that the risk of pregnancy loss attributable to amniocentesis is small; a figure of 0.5% is often used to represent this excess risk (Simpson et al., 1980). If the figure of 0.5% is accepted as the risk for amniocentesis-related pregnancy loss, then performance of the procedure on a group of pregnant 35-year-old women will result in the loss of two fetuses for every Down syndrome fetus detected.

The United Kingdom Medical Research Council study also identified an increase in respiratory problems in children born after amniocentesis; however, a report on children at age 5–7 years showed no increase in the incidence of neurological or other physical problems attributable to amniocentesis (Gillberg et al., 1982).

There is a concern that the trauma associated with the technique of CVS may lead to abnormal intrauterine development of the conceptus or may result in other poor pregnancy outcomes. Anecdotal examples of pregnancy continuation following attempted voluntary interruption of pregnancy during the first trimester have appeared, but controlled studies of pregnancy outcome in such instances are not available.

In the absence of data, a few theoretic considerations may be in order. Let us assume that the chorion basalis at 10 menstrual weeks of pregnancy is 1 cm thick and is round with an approximate diameter of 4 cm. The

Portex cannula is 19 cm long and has an inside diameter of 1.0 mm. The maximum volume of chorion basalis sampled at one time is limited by the volume of the cannula; that is, 14.915 mm^3. This volume is about 2% of the total volume of the chorion basalis at 10 menstrual weeks. It is not known at this time whether the villi regenerate or whether fibrous-like tissue will cover the sampling site. It has been proposed that impoverishment of villi and consequent insufficient placental function may impair intrauterine development. In any event, the volume of missing chorion appears to be numerically too small to support impoverishment of villi as a mechanism by which CVS may lead to poor pregnancy outcome. On the other hand, a temporary functional disturbance of the newly formed placenta may be construed as a possible teratogenic stimulus in spite of the minimal anatomic damage induced by the sampling. Although reported experience with CVS in animals and humans cannot be considered conclusive to date, there have been no data supporting any mechanism of sampling-related injury as a cause of poor pregnancy outcome.

INFECTION

Another area of concern relates to the possibility of CVS-induced infection. It has been suggested that because of the transcervical approach of CVS, microbial intrauterine colonization may occur. This in turn might lead to intrauterine infection with consequent morbidity for the mother and/or the conceptus. It is at least theoretically possible that infection of the embryo or the placenta may result in the production of anomalies comparable to the congenital rubella syndrome. Although experience in this respect is still limited, it is somewhat reassuring that so far reports describing maternal and fetal morbidity from organisms that may be present in the vaginal–cervical canal have been limited to instances of gonococcal infection.

Information on endocervical microbial colonization at the time of CVS has been reported (Scialli et al., 1985). Microorganisms commonly inhabiting the first-trimester endocervix include gram-positive and gram-negative bacteria and mycoplasma. Chlamydia may also be encountered. Many of these organisms may also be cultured from the Portex cannula after CVS, and it is presumed that seeding of the chorion is possible. How often such seeding results in clinically significant infection is unknown. Possible consequences of chorion infection include pregnancy loss, impairment of chorionic function, and infection of the embryo. That such complications occur is undocumented; however, future investigations into the potential adverse pregnancy effects of CVS will have to consider these possibilities.

REFERENCES

1. Au, W. W., Obergoenner, N., Goldenthal, K. L., Corry P. M., and Willingham, V. (1982). Sister-chromatid exchanges in mouse embryos after exposure to ultrasound in utero. *Mutat. Res. 103*:215–320.
2. Buckton, K. E. and Baker, N. V. (1972). An investigation into possible chromosome damaging effects of ultrasound on human blood cells. *Br. J. Radiol. 45*:340–342.
3. Gillberg, C., Rasmussen, P., and Wahlstrom, J. (1982). Long-term follow-up of children born after amniocentesis. *Clin. Genet. 21*:69–73.
4. Haupt, M., Martin, A. O., Simpson, J. L., Iqbal, M. A., Elias, S., and Sabbagha, R. E. (1981). Ultrasonic induction of sister chromatid exchanges in human lymphocytes. *Human Genet. 59*:221–226.
5. Hellman, L., Duffus, G., and Donald, I. (1970). Safety of diagnostic ultrasound in obstetrics. *Lancet 1*:1133–1135.
6. Ikeuchi, T., Sasaki, M., Oshimuoa, M., Azurni, J., and Tsuyi, K. (1973). Ultrasound and embryonic chromosomes. *Br. Med. J. 1*:112.
7. Lamb, M. D. (1975). Gangrene of a fetal limb due to amniocentesis. *Br. J. Obstet. Gynaecol. 82*:829–830.
8. Liebeskind, S., Bases, R., Mendez, F., Elequin, F., and Koenigsberg, M. (1979). Sister chromatid exchange in human lymphocytes after exposure to diagnostic ultrasound. *Science 205*:1273–1275.
9. National Council on Radiation Protection and Measurements (1983). Biological Effects of Ultrasound: Mechanisms and Clinical Implications, NCRP Report No. 74, NCRPM, Bethesda.
10. NICHD National Registry for Amniocentesis Study Group (1976). Midtrimester amniocentesis for prenatal diagnosis. Safety and accuracy. *J. Am. Med. Assoc. 236*:1471–1476.
11. Pizzarello, D. J., Vivino, A., Madden, B., Wolsky, A., Keegan, A. F., and Becker, M. (1978). Effect of pulsed low-power ultrasound on growing tissues. I. Developing mammalian and insect tissue. *Exp. Cell Biol. 46*:179–191.
12. Rickwood, A. M. (1977). A case of ileal atresia and ileocutaneous fistula caused by amniocentesis. *J. Pediatr. 91*:312.
13. Scheidt, P. C., Stanley, F., and Bryla, D. A. (1978). One-year follow-up of infants exposed to ultrasound in utero. *Am. J. obstet. Gynecol. 131*:743–748.
14. Scialli, A. R., Neugebauer, D. L., and Fabro, S. (1985). The microbiology of

the endocervix in patients undergoing chorionic villus sampling. *J. Human Genet.* (in press).

15. Selman, G. G., and Counce, S. J. (1953). Abnormal embryonic development in *Drosophila* induced by ultrasound treatment. *Nature (London) 172*:503–504.
16. Shepard, T. H. (1983). *Catalog of Teratogenic Agents,* 4th ed. The Johns Hopkins University Press, Baltimore.
17. Simpson, N. E., Dallaire, L., Miller, J. R., Siminovich, L., Hamerton, J. L., Miller, J., and McKeen, C. (1976). Prenatal diagnosis of genetic disease in Canada: Report of a collaborative study. *Can. Med. Assoc. J. 115*:739–746.
18. Simpson, N. E., Turnbull, A. C., Alexander, D., Bantok, H., Czerski, P., Doran, T. A., Kaback, M., Lindgren, S., Murken, J. D., Ogita, S., Seigal, D., and Sutherland, I. (1980). Genetic amniocentesis. *Prenat. Diag., Spec. Iss., Dec.:* 5 – 10.
19. Stark, C. R., Orleans, M., Haverkamp, A. D., and Murphy, J. (1984). Short- and long-term risks after exposure to diagnostic ultrasound in utero. *Obstet. Gynecol. 63*:194–200.
20. Stewart, H. F. and Stratmeyer, M. E. (1982). *An Overview of Ultrasound: Theory, Measurement, Medical Applications, and Biological Effects,* United States Department of Health and Human Services, Rockville.
21. United Kingdom Medical Research Council Working Party of Amniocentesis (1978). An assessment of the hazards of amniocentesis. *Br. J. Obstet. Gynaecol. 85* (Suppl. 2):1–41.
22. Wegner, R. D., Obe, G., and Meyenburg, M. (1980). Has diagnostic ultrasound mutagenic effects? *Human Genet. 56*:95–98.
23. WHO (1982). *Ultrasound.* Environmental Health Criteria 22, WHO, Geneva.

13

Surveillance of Risks in First Trimester Prenatal Diagnosis

LAIRD G. JACKSON
Jefferson Medical College, Thomas Jefferson University, Philadelphia, Pennsylvania

INTRODUCTION

The development of first-trimester prenatal diagnosis has evolved slowly over the past 16 years since the first reportes of Mohr (1) and other Scandinavian researchers (2,3). Until 1983, there was little collaboration or communication among the few workers interested in this approach. Partly as a result, the relative safety of the Chinese experience of the early 1970s (4) went largely unnoticed until just recently. Wider application of the critical observation of the Soviet group headed by Kazy, that real-time ultrasound could greatly improve the sampling procedure, was delayed fully 3 years from its initial publication (5). The appearance of the group's report in an English-language journal finally drew attention to this approach (6). Even the more recent resurgence of interest in first-trimester prenatal diagnosis fostered first by the British (7) and then the Italians (8) drew attention only slowly among geneticists and obstetricians. This became evident to us in our early exploration of the method in late 1982, when our initial information came entirely from molecular biologists! Even after our early work with chorionic villus sampling (CVS), it was apparent that only a few pioneers were aware of the significant potential, diagnostic advantages, and unresolved procedural and laboratory risks of this approach. Therefore, in June of 1983 after discussions with Professor Mahoney of Yale University and others in attendance at the 1983 meeting of the Fetal Medicine and Surgery group in Aspen, Colorado, a newsletter was initiated to foster communication among CVS investigators. The newsletter, informally dubbed the *CVS Latest News* was initially circulated to a small group of known active investigators, which included the members of the International Cooperative Research Group on Prenatal Diagnosis and Fetal Therapy (formerly known as the Fetoscopy Club). The intent was to circulate information on the progress of investigations using the new procedure and to serve as a common international collection point for data on the number of procedures attempted, diagnostic results, and problems with either the patients or their pregnancies. All data are contributed voluntarily by the collaborating investigators. To date, eight issues of the newsletter have been circulated to a growing list of recipients that now number over 400. The newsletter is compiled by the prenatal diagnosis group at the Division of Medical Genetics, Thomas Jefferson University, Philadelphia, Pennsylvania. It is supported by grants from the World Health Organization's Heritable Diseases Program (Anver Kuliev, director) and from the March of Dimes Birth Defects Foundation.

Although an important initial function of the newsletter was to circulate a complete and contemporary bibliography and notes on procedural and laboratory protocols, its most important role was to initiate a registry of first-trimester diagnostic attempts in pregnancies intended to continue. A simple reporting format was used that documented the total number of patients in which prenatal diagnosis was attempted in the first trimester by chorionic villus sampling. The number of patients in whom a successful diagnostic sample was obtained, number of therapeutic pregnancy terminations, number of pregnancies intended to continue after diagnosis, number of fetal losses, and total deliveries were also recorded (Table 1). The resulting figures are tabulated and listed by individual center as are the totals for all centers participating. Revised tables are circulated with each newsletter, and interim tables are available upon request. In addition, a set of forms has been devised to record pertinent information about each patient in whom a first-trimester prenatal diagnosis is attempted. The forms are kept as simple as possible and were developed collaboratively by our staff and members of the WHO Working Group on Hereditary Diseases (9). These forms are divided into two principal parts: the first containing demographic information about the patient and her past reproductive history and the second containing the data on the diagnostic sampling procedure, complications including fetal loss, laboratory results, and outcome with confirmation of the diagnosis and evaluation of the

Table 1 Fetal Loss[a]

Case load	No. of centers	Total No. of patients	Failed sample	Therapeutic abortion	Continued pregnancy	Loss max	Loss max (%)	Delivered
1–10	13	81	8	18	63	2	3.2	2
10–50	14	288	7	37	251	13	5.2	39
50–100	9	343	12	50	293	21	7.2	108
100–200	3	488	26	70	418	21	5.0	84
300–500	4	1697	32	116	1581	52	3.3	471
Total	(43 centers)	3194	86	323	2871	118	4.1	703

[a]Note: In those centers reporting 10 or less procedures, most pregnancies will not have advanced very far so that potential losses may not yet have been experienced. This may give a falsely low loss rate at first.

INTERVIEW ULTRASOUND-CRL_____mm RANDOM ALLOCATION????
Date:MM___DD___YY___ Date:WW___D__ CVS --
Record no.__________ FH? +(2) -(1) Amniocentesis--

REPRODUCTIVE HISTORY Total prior pregnancies:______
spontaneous abortions___ stillbirths______
therapeutic abortions___ livebirths______
Other preg or delivery problem(list)____________________

INDICATION FOR PROCEDURE(Circle one number)
1. Maternal age
2. Parent chromo rearrangment
3. Elevated Mat Serum AFP
4. Prior chromosome anomaly
5. X-linked disease(sexing)
6. Prior child mult malform.
7. Metabolic disease
Other
8. Hemoglobinopathy
9. History Neural Tube Defect
10. Other DNA diagnosis

CHORION VILLUS SAMPLING:Use pre-registered sampling method or file current method.
Date: MM___DD___YY___ Bleeding before sampling: No(1) Yes(2)

Uterus position:(circle one)
1.anteverted
2.mid-position
3.retroverted
4.retroflexed

Placental location:
1. Ant 4.low
2. Post 5.lat
3. Fund 6.other

Ultrasound
CRL_____mm
Date: WW___D___
No. fetuses (1) ()1)describe

DESCRIPTION OF PROCEDURE SHADE PLACENTA
No. of insertions____
Estimated wt of sample(mg)_______
Difficult procedure? No(1) Yes(2)
Successful procedure? No(1) Yes(2)

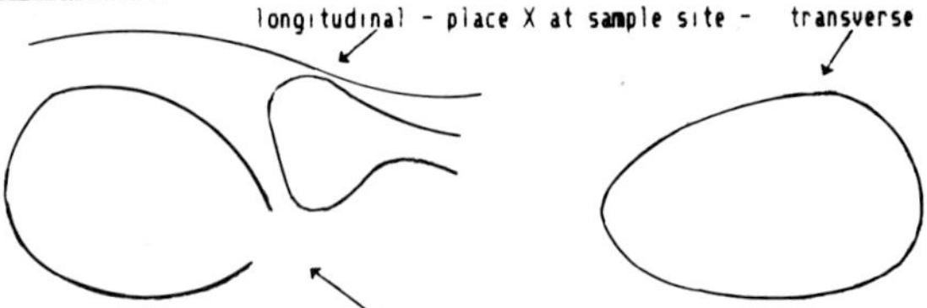

COMPLICATIONS: FOLLOWING SAMPLING
1.bleeding No(1) Yes(2) 3.discharge No(1) Yes(2) 5.pain No(1) Yes(2)
2.spotting No(1) Yes(2) 4.fever NO(1) Yes(2) 6.amnio fl leak No(1) Yes(2)
Describe time and duration if appropriate____________________

ULTRASOUND AT 16 WEEKS - DATE:MM___DD___YY___ BPD___.__

DELIVERY: livebirth surviving (1) / Neonatal death (3)
date: MM___DD___YY___ Infant:sex: M(1) F(2)
type____________________ weight(gm)_________
Infant abnormalities(describe-0 if none)

Placenta: abnormalities(describe - 0 if none)

FETAL LOSS:(2)
1-miscarriage(SAB) 4-abortion(social etc) 7-stillbirth(>28wks)
2-ther abortion(fetal anom) 6-intrauterine death(<28wks)

LABORATORY:- = normal;+ = affected;circle (fail) if failure to obtain result

Figure 1 Fetal diagnosis registry.

newborn child. Several versions of these forms have been circulated to the recipients of the newsletter as they have evolved. The final version has been simplified further to use yes or no (+/−) responses where possible and is shown in Figure 1. Response to both the newsletter and the registry and data forms has been encouraging. Over 2000 diagnostic cases had been recorded by the end of the first year of the newsletter circulation, and a considerable amount of information about fetal loss following the procedure has been accumulated.

METHOD AND RESULTS

The registry lists the center doing CVS trials and the investigator performing the procedure, the total number of procedures attempted, the number of failed procedures, terminations of pregnancy for diagnostic reasons, pregnancies intended to continue (total less terminations), number and percentage of fetal losses, and number of delivered pregnancies. A total of 43 centers contribute data to the registry. These centers are located in Europe (27), North America (15), and the Peoples Republic of China (1). In the total list of contributing centers, there are 13 with 10 or less procedures completed, 14 with 11 to 50 attempts, 9 with 51–100, 3 with 101–200, and 4 with more than 400 procedures in their experience. This represents a fairly wide range of experience among the contributing centers and must be taken into account as the data are reviewed and interpreted. In addition, the data include the experience of each of the investigators from their earliest studies and so reflects the average of that experience with the procedure over a period of learning and probable improvement. This experience is not all with the same method of obtaining the chorionic tissue. The majority of the operators use a fairly standard technique in which a soft 1.5-mm polyethylene cannula, stiffened by a malleable stainless-steel obturator, is gently inserted via the vagina and cervix into the body of the placenta (7). This method generally uses the commercially available catheter manufactured by the Portex Co. Three of the operators use the system pioneered by Dumez in Paris (10) in which straight metal biopsy forceps of 2.2-mm diameter is inserted transcervically under ultrasound guidance. Gustavii in Lund, Sweden has altered this approach slightly to guide the forceps by inserting them through a sidearm of an optical fetoscope which is inserted transcervically and guided to the sampling site by ultrasound (11). Final selection of the sampling site and sample is done under direct vision. Gustavii and one other investigator use this method. Two investigators use a variation of the soft catheter in which a stiffer plastic or metal cannula is used (12). In both, the instrument is resterilized either as the entire metal cannula and obturator, or the obturator alone is resterilized. There is a minor difference in the smoothness of the instrument after being recurved more than once. And one investigator enters the uterus via a transabdominal puncture and ultrasound guidance of a needle through the myometrium to the placental site (13). A smaller sampling needle is then inserted through the guide needle for actual aspiration sampling of the chorion. This method avoids passage throught the vagina and the unknown risk of microbial contamination associated with that approach. Finally, although the data include all sampled pregnancies and not just completed ones, all of the pregnancies are beyond the sixteenth week of gestation, and the majority are beyond the twenty-eighth gestational week.

The overall registry data show that a total of 3194 patients have had CVS attempted. There have been 86 failed attempts in this total. Of the total, 323 patients voluntarily terminated their pregnancies, leaving 2866 women continuing their pregnancies. Most of the terminations were for confirmed genetic diagnoses, although a small number (estimated at less than 2%) were terminated for sex preference or on social grounds. This therapeutic abortion rate for successful samplings is 10.4%, and after discounting the terminations for sex preference or social reasons would still be approximately 10%. In the continuing pregnancies, 118 fetuses were lost or 4.1% of the total. There have been 703 deliveries in the experience of the contributing investigators. The overall fetal loss figure requires some clarification. Early in the experience of several of the pioneer investigators, it was not possible to split chorion samples for more than one diagnostic test. Therefore, some samples did not have cytogenetic assessment when the principal test desired was one of the metabolic enzyme assays. Several instances of fetal loss from cases without diagnostic villus karyotypes have subsequently been shown to be aneuploid at spontaneous abortion. In addition, a few laboratories rely upon tissue culture diagnoses and have experienced loss of aneuploid fetuses at or just prior to completion of karyotyping. Because most parents would have electively terminated such pregnancies when the karyotype result was known with 48 hr, it was decided to eliminate all aneuploid cases from the loss column in the registry and treat them as terminated cases. The registry data are presented in this manner in Table 1.

In attempting to utilize this registry as a tool for evaluation of the CVS procedure, a number of questions may be asked. The first concerns the success of the procedure in actually achieving first-trimester fetal diagnosis. The registry data do not completely answer this as the data only document failures to achieve any fetal tissue sample. These failures are infrequent, occurring in 2.7% of attempted samplings. This ranges from a high of 10.6% from one center with considerable experience to a low of 0.8% in one center and 0 in another center with more than 100 cases. The data suggest that the variation is due to the two factors of relative aggressiveness in seeking an analyzable sample and the method of sampling used. The highest failure rates comes from a group that adheres to a rule of using no more than two attempted insertions regardless of circumstances, and the 0 rate comes from an investigator experienced in the use of the solid biopsy forceps. Further information is anecdotal, but indicates that few patients are subjected to repeat samplings in a second session (as opposed to repeat insertions of the sampling instrument in the same session), and few patients are rejected for reasons of unsuitable pelvic anatomy (stenosed cervical canal, severely retroflexed uterus, etc.). Thus, the data indicate that the procedure is applicable to almost all candidate patients and that a high percentage of sampling attempts will be successful in experienced hands. The risk of failure therefore appears to be slight.

More significant questions of risk involve the safety of the procedure for the mother, her fetus, and her newborn and developing child. The first two of these issues appear to provide reasonably good assurances from the data collected thus far. It is too early to expect anything but crude information regarding the last issue. Of the 700 children delivered, none have been reported to have malformations or problems attributed to the procedure. Less than 1% have had congenital malformation syndromes, and these were not conditions that would have been discoverable by prenatal diagnosis. No information is available on the developmental progress of any of these children. The available data on maternal health are also slim. No instances of maternal death have been reported. Although vaginal bleeding is a frequent minor complication, occurring in 30–40% of patients, it is largely confined to spotting or to amounts less than a usual menstrual flow. Occasional patients have repeated short periods of heavy bleeding, but no one has required treatment other than bed rest and mild sedation. Vaginal infections and chorioamnionitis have occurred in 10 patients, including at least three requiring therapy. Again

Table 2 Fetal Loss: Alternate Sampling Methods

Method	No. of centers	Total No. of patients	Failed sample	Therapeutic abortion	Continued pregnancy	Loss max	Loss max (%)	Delivered
Reusable cannula	2	141	3	26	115	11	9.6	34
Forceps	3	261	4	58	203	9	4.4	31
Optical + forceps	2	111	2	11	100	6	6.0	21
Transabdominal	1	85	0	4	81	0	0.0	26

no serious maternal sequelae have been reported. Most patients experience no more physical difficulties than the usual amniocentesis patient.

The most frequently cited risk of the CVS procedure is the risk of fetal loss by spontaneous abortion. Initial reports suggested that this loss might exceed 10% (14), but subsequent data indicate that this estimate was much too high. The registry data reveal a clear preliminary picture of the risk of fetal loss. The rate of fetal loss for a large number of cases is 4.1%, and this figure represents a conservative average of those centers with a significant amount of clinical experience. A comparison of those centers with the most experience and those with the least shows a striking difference in rates of fetal loss. The loss rate in the 36 centers with 100 or less procedures each is 5.93%, while in the four centers with more than 300 tests each it is 3.27%, a 55% difference (Table 1). There is also some interest in comparing the loss experience with the different methods of sampling (Table 2). The most popular method is the use of the soft catheter whose operators show a loss rate of 3.88% (2371 cases). Two operators use either a reusable metal cannula or a stiff plastic cannula with a reusable metal obturator and have an aggregate loss rate of 9.57% (115 cases). Two operators use an optical instrument similar to a fetoscope, allowing direct vision of the chorion sampling via an inserted biopsy forceps with a loss rate of 6% (100 cases). Three of the investigators use the thin straight biopsy forceps alone with ultrasound guidance and have a 4.46% loss rate (224 cases). A final investigator is the only operator using a transabdominal, as opposed to a transcervical, approach, and his loss rate is 0% (81 cases).

DISCUSSION

The registry data are clearly insufficient to provide a real judgment on the safety of the CVS procedure or a clear assessment of any of the risks. They do show significant trends in at least two areas. There is the risk of failure of the procedure to either obtain a sample of fetal tissue adequate for laboratory analysis or the risk of fetal loss subsequent to the procedure. As stated above, the risk of failure of the procedure appears to be slight. The centers with major experience have less than a 2% failure rate, and their more recent experience suggests an even lower rate is achievable. It appears that some patients will have a uterine or placental position (or combination thereof) that will not be safely approached. The percentage of such patients is obviously small, and it is likely that it will diminish with further experience.

The fetal loss experience is probably the most important question to be addressed by the registry data. Here the data provide at least a useful early statement of the experience of the investigators, which is reassuring for the future development of this procedure. The 4.1% fetal loss rate would appear to be an extremely low rate of pregnancy loss when compared to predicted rates of pregnancy loss from the eighth to tenth week of pregnancy onward (15). However, such rates were obtained from data collected before pregnancy evaluation by ultrasound was possible. More recently, data have been obtained with ultrasound verification of pregnancy viability by determining fetal cardiac activity together with normal crown–rump length of the fetus for gestational age with matching gestational sac size. These data are somewhat difficult to use for comparative purposes as each report provides assessment of the loss experience in different ways with different populations, and each utilizes different end points of gestation for observation. Nevertheless, they provide some insight suggesting a far lower than expected rate of pregnancy loss from normal pregnancies than had been previously thought. In one group of women whose pregnancies were evaluated by ultrasound at 8–10 weeks of gestation as controls for a collaborative study of diabetic pregnancies, there were 2 pregnancy losses in the group of 225 women observed through 12 weeks—a 0.9% loss rate. The same group, followed to term, experienced 6 more losses for an overall rate of 3.7% (16). In another group from the Netherlands, patients seen at a university obstetrics service were followed after ultrasound evaluation of the pregnancy at 8–10 weeks of gestation (17). Here 274 patients were seen, with 9 pregnancy losses at 16 weeks gestation—a loss rate of 3.3%. Only 236 of these were patients from the normal clinic population, the others having been referred for ultrasound evaluation for (presumably) some suspected difficulty. In the smaller group, there were only 5 losses for a rate of 2.1%. In both of the above studies, the average maternal age was below 35 years. In contrast, the group at the University of British Columbia retrospectively evaluated a large series of ultrasounds and found 796 women having scans at 7–12 weeks of gestation whose pregnancies would be evaluated through 20 weeks of gestation (18). There were 17 losses in the group, for a rate of 2.13%. These could be further subdivided by maternal age into a group under 30 years (347) with 5 losses (1.5%), the group from 30 to 34 years (238) with 6 losses (2.5%), and a group over 35 years (149) with 6 losses (4%). Actually, the latter group had 133 women between 35 and 39 years of age with 4.5% loss and a group over 40 years of age with no losses that was too small to analyze. It is of some interest that in the last study, only 27.3% of the normal deliveries during the time of the study had ultrasounds done for "spotting", whereas 65% of the spontaneous abortion group was evaluated for this complaint. This suggests that even these rates of pregnancy loss may be too high when stricter ultrasound and clinical criteria for "normalcy" are developed. Using the reported experience of one large amniocentesis series, another instructive comparison may be made. Golbus et al. (19), in reviewing 3000 amniocenteses (performed mainly for advanced maternal age of 35 and over), noted a combined pregnancy loss in the week prior to the procedure (usually gestational weeks 16–17) of 2.4%. Following the procedure, there was a 1.4% loss of pregnancies through week 28 of gestation. All of these figures are remarkably close to the loss experience of the larger CVS series and suggest that their losses, especially in the later group of patients where the procedure was performed after the initial learning phase at these centers, may be largely associated with normal causes of spontaneous abortion, and few are directly related to the procedure. Assuming that the majority of patients in the CVS registry are 35 and over, the 4% loss figure from the registry data may represent no more than 0.5%–1.5% added risk over background loss.

Unfortunately, the registry does not provide control data for comparison of fetal loss rates within the same centers performing the CVS procedures. Neither case control nor random or unselected controls are available in any center reporting. Nevertheless 100 of the 118 reported CVS losses have been documented with some details of their dates of sampling, date of pregnancy loss, and ultrasound and clinical findings. These data allow some examination of the experience with an intent to find associations between the CVS procedure and the event of fetal loss. Most samples were taken in a narrow time period between the beginning of the ninth week and the middle of the eleventh week of gestation. This concentration of the sampling "window" happened early enough that few losses occurred to patients sampled before or after this time period, and so it is not possible to draw conclusions about the safety of the sampling time with any numerical support. It is obviously the conclusion of the investigators that a combination of increased ease of ultrasound visualization of the sampling site, ease of insertion of the sampling device, and a perceived lowering of complications led to the choice of this gestational time for sampling. The fetal losses occurred as early as the first 24 hr post-CVS and as late as 36 weeks of gestation. (These should not be included as fetal loss per se.) However, all but two losses did occur prior to the completion of 28 weeks. Of these, 75% (or 3.1% fetal loss) occurred by 16 weeks of gestation, and only 25% (1.1% fetal loss) after 16 weeks and up to 28 weeks. This suggests that few losses after 16 weeks may be attributable to the procedure, but that 1–1.5% of the earlier 3% loss may be affected by the sampling. The distribution in the first 6 weeks following sampling is of interest, with 19% of the total losses occuring by 7 days post-CVS, 40% by 14 days, 68% by 28 days, and 78% by 42 days. The majority of the losses within the first 2 weeks may very well be procedurally related. A history of fever or excessive bleeding in these patients occurs more frequently than in those with later losses, which also supports this supposition. Ten to 15% of the total of 100 losses had a history of fever or actual infection. Most of these occurred with a history of loss within 15 days of the procedure. In contrast, a history of bleeding was found in later losses as well as in patients with no loss. In this regard, it is of interest to note that the single investigator using the transabdominal approach has a reasonable sample size of 81 continuing pregnancies, all of them beyond 16 weeks of gestation with no pregnancy losses reported. The transabdominal approach is the only technique in use that completely avoids the possibility of introduction of vaginal contamination into the sampling area by the procedure itself. Clearly, the question of infection is one of concern regarding both the potential for fetal loss and maternal morbidity. Further evaluation will need careful development of techniques to monitor the procedure by microbiological and pathological means. In the meantime, care in performance of the procedure appears to offer reasonable safety to the patient and her pregnancy.

In summary, the CVS registry has managed to accumulate a significant amount of information about this new procedure in a short period of time. These data suggest strongly that the procedure has no inherent risks that would preclude its further development. Further assessment of the risks of the procedure to mother, pregnancy, and developing child must await the design and implementation of controlled clinical trials involving the collaboration of many investigators.

ACKNOWLEDGMENTS

The author wishes to thank the researchers associated with the CVS registry. This work was made possible by data from the following contributors: A. Antasklis, Athens; J. Apuzzio, Newark; R. Benzie, Toronto; K. Blackmore, New Haven; B. Brambati, Milan; R. Carpenter,

Houston; J. Crane, St. Louis; F. Duffos, Paris; Y. Dumez, Paris; S. Elias, Chicago; G. Ghirardini, Montechio Emilia; D. Gilmore, Glasgow; N. Ginsburg, Chicago; M. Golbus, San Francisco; J. Goldberg, New York; B. Gustavii, Lund; N. Hahnemann, Aalborg; P. Harper, Cardiff; Z. Intody, Budapest; M. Jahoda, Rotterdam; C. King, Kansas City; J. Larsen, Washington, D.C.; R. Lilford, London; I. Mackenzie, Oxford; F. Mariona, Detroit; L. Marsk, Stockholm; G. Monni, Cagliari; A. Oldrini, Milan; A. Pachi, Rome; T. Perry, Montreal; J. Phillip, Copenhagen; E. Porro, Genoa; R. Rauskolb, Northeim; F. Redwine, Richmond; C. Rodeck, London; F. Rodesch, Brussels; J. Scrimgeour, Edinburgh; F. Sondergaard, Copenhagen; N. Sun, Beijing; E. Szabo, Szeged; R. Wapner, Philadelphia; R. Ward, London; J. Watson, Denver; A. Zwinger, Prague;

Work reported here was supported in part by grants from the March of Dimes Birth Defects Foundation and the Hereditary Diseases Program, WHO.

REFERENCES

1. Mohr. J. (1968). Foetal genetic diagnosis: Development of techniques for early sampling of foetal cells. *Acta Pathol. Microbio. Scand. 73*:73–77.
2. Hahnemann, N. (1974). Early prenatal diagnosis; a study of biopsy techniques and cell culturing from extraembryonic membranes. *Clin. Genet. 6*:294–306.
3. Kullander, S. and Sandahl, B. (1973). Fetal chromosome analysis after transcervical placental biopsies during early pregnancy. *Acta Obstet. Gynecol. Scand. 52*:355–359.
4. Department of Obstetrics and Gyneacolgy (1975). Tietung Hospital, China. Fetal sex prediction by sex chromatin of chorionic villi cells during early pregnancy. *Chin. Med J. 1*:117–126.
5. Kazy, Z., Bakharev, V. A., and Stygar, A. M. (1979). Value of the ultrasonic studies in biopsy of the chorion, according to genetic indicators. *Akush-Ginekol. (Mosk) 8*:29–31.
6. Kazy, Z., Rozovsky, I. S., and Bakharev, V. A. (1982). Chorion biopsy in early pregnancy: A method of early prenatal diagnosis for inherited disorders. *Prenatal Diag. 2*:39–45.
7. Ward, R. H. T., Model, B., Petrou, M., Karagozlu, F., and Douratsos, E. (1983). A method of chorionic villus sampling in the first trimester of pregnancy under real time ultrasonic guidance. *Br. Med. J. 286*:1542–1544.
8. Simoni, G., Brambati, B., Danesino, C., Rossela, F., Terzoli, G. L., Ferrari, M., and Fraccaro, M. (1983). Efficient direct chromosome analyses and

enzyme determinations from chorionic villi samples in the first trimester of pregnancy. *Hum. Genet. 63*:349–357.
9. WHO. Report of a WHO working group on fetal diagnosis of hereditary diseases (1983). WHO Document HMG/WG/83.2.
10. Goosens, M., Dumez, Y., Kaplan, L., Lupker, M., Chabret, C., Henrion, R., and Rosa, J. (1983). Prenatal diagnosis of sickle cell anemia in he first trimester of pregnancy. *N. Engl. J. Med. 309*:831–833.
11. Gustavii, B. (1983). First-trimester chromosomal analysis of chorionic villi obtained by direct vision technique. *Lancet ii*:507–508.
12. Rodeck, C. H., Morsman, J. M., Nicolaides, K. H., McKenzie, C. M., Gosden, C. M., and Gosden, J. R. (1983). A single-operator technique for first-trimester chorion biopsy. *Lancet ii*:1340–1341.
13. Schmidt-Jensen, S., and Hahnemann, R. (1984). Transabdominal fine needle biopsy from chorionic villi in the first trimester. *Prenatal Diag. 4*:163–169.
14. Hobbins, J. C. Consequences of chorionic biopsy. (1984). *N. Engl. J. Med. 310*:1121
15. Harlap, S., Shiono, P. H., and Ramrachan, S., (1980). A life table of spontaneous abortions and the effects of age, parity and other variables. In *Human Embryonic and Fetal Death,* (I.H. Porter and E. B. Hook, eds.), pp. 145–158. Academic Press, New York.
16. Simpson, J. L. (1984). Low fetal loss after normal ultrasound at 8 weeks gestation. Implications for chorionic villus sampling (CVS). The Diabetes in Early Pregnancy Project NICHD. *Am. J. Human Genet. 36*:197S.
17. Christaens, G. C. M. L., and Stountenbeek, P. P. H. (1984). Spontaneous abortion in proven intact pregnancies. *Lancet ii*:571.
18. Wilson, R.D., Kendrick, V., Wittman, B.K., and McGillivray. B.C. (1984). Risk of spontaneous abortion in ultrasonically normal pregnancies. *Lancet ii*:920–1.
19. Golbus, M. S., Loughman, W. D., Epstein, C. J., Halbach. G., Stephens, J. D., and Hall, B. D. (1979). Prenatal diagnosis in 300 amniocenteses. *N. Eng. J. Med. 300*:157–163.

14

Methodologic Problems in Determining Fetal Loss Rates

JOE LEIGH SIMPSON
Northwestern University Medical School, Chicago, Illinois
JAMES L. MILLS
National Institute of Child Health and Development, National Institutes of Health, Bethesda, Maryland

METHODOLOGIC PROBLEMS IN DETERMINING FETAL LOSS RATES

In humans, fetal loss rates have been estimated by a variety of approaches: retrospective (historical) and prospective clinical and laboratory [based upon positive human chorionic gonadotropin (hCG) assays]. However, the precise frequency of losses is still uncertain, especially by specific gestational intervals. This is unfortunate because precise information on background loss rates is crucial for assessing the safety of chorionic villus sampling (CVS). Clinical studies considered by some investigators (Lippman, 1983; Gustavii, 1984) to be useful for assessing CVS safety are actually not appropriate because they include only early registrants (self-selection) and because they do not take into account asymptomatic deaths. Such flaws will make fetal losses after 8–10 weeks gestation seem higher. Spuriously high estimates for loss rates will make CVS seem safer than it is. Some procedure-related losses will be falsely attributed to background losses. Using a population with a spuriously low estimated loss rate for comparison would, conversely, result in CVS being falsely blamed for some fetal losses.

This chapter will address several issues that must be considered in designing studies to assess the safety of CVS. First, we shall review existing data pertaining to fetal loss rates in the human and discuss how they were derived. Second, we shall consider methodologic problems that invalidate many of the commonly cited loss rate estimates.

TRADITIONAL METHODS FOR EXISTING FETAL LOSS RATE ESTIMATES

Three sources of data have traditionally served as the basis for calculating fetal loss rates: (a) losses following positive beta human chorionic gonadotropin (β-hCG) assays early in gestation; (b) losses surmised from morphological appearances of early embryos; and (c) losses determined on the basis of clinically recognized pregnancy. Overall, fetal loss rates have been estimated either on the basis of the first source alone or by extrapolating on the basis of information derived from the second and third sources combined. Either approach is subject to error.

Beta Human Chorionic Gonadotropin Studies

Miller et al. (1980) studied 197 women through 623 cycles. Beginning 21 days after the previous menses and continuing until menstruation or pregnancy, urinary β-hCG assay was performed on alternate days. Pregnancy was defined as either a single value of 5 μg/liter or 2 values of 2 μg/liter. In 152 of the 623 cycles, β-hCG was sufficiently elevated to justify the diagnosis of pregnancy. However, in only 102 of the 152 (67%) was pregnancy appreciated clinically. Of the 102 conceptions showing clinical evidence of pregnancy, 14 were later lost (14%). The overall frequency of losses (clinical and subclinical) was 43%.

Edmonds et al. (1982) diagnosed pregnancy with a urine radioimmunoassay for β-hCG, a value of 56 IU/ liter being considered positive. Testing began 21 days after the last menstrual period. Of 198 ovulatory cycles, 118 showed a raised hCG. Only 51 of the 118 showed clinical evidence of pregnancy; 6 of the 51 (12%) experienced clinically recognized abortions. No positive β-hCG assays were observed in a concurrent series of women who had previously undergone sterilization, suggesting that false positive results were not a serious problem.

Whittaker et al. (1983) studied 226 cycles, performing β-hCG serum radioimmunoassay approximately 25 days after the previous menses. Pregnancy was diagnosed if β-hCG was 16 mU/ml or greater. Neither women in the follicular phase nor men showed values over 4 mU/ml. Of the 226 cycles, 92 showed elevated β-hCG and 85 had a clinically recognized pregnancy. Of the 85, spontaneous abortions occurred in 11 (13%). The clinically recognized loss rate in this study was very similar to that found by Miller et al. (1980) and Edmonds et al. (1982). However, the unrecognized loss rate was much lower in the study of Whittaker et al. (1983). The differences presumably reflect the higher cut-off required for diagnosing pregnancy in the study by Whittaker et al. and perhaps also reflect differences in the ability to detect β-hCG in serum versus urine.

Early Morphological Studies

Hertig and Rock (Hertig et al., 1956, 1959; Hertig and Rock, 1973) examined the fallopian tubes, uterine cavities, and endometria of women undergoing elective hysterectomy. Prior to surgery, the date of ovulation was deduced on the basis of basal body temperature elevations. Coital times were recorded. All women were of proved fertility, and their mean age was 33.6 years. Over a series of many years, eight preimplantation embryos were recovered. Four of the eight preimplantation embryos (less than 6 days conception) were morphologically abnormal. Until recently, the assumption has been that the four abnormal embryos probably would not have implanted. Moreover, it was assumed that had they implanted, they would not have survived very long after implantation. Similarly, 9 of 26 implanted embryos (6–14 embryonic days) were morphologically abnormal, and it was likewise assumed that they would not continue to develop.

Studies utilizing in vitro fertilization (IVF) techniques are now casting doubt on some of these assumptions. Angell et al. (1983) performed cytogenetic studies on 11 human conceptions fertilized in vitro. All conceptions appeared morophologically normal. However, two of the three successfully karyotyped embryos were abnormal: one haploid (22,X,−15) and one trisomic (47,XY,+D). Another morphologically normal embryo also was haploid, but could not be karyotyped. In addition, IVF centers now routinely observe normal pregnancies after reimplanting morphologically abnormal embryos (Edwards et al., 1984). Thus, fetuses that show cytogenetic abnormalities need not show morphological abnormalities at this stage, whereas embryos that appear abnormal may develop into normal children. Of course, in vitro and in vivo selection against abnormal embryos may not be comparable. Moreover, preimplantation and early implantation stages are known to be those stages in which mouse monosomies and trisomies cease to develop (Gropp 1973, 1975). Nonetheless, available data suggest that caution should be exercised in correlating morphological appearance of an embryo with its likelihood of survival.

Studies of Hertig and Rock are relevant to the issue of CVS safety because the high loss rates derived on the basis of their data have been extrapolated to other populations. Accepting the assumption that subclinical loss rates are high leads one to conclude that most conceptions would be lost prior to clinical recognition. However, the sample of Hertig and Rock is small (N=34), gathered over many years, and is perhaps unrepresentative in that the women were older, had gynecologic disorders warranting surgery, and had had multiple pregnancies.

Clinically Recognized Losses

A third traditional method for determining loss rates involves tabulating clinically recognized losses. We shall later see that a shortcoming in such studies has been such that the time at which a loss occurred was determined on the basis of clinical criteria, namely, bleeding or passage of tissue. Furthermore, most studies assessing clinically recognized losses were performed when pregnancy tests could have failed to detect pregnancies before 6–7 weeks gestation. Because common clinical practice at the time usually dictated attempts to confirm pregnancy only after a second missed menstrual period, many, if not most, of the clinically recognized losses in the earlier literature must be assumed to have occured at least 8 weeks beyond the last menstrual period. Neither retrospective nor prospective studies would have identified earlier losses on the basis of clinical criteria.

Despite potential shortcomings, most earlier studies consistently reported clinical fetal loss rates around 12–15% (Yerushalmy et al., 1956; Tietze and Martin, 1975; Reed and Kelly, 1958; Stevenson et al., 1959; French and Bierman, 1962; Erhardt, 1963; Warburton and Fraser, 1964; Bierman et al., 1965; Shapiro et al., 1971; Naylor, 1974; Royal College of General Practitioners, 1976; Leridon, 1977).

Some of the more widely cited studies are summarized in Table 1. Many are retrospective, not surprisingly because such an approach accumulates data rapidly. Pregnant as well as nonpregnant populations have been studied. In studying pregnant populations retrospectively, it is necessary to exclude the current pregnancy because women with bad outcomes (early abortion) are less likely to be registered and counted. Omitting the current pregnancy eliminates this obvious source of bias, but other sources exist as well. One alternative is sampling a nonpregnant population at random, in which case a larger population is needed because many subjects will not have attempted pregnancy.

Examples of retrospective studies on nonpregnant populations were

Table 1 Clinical Loss Rates[a]

Investigator	Clinically recognized pregnancies	Ascertained during pregnancy	Method	Fetal losses %
Reed and Kelly (1958)	479	No	Retrospective, using sample first identified in 1934	17.3
Stevenson et al. (1959)	9,526	No	Retrospective, record search involving women identified at delivery	11.8
Erhardt (1963)	2,573	No	Retrospective, data of obstetricians	9.1
Warburton and Fraser (1964)	6,835	No	Retrospective study of mothers identified in pediatric clinic	14.7
Shapiro et al. (1971)	11,630	Yes	Prospective, health maintenance organization	12.6
Naylor (1974)	33,255	Yes	U.S. Collaborative Perinatal Project sample, previous obstetric history	12.6
Royal College of General Practitioners (1976)	10,986	No	Prospective, ascertained before pregnancy	13.4
Leridon (1977)	5,672	No	Retrospective, geographically defined (Martinique)	12.1
Miller et al. (1980)	102[b]	No	Prospective (β-hCG)	14.0
Edmonds et al. (1982)	51[b]	Yes	Prospective (β-hCG)	13.0
Whittaker et al. (1983)	85[b]	Yes	Prospective (β-hCG)	12.0

[a]Representative surveys showing crude fetal loss, uncorrected for maternal age and other variables, to be 12–15%. Other surveys also exist, as reviewed by Leridon (1977). However, those surveys especially seem biased by including induced abortions or full-term stillbirths, or by memory bias.

[b]Sample restricted to *subset* of women showing clinically recognized pregnancies and losses.

those of Tietze and Martin (1958) and by Leridon (1977). Tietze and Martin studied patients analyzed for the Kinsey report. The loss rate was only 9.1%, but the sample is not necessarily representative of the general population. Leridon's study revealed a 12.1% loss rate in Martinique, an island whose inhabitants may or may not be exposed to environmental agents comparable to those of the United States or continental Europe. Genetic differences may exist as well. Warburton and Fraser (1964) is another frequently cited retrospective study, one involving women ascertained in a pediatric clinic. A bias inherent in this latter approach is that such women must have at least one live-born infant in order to be attending the clinic. This is relevant because fetal loss rates are higher in couples with no live-born infants, at least among samples of repetitive aborters (Poland et al., 1977). Another type of retrospective study is that of Naylor (1974), who analyzed pregnancy history in the sample of pregnant women registering in the U.S. Collaborative Perinatal Project. In the 13-hospital survey, there were 33,255 previous pregnancies and 12.6% fetal losses. The rate was age dependent, as will be discussed below (see section on nongenetic confounding variables).

Prospective studies would seem preferable to retrospective studies for some of the reasons outlined above. A prospective design would involve determining fetal loss rates by identifying and following a nonpregnant population over many years. However, a major problem is the low yield (inefficiency) of such an approach. Another problem is failure to identify pregnancies in women under surveillance.

One relevant study is the control sample in the Royal College of General Practitioners study designed to investigate pregnancy outcome following cessation of oral contraceptives. Of 10986 control women ascertained before pregnancy, 1475 had a spontaneous abortion (13.4%).

Prospective studies have also been conducted in women ascertained after they become pregnant. There are several potential problems. First, women in such samples may be unrepresentative of the general population, especially if identified in a selected referral population, as is generally the case in a university. Second, loss rates in populations recruited during pregnancy are likely to be spuriously depressed because those women who abort before registration cannot be included. On the other hand, the motivations for registering early in pregnancy are uncertain, perhaps reflecting prior obstetric complications (e.g., bleeding).

One frequently cited study involves all inhabitants of Kauai, Hawaii. Investigators attempted to identify all pregnant women, and determine subsequent loss rates. The overall loss rate was 9.1% (French and

Bierman, 1962; Bierman et al., 1965). However, only 19% of Kauai pregnancies were identified prior to 8 weeks, indicating failure to identify some losses. Studies involving prepaid health maintenance organizations should minimize the liklihood that women experiencing early losses avoid medical attnetion for financial reasons. Indeed, Shapiro et al, (1971) observed a 12.6% fetal loss rate (N=11,630). As in other studies, the loss rate was directly correlated with age.

Difficulties of detecting early losses should be obviated by prospectively studying ovulating women on whom β-hCG radioimmunoassays are performed in each tycle. Three studies adhering to this design have already been cited. Although data remain limited, the clinically recognized loss rates were quite similar: 14% in Miller et al. (1980), 13% in Whittaker et al. (1983), and 12% in Edmonds et al. (1982). Incidentally, clinical losses in these studies might have occurred ealier than in the more traditional studies cited in this section.

Two other aspects of the problem of clinical loss rate calculations deserve mention: (a) age and (b) loss by gestational interval. First, in all studies, older women consistently showed higher loss rates. In the 30–34 age group, loss rates are approximately 15%, 17–18% between ages 35 and 39, and 25% above age 40. Second, loss rates have been calculated by gestational intervals, obviously of great relevance of CVS. Unfortunately, studies based upon clinical criteria for fetal loss rarely provide data on those losses occurring earlier than 8 weeks after the last menstrual period. For example, Stevenson et al. (1959) reported that about 45% of all losses occurrred between 7 and 11 weeks, and about 30% between 12 and 15 weeks. To address the reality that subjects present at different stages of gestation, various life table analyses have been derived. One frequently cited study is the Kauai study of French and Bierman (1962) and Bierman et al. (1965). Life table estimation of total loss rate was 23.7%, with a 7% loss rate in the 8- to 12-week interval. Such calculations have been used for comparison with loss rates following CVS. As we shall discuss, such assumptions are fallacious because the calculations fail to take into account fetal deaths occurring weeks before clinical manifestation of problems.

PROBLEMS ESTIMATING FETAL LOSS RATES

Beta Human Chorionic Gonadotropin Assays

Assaying hCG or its beta subunit can be performed on either serum or urine. The consensus is that β-hCG is not detectable before implantation, a process that usually occurs 8–10 days after fertilization (Lenton et al., 1982). However, Saxena (1983) believes that β-hCG can be detected as early as 6 days after fertilization. Production of β-hCG is also variable. In one group of normal conceptuses, 5.3% produced measurable β-hCG 8 days after the LH peak, 15.8% after 9 days, 53.2% after 10 days, and 100% after 11 days (Lenton et al., 1982). Although β-hCG levels progressively increase, pregnancy is difficult to establish until approximately 10 days after conception. Detection may prove especially difficult if the conceptus is abnormal because in such cases β-hCG production is often subnormal (Braunstein et al., 1978; Lenton et al., 1982; Saxena, 1983). Thus, β-hCG levels are not only low early in normal pregnancy, but even lower in abnormal conceptuses. For both of these reasons it is essential to utilize an assay capable of detecting very small amounts of the hormone.

One problem in assaying β-hCG is that both radioreceptor assays and radioimmunoassays have difficulties detecting low levels of the hormone because of "noise." Some radioimmunoassays have difficulty with luteinizing hormone (LH) cross-reactivity as well. Recall that glycoprotein hormones (e.g., hCG, LH, FSH) share a common α-chain of virtually identical amino acid sequences. It is the β chain that determines hormonal specificity. In addition, β-chain hCG is similar to α-chain LH. Of their first 115 amino acids, 89 are identical; only the 30 C-terminal amino acids are unique (Tyrey, 1982). Receptor assays must overcome the problems posed by these hormonal similarities. Because cross-reactivity exists between LH and β-hCG, inadvertently measuring LH can be a serious problem in attempting to diagnose early pregnancy. An erroneously timed measurement may in some assays measure both LH surge as well as hCG, resulting in a false-positive diagnosis of pregnancy. An assay attempting to detect only a very small amount of hCG is relatively more vulnerable to the effects of erroneously measured LH. Although hCG assays directed against the entire compound may show considerable cross-reactivity with other glycoprotein hormones, β-subunit assays should be able to distinguish LH from hCG if the antibody is formed against a portion of the β-chain characterized by a unique amino acid sequence.

These difficulties in hCG identification should be recalled when assessing studies of early pregnancy loss rates. Designating a very low level of hCG as evidence of pregnancy will almost inevitably result in a spuriously high "loss" rate. Such designation would confer a relatively higher risk that "noise" or LH will be measured as hCG, resulting in women with a normal menstrual period being diagnosed as having had an early fetal loss. Conversely, insisting upon a high β-hCG level as diagnosis of pregnancy will result in a spuriously low loss rate (Fig. 1). True pregnancies ending in early abortion may never generate sufficient hCG for identification, especially if abnormal.

For all these reasons, independent confirmatory tests are needed to diagnose pregnancy. Of course, a confirmatory test is not essential if prengnacy proceeds to produce anatomical evidence, e.g., products of conception. However, lack of confirmation is a problem in those pregnancies (or false pregnancies) in which a brief transient rise in hCG is followed by bleeding around the time of the expected menstrual period. Use of a pregnancy-specific protein, such as pregnancy-specific β^1-glycoprotein (SP1), may be of interest in this regard. This particular glycoprotein appears specific for pregnancy, is secreted by the syncytiotrophoblast, and is present in maternal serum in increasing amounts beginning early in pregnancy (Ahmed and Klopper, 1983). Pregnancy-specific β^1-glycoprotein has the advantage of not being similar in structure to any pituitary hormone. Depending on the minimum detection limit set, SP1 has been found in maternal blood as early as 20–24, 18–23, 10, or 6–14 days after ovulation (See Ahmed and Klopper, 1983). If its early detectability proves consistently reproducible, SP1 may not only become competitive with β-hCG as a pregnancy test but could almost certainly serve to validate early pregnancies suspected by low yet detectable β-hCG levels.

Retrospective Analyses

Inquiring about a woman's previous pregnancy outcomes is less than an ideal way to estimate abortion rates. First, there is difficulty in determining the significance of a "missed period." Because most losses occur early in pregnancy, a "missed" or "late" period could either represent an undetected fetal loss or it might merely indicate an anovulatory cycle. Second, induced abortions may be misclassified, perhaps even subconsciously. Below we shall comment further on the frequency of illicit abortions. Here we note only that women may choose to classify an induced abortion as spontaneous because of the social stigma sometimes attached to induced terminations. If the obstetrical history surveyed an interval when induced abortions were illegal, there is likely to be even greater reluctance to admit having had such a procedure Failing to classify induced abortions accurately will spuriously increase

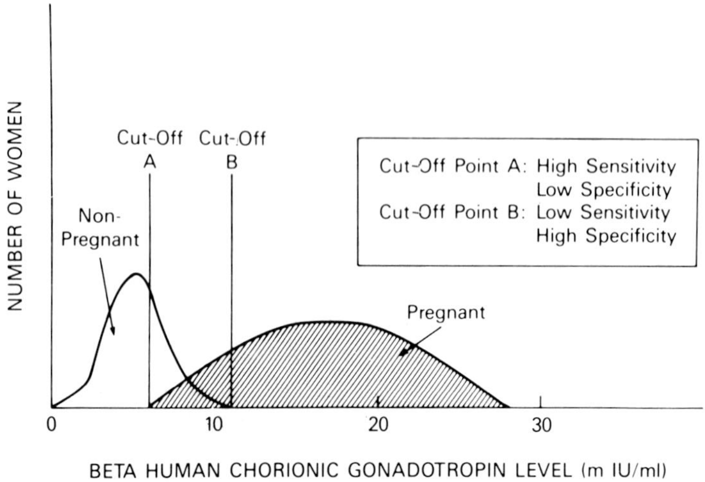

Figure 1 Diagrmatic representation of the problem in choosing a specific value (cut-off) as indication of a pregnancy test being either positive or negative. Choosing point A as the cut-off would ensure that a very high percentage of those who were actually pregnant identified as pregnant by the test; thus, there would be a high sensitivity (true positive)/(true negative + false positive). However, the price for this high sensitivity would be low specificity (true negative)/(true negative + false positive). Thus, many nonpregnant women would be called pregnant. On the other hand, choosing point B as the cutoff produces the opposite result. Many pregnant women would be called nonpregnant, but few nonpregnant women would be called pregnant. The amount of overlap between the test results of the pregnant and nonpregnant groups is a measure of the accuracy of the test. In practice, a study using a very low level of hCG as the cutoff for pregnancy may or may not have actually had high loss rates because the assay might have detected either marginal pregnancies that are destined to abort and can produce only small amounts of hCG or nonpregnant women whose late (anovulatory) menstrual period was mistaken for abortion. Reproduced from Simpson and Mills (1985).

the rate of fetal losses if induced terminations are recorded as spontaneous. Third, poor memory may be a problem in eliciting an obstetrical history. Women who have completed their child-bearing may fail to recall events that transpired many years earlier. On the other hand, it is important to interview women who have passed the child-bearing age because the rate of pregnancy wastage increases with maternal age (Shapiro et al., 1971). Interviewing only women in their early or middle reproductive years will yield a lower estimate of losses than interviewing the same women at the end of their child-bearing years. For all the above reasons, retrospectively estimating fetal loss rates is unsatisfactory for anything but a rough estimate.

Time of Registration and Life Table Analysis

The time at which women register for prenatal care is crucial in determining fetal loss rates. As noted above, the risk of pregnancy loss is greater at the start than at the end of pregnancy. Many women abort early, never even registering for care and thus not being counted as pregnant. An experimental design utilizing early pregnancy diagnosis would be necessary to ensure both higher loss rates and more accurate assessments. Because the diagnosis of pregnancy is usually made relatively late in gestation, life table analysis has been proposed to compensate this shortcoming (French and Bierman, 1962; Shapiro et al., 1971; Harlap et al., 1980b). Life tables calculate the probability that an event, such as abortion, will occur during successive time intervals, e.g., weeks or months of pregnancy. The probabilities of survival over each interval can be multiplied together to derive a cumulative probability of surviving the entire period (i.e., pregnancy). A modified cohort life table is used for pregnancy wastage studies. Such an approach theoretically allows inclusion of subjects followed for different lengths of time, namely, those registering for prenatal care at different times.

Life table methods for estimating fetal losses are ill-advised for several reasons. In most studies, there are almost no observations in the first month of pregnancy, making it impossible to calculate a survival rate for this critical period of pregnancy. Relatively few additional women register for care over the next 1–2 months. Most pregnant women are thus not represented in calculations, for which reason early rates must be viewed with some suspicion. The direction of bias is not even certain. A disproportionate number of women with bleeding or threatened abortion might register for obstetrical care in the second gestational month, whereas women with uncomplicated pregnancies might not bother to register so early. The result would be an overestimation of the risk of fetal loss. Conversely, early registrants may be very health conscious and thus at "low risk." The result would be an underestimation of actual loss rates. Inasmuch as the life table approach requires multiplying the probabilities of having a loss each month to arrive at an overall loss rate, missing information or biased rates early in pregnancy could distort and, hence, invalidate the overall results. In fact, standard texts (Mausner and Bahn, 1974) caution against using life tables when a substantial proportion of the cohort is lost to follow up. Such a situation is analogous to pregnancy. In pregnancy, however, the events of interest are actually occurring before a potential subject enters the cohort, rather than after withdrawal.

Failing to register all subjects at the onset of pregnancy also makes it more difficult to assess the importance of agents thought to cause abortion. Suppose, for example, that heavy alcohol consumption caused early losses. Too few pregnancies in heavy drinkers might persist long enough for women to register and, hence, for the alcohol to be identified. Conversely, should alcohol delay abortion, drinkers would abort later than nondrinkers; thus, more drinking women would be identified as pregnant. In this case the ostensible conclusion—alcohol promotes abortion—would actually be the erroneous conclusion, the true conclusion that alcohol delays abortion not being drawn.

In summary, lack of information about very early pregnancy makes estimating loss rates difficult. The unpredictable manner in which women present for pregnancy diagnosis makes life table analysis hazardous.

Induced Abortion

Unwittingly recording induced (illicit) abortions as spontaneous has doubtless contributed to spuriously high fetal loss rates in many studies. Illicit abortions probably occurred very frequently prior to liberalized abortion laws in the United States (1971–1972). Leridon (1977) also observed the phenomenon in Paris. In our opinion, the phenomenon of unrecognized illicit abortions casts suspicions upon almost all loss rates derived from data gathered prior to legalized abortion. Indeed, there is considerable evidence that induced abortions occurred much more frequently than generally appreciated. In the Kinsey report, 10% or more of American women admitted having induced abortions in the 1950–1959 decade (Gebhard et al., 1959). Even more revealing, the number of uterine curettages performed for incomplete abortion was far greater prior to legalization than only 1 year later. In New York City municipal hospitals, curettages for this purpose decreased over 50% in the year following legalization (Pakter, 1975). Physicians obviously did not suspect they were "completing" an abortion initiated illegally by a third party; however, in retrospect precisely such an event must have occurred.

Unwittingly recording induced abortions as spontaneous abortions may influence other calculations as well. In some cultures, older women may be more likely than younger women to have the financial means and social contacts to acquire illicit abortions. The accepted increase in fetal losses in older women could thus in part be artifactual, although persistence of the age effect in New York City data collected after legalization (Stein et al., 1980) suggests that this is not the case. Greater availability of illicit abortions to older women might also play a part in the apparent increase in fetal loss observed with increasing gravidity. Another troublesome issue is that, with the passage of time, women may increasingly be likely to consider induced abortions as spontaneous. Certainly there would be little incentive to volunteer incriminating information for purposes of an investigation. Thus, retrospective studies would show the bias of inadvertently counting illicit abortions as spontaneous.

Missed Abortion

Failure to determine precisely the time at which fetal loss occurred is a pivotal, albeit inevitable, error in using fetal loss rate calculations to assess CVS safety. The problem reflects the fact that pregnancy losses were until recently diagnosed solely on the basis of clinical symptoms, e.g., passage of tissue or blood and opening of internal cervical os. Fetal demise could have occurred days or even weeks earlier.

Most first-trimester losses are recognized after 8 weeks of gestation. If viability persists until shortly before maternal clinical symptoms (e.g., bleeding), those fetuses aborting during the 9- to 12-week interval should show a normal ultrasound at 8 weeks of gestation. If so, loss rates following ultrasonographic confirmation of viability would be comparable to the actuarial (life table analysis) calculations of Leridon (1977) and others. Indeed, it is this assumption that presumably justifies calculations by Lippman (1983) and Gustavii (1984) concerning loss rates to be expected following CVS.

Suppose, on the other hand, the fetal viability ceases weeks before maternal symptoms appear? Suppose fetuses aborting at 10–12 weeks actually died weeks previously. If so, aborting pregnancies would not be normal by ultrasound at 8 weeks. Because all subjects undergoing CVS have a viable fetus, the suitable control comparison for studies evaluating safety must then be pregnancies with viable fetuses of comparable gestational age. Data from ourselves and others are now suggesting that missed abortion is, in fact, the rule rather than the exception. Most first-trimester deaths occur before 8 weeks gestation.

Confounding Genetic Variables

Excluding confounding genetic variables in assessing safety of a procedure (CVS) developed for genetic testing may seem unnecessary. However, recall that a variety of different genetic mechanisms exist, and further recall that some genetic abnormalities are more readily detected than others. Some genetic abnormalities (e.g., balanced translocations) confer upon couples having them an increased a priori risk for suffering a fetal loss. Increased fetal loss rates in such women who undergo CVS might thus not be the result of the procedure but rather the result of an increased background loss rate.

Genetic variables necessary to take into account include cytogenetic as well as gene-mediated (mendelian or polygenic) factors. Unfortunately, identification of couples who are genetically predisposed to losses is not always easy. In fact, it is sometimes impossible. Cytogenetic variables include both numerical as well as structural factors.

Recurrent Aneuploidy

Half of all first-trimester losses show chromosomal abnormalities. It is of great importance to understand that recurrent numerical chromosomal abnormalities (aneuploidy) may be responsible for recurrent fetal losses. Excluding the (uncommon) parental rearrangements, the complements of two successive abortuses in a given family are usually either both normal or both abnormal. That is, abortuses are nonrandom with respect to chromosomal complements (Hassold, 1980). If the complement of the first abortus is normal, the likelihood of the complement of the second abortus also being normal is 70%. If the complement of the first abortus is abnormal, the likelihood of the complement of the second abortus also being abnormal is 80%. The recurrent aneuploidy usually is trisomy, but it may also be monosomy or polyploidy. Such data suggest that certain couples are predisposed toward production of chromosomally abnormal conceptions, most of which result in spontaneous abortion. Part of this effect may result from maternal age. Nonetheless, the possibility of unwitting selection bias due to inclusion of disproportionate numbers of subjects with recurrent aneuploidy is real. This may especially exist if previous trisomy is a frequent indication for CVS in a given series.

Adding to the uncertainty is the question of whether a previous trisomic abortus increases the risk for subsequent trisomic live-born infants. By contrast, a previous trisomic live-born definitely confers increased risk for additional trisomic live-borns. However, the effect is greatest when the mother was relatively young when her trisomic infant was born (Stene et al., 1984). Above age 29 or so the risk is little increased over the risk for the general population of that age. Whether trisomic abortions increase the risk for trisomic live-borns is uncertain, although several studies suggest a relationship (Alberman, 1981; Warburton et al., 1982). Whether a trisomic live-born increases the risk for a subsequent abortion is also unclear. It is surprisingly difficult to identify and deal with this problem in a CVS-fetal loss rate study.

In summary, it is clear that aneuploidy must be considered when designing studies of CVS safety. First, studies assessing fetal loss rates in CVS subjects versus controls are much cleaner if aneuploid abortuses are excluded. That is, analysis is preferable if restricted to euploid losses. Second, recurrent aneuploidy and its relationship to live-born trisomy remains to be elucidated. However, any existing effect would seem most relevant to subjects who present for CVS because of previous trisomic offspring, especially live-borns. Chorionic villus samples containing disproportionate numbers of subjects with this indication would be at spuriously increased risk for fetal losses, strongly justifying the monitoring of cytogenetic status of all abortuses occurring after CVS.

Translocations

A confounding genetic variable that can be addressed is that of parental chromosomal rearrangements—translocations and inversions. These arrangments are not common. Incidence of the former is about 1 per 1000 live-borns in its balanced form (Hook and Hamerton, 1977). The incidence of inversions is even lower. However, couples with such rearrangements may seek prenatal diagnosis. Thus, the proportion of women undergoing CVS for these indications should be monitored to assure that the study group is not at unusually high risk for abortion because of disproportionate numbers of subjects undergoing CVS for these reasons. This would be essential if cytogenetic studies are not performed routinely on all fetal losses occurring after CVS.

Individuals with balanced translocations are phenotypically normal. However, gametes may, as a result of normal meiotic segregation, show chromosomal duplications of deficiencies, which produce abortuses or anomalous live-borns. Balanced translocations are usually detected because cytogenetic studies were initiated in a family experiencing an anomalous live-born or in couples experiencing repetitive abortions. In a rigorous study of CVS safety, translocations should be excluded in all couples. This is not likely to prove feasible, but all repetitive aborters should be karyotyped. Indeed, about 5% of couples experiencing at least two abortions have a balanced translocation (Simpson et al., 1981; Simpson, 1985). Females are twice as likely as males to show a translocation, but screening both males and females is appropriate.

Inversions

An inversion is a less common cause for fetal losses than a translocation. In inversions, an intrachromosomal rearrangement occurs in which the order of genes is reversed from the original. Inversions are usually caused when two chromosomal breaks are followed by reinsertion (in reverse order) of the temporarily free chromosomal segment. Inversions in which break points are on opposite sides of the centromeres are pericentric; those in which break points are on the same side of the centromere are paracentric. Heterozygotes for either type may be normal if genes are neither lost, gained, nor altered as result of the breaks leading to the inversion.

Unbalanced products result in either abortuses or, less often, anomalous live-born offspring. As shown in Figure 2, the abnormal consequences associated with inversions occur as a result of crossing-over within the meiotic loop that occurs due to the inversion. This complex subject is discussed elsewhere (Simpson, 1981).

The prevalence of inversions is low, but when present they clearly increase the likelihood of fetal loss. Pericentric inversions lead to increased rates of abortions and anomalous live borns. Paracentric inversions result only in increased rates of abortions. Inversions thus occur with increased frequency in couples experiencing repeated abortions or having anomalous offspring. Parental chromosomal studies may be necessary to exclude inversions, as they may be to exclude balanced translocations.

Genes

Finally, it would be quite reasonable to hypothesize the existence of lethal recessive genes, given the frequency with which mutant recessive genes cause neonatal deaths. However, almost nothing is known in this area.

Nongenetic Confounding Variables

A host of population and environmental variables influence fetal loss rates. Absolute loss rates will vary according to age and according to presence or absence of such toxins as alcohol or cigarettes. Estimating CVS safety must take these variables into account in order to assure that control subjects are comparable to CVS subjects.

Maternal Age

The well-known relationship between fetal loss and advancing maternal age has already been noted. The explanation is unknown. It is known that trisomic fetuses occur more commonly in older women and that most are aborted. It is not so widely appreciated that older women are also at greater risk of aborting a chromosomally normal fetus.

Hassold and co-workers (1980) performed cytogenetic studies on 1000 spontaneous abortions in a single hospital in Honolulu. In comparison with women bearing live-born infants, maternal age was significantly increased not only in those bearing chromosomally abnormal abortuses, but as well in those showing chromosomally normal abortuses. Because there is a tendency for couples to have repeated chromosomally normal abortuses (see section on confounding genetic variables) and because this could raise the mean maternal age of the chromosomally normal abortus group, the authors removed all women who had had two or more chromosomally normal abortuses. The mean maternal age for the remaining subjects with chromosomally normal abortuses was still significantly higher than that of the group with live-born infants.

The relationship between maternal age and chromosomally normal abortuses has also been examined by Stein and colleagues (1980) at three New York City hospitals. They examined data on 1417 spontaneous abortions and 11,184 live births. As in the Honolulu study, the mean maternal age was significantly greater in those women producing euploid abortuses (26.8 years) than those producing live births (25.8) years.

As shown in Fig. 3, the estimated rates of spontaneous abortion increased impressively beginning around age 35. The rate for euploid abortuses shows almost the same pattern as the rate for trisomic abortuses. These studies clearly indicate that the association between maternal age and abortion is due to an increasing risk of aborting chromosomally normal as well as chromosmally abnormal fetuses.

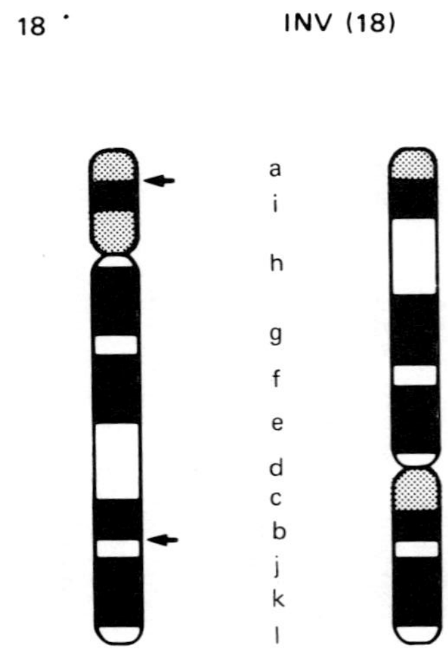

PARENTAL
HOMOLOGUES

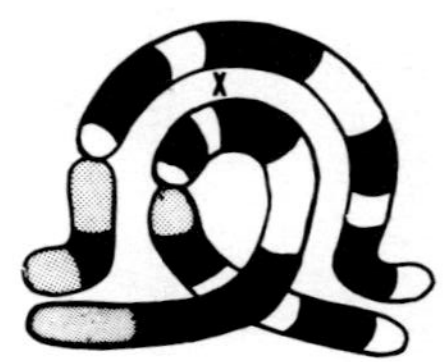

PAIRING* AT MEIOSIS,
SINGLE CROSSOVER
WITHIN INVERSION

*Only two of the four strands are shown.

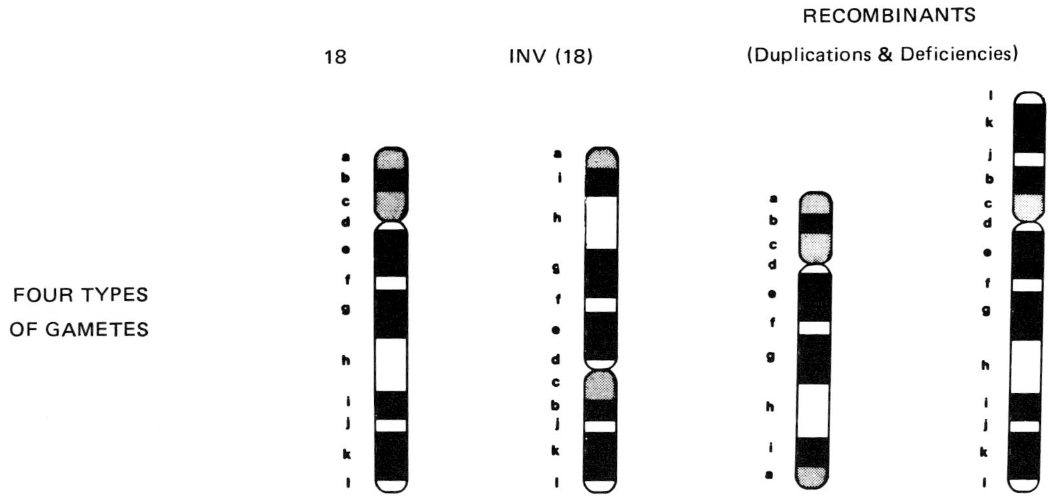

Figure 2 Effects of a single crossing-over within a pericentric inversion loop. In the top portion of the figure, the inversion chromosome is shown to the right, with the new order of chromosomal regions (*aihgfedcbjkl* in lieu of the original *abcdefghijkl*). After crossing-over at meiosis I, the four products are shown in the bottom of the figure. Two of the four gametes are abnormal. From Simpson (1981).

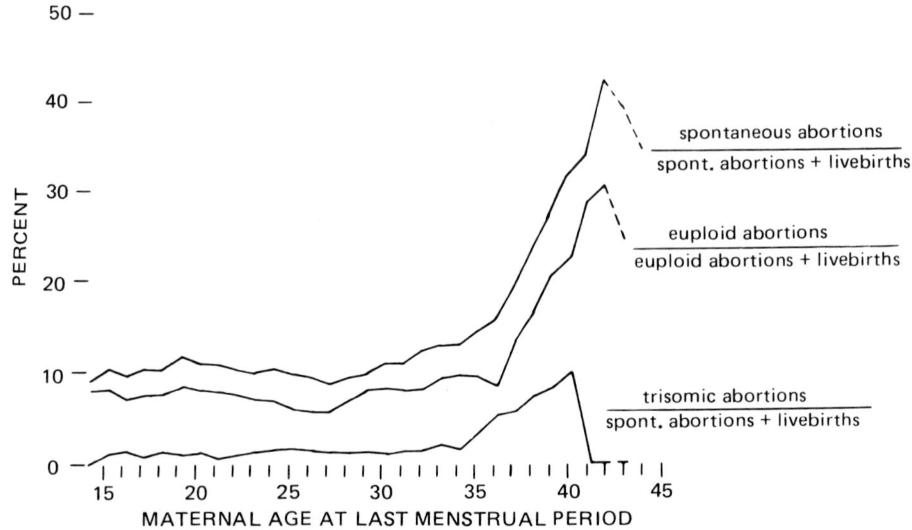

Figure 3 Estimated rates of euploid and aneuploid (trisomic) abortuses by maternal age. Curves were smoothed by estimating rates at each maternal age using the number of events observed at each age and the two adjacent ages. Dotted line (-----) indicates denominator less than 25. From Stein et al. (1980).

Gravidity

Superficial analysis suggests that the risk of fetal loss increases with increasing gravidity. (See Naylov and Warburton, 1979). The true effect of gravidity, however, is extremely difficult to assess for several reasons. First, women with repeated bad outcomes may continue to try to achieve a normal pregnancy. Second, increasing gravidity is inexorably linked to increasing maternal age, a well-established risk factor. Because of these problems, it is necessary to control for age and prior spontaneous abortions in assessing the effect of gravidity.

Roman and Alberman (1980) used a postal questionnaire to obtain pregnancy information on all women in the 1975 British Medical Register. Of 5700 respondents, 3502 had had a pregnancy. From these responses, the authors were able to analyze abortion risks by pregnancy order in women of varying gravidity. The results, shown in Fig. 4, indicate that for all gravidities, the lowest rate of abortion occurs in the last pregnancy. The trend is highly significant ($p < 0.0001$). When only women likely to have completed their families (i.e. those over age 35)

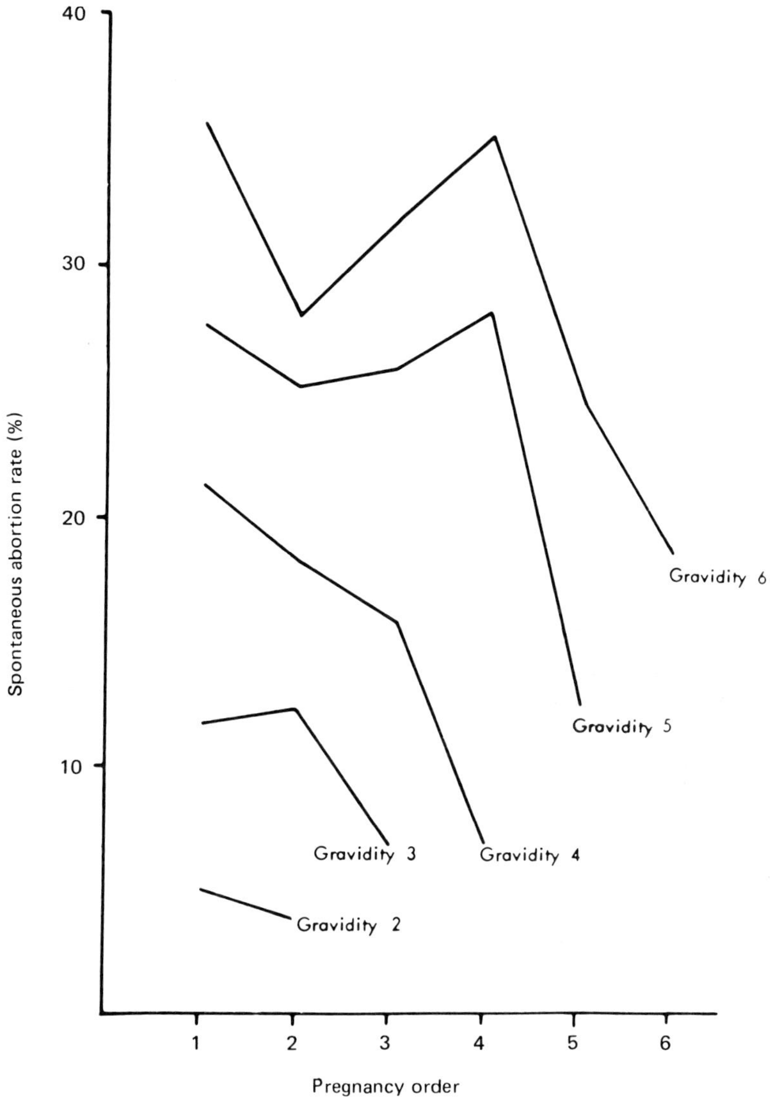

Figure 4 Percentage of spontaneous abortions by pregnancy order. From Roman and Alberman (1980).

were examined, the results remained similar. In this study, the apparent effect of gravidity is explained, at least in part, by those experiencing bad outcomes continuing to have additional pregnancies. These data also support the hypothesis that a woman is more likely to stop trying to become pregnant after a successful than after an unsuccessful pregnancy.

Kline et al. (1978) used a case-control approach to evaluate the effect of gravidity. They concluded that spontaneous abortion was not related to gravidity, independent of maternal age and previous abortion history. In a companion paper, Kline (1978) provided an interesting review of the problems in assessing gravidity effects.

In summary, the apparent association between gravidity and spontaneous abortion is, in reality, merely an effect of maternal age and compensation for previous bad pregnancy outcomes.

Cigarettes

Maternal smoking during pregnancy has been associated with spontaneous abortion. Kline and co-workers (1980) and Kline and Stein (1984) found increased abortion rates in smokers, independent of maternal age and alcohol consumption. Alberman and colleagues (1976) reported that smokers had a higher (although not significantly higher) proportion of abortuses with normal karyotypes, suggesting that smoking affects the conceptus directly rather than by causing chromosomal abnormalities.

Alcohol

Two major studies have reported an association between alcohol consumption during pregnancy and fetal losses. In a case-control study (Kline et al., 1980), 616 women suffering spontaneous abortions were compared with 632 women delivering at 28 gestational weeks or more. Among the women whose pregnancy ended in abortion, 17.0% drank at least twice per week, compared to 8.1% of the control women. After adjusting for potential confounding facts (e.g., smoking, age, and prior abortions), the association between alcohol and abortion remained significant. In a prospective study (Harlap and Shiono, 1980) of 32,019 women interviewed at their first prenatal visit, alcohol was also associated with significantly increased second-trimester fetal loss rates. The relative risks of spontaneous abortion were 1.03 (not significant), 1.98 ($p < 0.0001$), and 3.53 ($p < 0.01$) in women taking less than 1, 1–2, and 3 or more drinks daily compared to nondrinkers. Furthermore, the effect was not explained by smoking, prior abortion, age, or other risk factors.

A slightly increased risk for aborting in the first trimester was found, but it did not reach statistical significance.

These studies suggest that alcohol drinking, perhaps even in modest quantities, increases the risk of spontaneous abortion. However, evidence is usually insufficient to implicate alcohol as the cause of abortion in an individual case.

Contraception

Does maternal contraceptive use, particularly if contraceptives are used after conception, increase the risk of spontaneous abortion? Data from the Oxford Family Planning Association (Vessey et al., 1979) and the NICHD-Kaiser-Permanente Birth Defects Study (Harlap et al., 1980a) indicate that women who discontinue oral contraceptives before conception are not at increased risk for fetal losses. In the Walnut Creek study (Harlap et al., 1979) women who experienced oral contraceptive failures had significantly higher loss rates in the first trimester than the study population in general. Higher loss rates after oral contraceptive failures were not found in Oxford, but the number of observations was too small to exclude an effect.

Prior exposure to an intrauterine device (IUD) does not appear to increase the risk of spontaneous abortion. Conception with an IUD in place, however, markedly increases the risk (Vessey et al., 1979; Harlap et al., 1980a). Spermicide exposure, either before or after conception, does not appear to increase the rate of spontaneous abortion (Harlap et al., 1980a; Vessey et al., 1979; Mills et al., 1985).

Induced Abortion

The Walnut Creek Birth Defects Study (Harlap et al., 1979) addressed the question of whether induced abortions increase the risk of spontaneous abortion in subsequent pregnancies. There proved to be no effect in parous women. Among nulliparae, the relative risk was 3.27 in those whose induced abortions were performed before 1973. In those performed later, however, there was no significant increase in risk. Increasing physician experience is probably responsible for more favorable prognoses after more recent abortions.

Other Factors

Several other risk factors for spontaneous abortion are frequently overlooked in large studies, although they would rarely be missed in the clinical setting. A number of infectious agents can cause fetal losses.

Cytomegalovirus, herpes simplex type I and II, rubella, rubeola, and Venezuelan equine encephalitis are all viral agents known or strongly suspected to cause abortion (Sever, 1979). Syphilis and *Toxoplasma gondii* may also cause fetal demise.

Severe malnutrition can result in both infertility and fetal death. The Dutch famine during World War II resulted in a dramatic reduction in live births (Susser and Stein, 1979). Both infertility and stillbirths were important factors.

Environmental Chemicals

Surprisingly little information is available on the effects of environmental chemicals on human reproduction. There are many possible explanations for this dearth of information. Many corporations attempt to keep women in the reproductive age group away from chemicals. If exposure occurs, there may be multiple agents, making it impossible to determine the effects of any specific one. Finally, abortion is a difficult outcome to monitor because losses are frequent, do not always come to the attention of the health care system, and are not usually disclosed by women to their colleagues.

In animal studies, many compounds have been shown to interefere with reproduction. In the human, however, there is woefully little evidence to refute or confirm most of these findings. Available data concerning reproductive hazards from environmental chemicals were thoroughly reviewed by Barlow and Sullivan (1982). They concluded that only seven agents were associated with human abortion or female infertility: anesthetic gases, aniline, arsenic, benzene, ethylene oxide, formaldehyde, and lead. Even for this small group, the evidence is far from overwhelming.

It follows that taking into account the confounding effects of fetal loss due to environmental toxins is difficult. Certainly, information on exposures should be collected in studies assessing CVS safety. However, analysis should be conducted with caution.

BACKGROUND FETAL LOSS RATES SUITABLE FOR ASSESSING CHORIONIC VILLUS SAMPLING SAFETY

Randomized clinical trials are accepted as essential for assessing the safety of CVS. However, until such trials are completed we must rely on other sources. We have outlined (in the preceding sections) those reasons why the preliminary assessment of CVS safety requires comparing CVS loss rates to rates of women diagnosed early in pregnancy and shown to have viable pregnancies at a specific time of gestation.

This requirement is not met by reports of outcomes of ultrasonographically viable pregnancies confirmed at initial obstetrical registration. Although not without interest, these studies suffer from certain methodological problems. One problem is the lack of precise information concerning time of conception. Another problem is potential selection biases. Are women presenting at 7–10 weeks of gestation unusually health conscious, and thus at spuriously low risk for abortion? Alternatively, are such women unusually concerned about their pregnancy, and thus at spuriously high risk? Of 274 women having a viable fetus at their first obstetrical visit ("before the end of the tenth week"), Christiaens and Stoutenbeek (1984) observed a loss rate of 3.3% prior to 16 weeks. Of 734 women having a viable fetus at their initial visit (7–12 weeks), Wilson et al. (1984) found a loss rate of 2.43% prior to 20 weeks. Loss rates were 1.5% in women under 30 years, 2.5% in those aged 30–34, and 4.5% in those over age 35.

The Diabetes in Early Pregnancy Study (DIEP) is a study whose experimental design meets almost all the objects raised previously. In this NICHD-funded collaborative study, five United States universities (Harvard, Cornell, Pittsburgh, Northwestern, and the University of Washington) and the sponsoring agency (NICHD) are addressing various questions relating to the effect of insulin-dependent diabetes mellitus on early pregnancy. The study design is described elsewhere (Mills et al., 1983). Briefly, control and diabetic women are recruited prior to conception, monitored to ensure prompt diagnosis of pregnancy by serum β-hCG within 21 days of conception, and monitored closely during pregnancy. Monitoring includes ultrasound examinations performed 8 and 12 weeks after the last menstrual period (6 and 10 weeks embryonic development). The control sample is well-educated, upper middle class, and has a mean age of approximately 30 years (Mills et al., 1983; Simpson, 1984). Our data (Simpson, 1984) on control subjects with a normal 8-week ultrasound is showing loss rates comparable to those found by Christiaens and Stoutenbeek (1984).

CONCLUSIONS

The 4–5% fetal losses observed following CVS are not corrected for a host of confounding variables. Although we still support the cautious introduction of CVS as a clinical service (Elias et al., 1985), limitations in assessing loss rates must be borne in mind.

As an example, one of the initial reasons for general approbation was the expectation that background loss rates should be relatively high because 12–15% of all pregnancies were believed lost in the first trimester and because most losses were not recognized clinically until after 8 weeks. However, this high (12–15%) loss rate was derived on the basis of studies in which pregnancy was diagnosed as lost solely on the basis of clinical findings. Clinical recognition of fetal loss was made on the basis of maternal bleeding, passage of fetal tissue, or failure of uterine enlargment. Fetal demise can now be diagnosed more accurately on the basis of ultrasonographic criteria, namely, absence of fetal heart motion. In contrast to the relatively high loss rates recognized clinically in the 8- to 12- week interval, a viable 8-week fetus (fetal heart motion, normal crown–rump length) is now being shown to be lost relatively infrequently (2–4%). This low rate further indicates that fetal demise usually occurs prior to 8 weeks. Those fetal losses recognized clinically during the 8- to 12-week interval are frequently pregnancies in which fetal death occurred much earlier (missed abortion).

The low loss rates observed after a viable fetus is detected on 8-week ultrasound is that rate most directly applicable to CVS. However, such rates must still be applied with caution. First, subjects in existing series are slightly younger than CVS patients. Second, our sample (Simpson, 1984) may be at low risk for fetal losses because they are sufficiently motivated to have volunteered for pregnancy diagnosis within 21 days of conception. Early obstetrical registrants, namely, those of Christiens and Stoutenbeek (1984) and of Wilson et al. (1984), may or may not similarly be at low risk. The nature of selection bias in samples of early obstetrical registrants is also unknown, as already discussed.

Definitive answers concerning safety of CVS await randomized trials, currently in progress. The low absolute loss rates observed following CVS are encouraging, but remain consistent with a procedure-related loss of 1–3%. The precise magnitude will be crucial in determining whether CVS is an alternative to amniocentesis.

REFERENCES

1. Ahmed, A. G., and Klopper, A. (1983). Diagnosis of early pregnancy by assay of placental proteins. *Br. J. Obstet. Gynaecol. 90*:604–611.
2. Alberman, E. D. (1981). The abortus as a predictor of future trisomy 21. In

Trisomy 21 (Down Syndrome) (F. F. de la Cruz and P. S. Gerald eds.) pp. 69–76. University Park Press, Baltimore.

3. Alberman, E., Creasy, M., Elliott, M., and Spicer, C. (1976). Maternal effects associated with fetal chromosomal anomalies in spontaneous abortions. *Br. J. Obstet. Gyaecol. 83*:621–627.
4. Angell, R. R., Aitken, R. J., van Look, P. F. A., Lumsden, M. A., and Templeton, A. A. (1983). Chromosome abnormalities in human embryos after in vitro fertilization. *Nature (London) 303*:336–338.
5. Barlow, S., and Sullivan, F. M. (1982). *Reproductive Hazards of Industrial Chemicals: An Evaluation of Animal and Human Data*. Academic Press, New York.
6. Bierman, J., Siegel, E., French, F. E., and Simonian, K. (1965). Analysis of the outcome of all pregnancies in a community. *Am. J. Obstet. Gynecol. 91*:37–46.
7. Braunstein, G. D., Karow, W. G., Gentry, W. C., Rasor, J., and Wade, M. E. (1978). First-trimester chorionic gonadotropin measurements as an aid in the diagnosis of early pregnancy disorders. *Am. J. Obstet. Gynecol. 131*:25–32.
8. Christiens, G. C. M. L., and Stoutenbeek, P. H. (1984). Spontaneous abortion in proven intact pregnancies. *Lancet 2*:572–573.
9. Edmonds, D. K., Lindsay, K. S., Miller, J. F., Williamson, E., and Wood, P. J. (1982). Early embryonic mortality in women. *Fertil. Steril. 38*:447–453.
10. Edwards, R. G., Fishel, S. B., Cohen, J., Fehilly, C. B., Purdy, J. M., Slater, J. M., Steptoe, P. C., and Webster, J. M. (1984). Factors influencing the success of in vitro fertilization for alleviating human infertility. *J. in Vitro Fertil. Embryo Transf. 1*:3–23.
11. Elias, S., Simpson, J. L., Sabbagha, R., Martin, A. O. Gerbie, A. B., and Keith, L. G. (1985). Chorionic villus sampling for first trimester prenatal diagnosis (Northwestern University) *Am. J. Obstet. Gynecol. 152*:204–210.
12. Erhardt, C. L. (1963). Pregnancy losses in New York City, 1960. *Am. J. Pub. Health 53*:1337–1352.
13. French, F. E. and Bierman, J. M. (1962). Probabilities of fetal mortality. *Pub. Health Rep. 77*:835–847.
14. Gebhard, P. H., Pomeroy, W. B., Martin, C. E., and Christenson, C. V. (1959). *Pregnancy, Birth and Abortion*. Heinemann, London.
15. Gropp, A. (1973). Fetal mortality due to aneuploidy and irregular meiotic segregation in the mouse. In *Les Accidents Chromosomiques de la Reproduction*, (A. Boué, C. Thibault Eds.), pp 255–268, INSERM, Paris.
16. Gropp, A. (1975). Chromosomal animal model of human disease. Fetal trisomy and developmental failure. In *Teratology* (L. Berry and D. E. Poswillo, eds.) pp. 17–35. Springer-Verlag, Berlin.
17. Gustavii, B. (1984). Chorionic biopsy and miscarriages in first trimester *Lancet 1*:562.

18. Harlap, S. and Shiono, P. H. (1980). Alcohol, smoking and incidence of spontaneous abortions in the first and second trimester. *Lancet 2*:173–176.
19. Harlap, S., Shiono, P., Ramcharan, S., Berendes, H., and Pellegrin, F. (1979). A prospective study of spontaneous fetal losses after induced abortions. *N. Engl. J. Med. 301*:677–681.
20. Harlap, S., Shiono, P., and Ramcharan, S. (1980a). Spontaneous fetal losses in women using different contraceptives around the time of conception. *Intern. J. Epidemol. 9*:49–56.
21. Harlap, S., Shiono, P., and Ramcharan, S. (1980b). A life table of spontaneous abortions and the effects of age, parity, and other variables. In *Human Embryonic and Fetal Death,* (I. H. Porter and E. B. Hook, eds.), pp 145–158. Academic Press, New York.
22. Hassold, T. H. J. (1980). A cytogenetic study of repeated abortions. *Am. J. Human Genet. 32*:723–730.
23. Hassold, T., Chen, N., Funkhouser, J., Jooss, T., Manuel, B., Matsura, J., Matsuyama, A., Wilson, C., Yamane, J. A., and Jacobs, P. A. (1980). A cytogenetic study of 1000 spontaneous abortions *Ann. Human Genet. 44*:151–164.
24. Hertig, A., and Rock, J. (1973). Searching for early fertilized human ova. *Gynecol. Invest. 4*:121–139.
25. Hertig, A. T., Rock, J., and Adams, E. C. (1956). A description of 34 human ova within the first 17 days of development. *Am. J. Anat. 98*:435–494.
26. Hertig, A. T., Rock, J., Adams, E. C., and Menkin, M. C. (1959). Thirty-four fertilized women ova, good, bad and indifferent, recovered from 210 women of known fertility: A study of biologic wastage in early human pregnancy. *Pediatrics 23*:202–211.
27. Hook, E. B. and Hamerton, J. L. (1977). The frequency of chromosome abnormalities detected in consecutive newborn studies—differences between studies—results by sex and by severity of phenotypic involvement. In *Population Cytogenetic Studies in Humans.* (E. B. Hook and I. H. Porter, eds.), pp. 63–79. Academic Press, New York.
28. Kline, J. (1978). I. An epidemiological review of the role of gravidity in spontaneous abortion. *Early Human Develop. 1*:337–344.
29. Kline, J. and Stein, A. (1984). Spontaneous abortion (miscarriage). In *Perinatal Epidemiology* (M. B. Bracken, ed.) Oxford University Press, New York.
30. Kline, J., Shrout, P. E., Stein, Z. A. Susser, M., and Weiss, M. (1978). II. An epidemiological study of the role of gradivity in spontaneous abortion. *Early Human Develop. 1*:345–356.
31. Kline, J., Shrout, P., Stein, Z., Susser, M., and Warburton, D. (1980). Drinking during pregnancy, and spontaneous abortion. *Lancet 2*:176–180.
32. Lenton, E. A., Neal, L. M., and Sulaiman, R. (1982). Plasma concentrations of human chorionic gonadotropin from the time of implantation until the second week of pregnancy. *Fertil. Steril. 37*:773–778.

33. Leridon, H. (1977). *Human Fertility*. University of Chicago Press, Chicago.
34. Lippman, A. (1983). Consequences of chorionic biopsy. *N. Engl. J. Med. 310*:1121.
35. Mausner, J. S., and Bahn, A. K. (1974). *Epidemiology*. W. B. Saunders, Philadelphia.
36. Miller, J. F., Williamson, E., Glue, J., Gordon, Y. B., Grudzinskas, J. G., and Sykes, A. (1980). Fetal loss after implantation: A prospective study. *Lancet 2*:554–556.
37. Mills, J. L., Rishl, A. R., Knopp, R. H., Ober, C. L., Jovanovic, L. G., and Polk, B. F. (1983). NICHD-Diabetes in Early Pregnancy Study. Malformations in infants of diabetic mothers: Problems in study design. *Prevent. Med. 12*:272–286.
38. Mills, J. L., Reed, G. F., Nugent, R. P., Harley, E. E., and Berendes, H. W. (1985). Are there adverse effects of periconceptional spermicide use? *Fert. Steril. 43*:442–446.
39. Naylor, A. F. (1974). Sequential aspects of spontaneous abortion: Maternal age, parity, and pregnancy compensation artifact. *Soc. Biol. 21*:195–205.
40. Naylor, A. F. and Warburton, D. (1979). Sequential analysis of spontaneous abortion II. Collaborative study data show that gravidity determines a very substantial rise in risk. *Fertil. Steril. 31*:282–286.
41. Pakter, J. (1975). Legal abortion: A half decade of experience. *Fam. Plan. Perspect. 7*:248–255.
42. Poland, B. J., Miller, J. R., Jones, D. C., and Trimble, B. K. (1977). Reproductive counseling in patients who have had a spontaneous abortion. *Am. J. Obstet. Gynecol. 127*:685–691.
43. Reed, T. E., and Kelly, E. L. (1958). The completed reproductive performances of 161 couples selected before marriage and classified by ABO blood group. *Ann. Human Genet. 22*:165–181.
44. Roman, E., and Alberman, E. (1980). Spontaneous abortion, gravidity, pregnancy order, age and pregnancy interval. In *Human Embryonic and Fetal Death* (I. H. Porter, and E. B. Hook, eds.), pp. 129–143. Academic press, New York.
45. Royal College of General Practitioners (1970). Oral Contraceptive Study. The outcome of pregnancy in former oral contraceptive users. *Br. J. Obstet. Gynaecol. 83*:608–616.
46. Saxena, B. B. (1983). Human chorionic gonadotropin. In *Endocrinology of Pregnancy* 3rd ed. (F. Fuchs and A. Klopper, eds.), pp. 50–72. Harper and Row, Philadelphia.
47. Sever, J. L. (1979). Infectious causes of human reproductive loss. In *Human Embryonic and Fetal Death*, 3rd ed. (I.H. Porter and E. B. Hook, eds.), pp. 169–175. Academic Press, New York.
48. Shapiro, S., Levine, H. S., and Abramowicz, M. (1971). Factors associated with early and late fetal loss. *Advan. Plan. Parenth. 6*:15–58.
49. Simpson, J. L. (1981). Pregnancies in women with chromosomal abnormali-

ties. In *Genetic Diseases in Pregnancy* (J. D. Schulman and J. L. Simpson, eds.), pp. 439–471. Academic Press, New York.

50. Simpson, J. L. (1984). Low fetal loss rate after normal ultrasound at eight weeks gestation: Implications for chorionic villus sampling (CVS). The Diabetes in Early Pregnancy Project NICHD. *Amer. J. Human Genet.* *36*:197S.
51. Simpson, J. L. (1985). Repetitive spontaneous abortion. In *Perinatal Genetics.* (I. H. Porter, ed.). Academic Press, New York.
52. Simpson, J. L., and Mills, J. L. (1985). Methodologic problems in determining fetal loss rates: Relevance to chorionic villus sampling. *Human Genet.* (in press).
53. Simpson, J. L., Elias, S., and Martin, A. O. (1981). Parental chromosomal rearrangements associated with repetitive spontaneous abortions. *Fertil. Steril.* *36*:584–590.
54. Stene, J., Stene, E., and Mikkelsen, M. (1984). Risk for chromosome abnormality at amniocentesis following a child with a non-inherited chromosome aberration. *Prenatal Diagn* *4*:81–97.
55. Stein, Z., Kline, J., Susser, E., Shrout, P., Warburton, D., and Susser, M. (1980). Maternal age and spontaneous abortion. In *Human Embryonic and Fetal Death* (I. H. Porter and E. B. Hook, eds.), pp. 107–127. Academic Press, New York.
56. Stevenson, A. C., Dudgeon, M. Y., and McClure, H. I. (1959). Observations on the results of pregnancies in women resident in Belfast II. Abortions, hydatidiform moles and ectopic pregnancies. *Ann. Human Genet.* *23*:395–414.
57. Susser, M., and Stein, Z. (1979). Prenatal diet and reproductive loss. In *Human Embryonic and Fetal Death* (I. H. Porter and E. B. Hook, eds.), pp. 183–196. Academic Press, New York.
58. Tietze, C., Martin, C. E. (1957) Fetal deaths, spontaneous and induced, in the urban white population of the United States. *Popul. Stud. (NY)* *11*:170–176.
59. Tyrey, L. (1982). Human chorionic gonadotropin: Structural, biologic and immunologic aspects. *Semin. Oncol.* *9*:163–173.
60. Vessey, M., Meisler, L., Flavel, R., and Yeates, D. (1979). Outcome of pregnancy in women using different methods of contraception. *Br. J. Obstet. Gynaecol.* *86*:548–556.
61. Warburton, D., Hutzler, M., Kline, J., Stein, Z., and Strobino, B. (1982). Recurrence risk for trisomy following a trisomic spontaneous abortion. Presentation at the Annual Meeting, American Society of Human Genetics, Detroit, September 28–October 2, 1982.
62. Warburton, D., and Fraser, F. C. (1964). Spontaneous abortion risks in man: Data from reproductive histories collected in a medical genetics unit. *Am. J. Human Genet.* *16*:1–25.

63. Whittaker, P. G., Taylor, A., and Lind, T. (1983). Unsuspected pregnancy loss in healthy women. *Lancet 1*:1126–1127.
64. Wilson, R. D., Kendrick, V., Wittman, B. K., and McGillivray, B. C. (1984). Risk of spontaneous abortion in ultrasonographically normal pregnancies. *Lancet 2*:920–921.
65. Yerushalmy, J., Bierman, J. M., Kemp, D. H., Connor, A., and French, F. E. (1956). Longitudinal studies of pregnancy on the island of Kauai, Territory of Hawaii. *Am. J. Obstet. Gynecol. 71*:80–96.

15

Some Social Implications of Early Fetal Diagnosis

B. MODELL
Faculty of Clinical Sciences, University College, London, England

THE UNIQUE FEATURES OF GENETIC COUNSELING FOR REPRODUCTIVE RISKS

The general sequence of interaction between the patient and the doctor summarized in Figure 1 (see p. 261) has special characteristics in genetics. The practice of medical genetics, particularly when it is concerned with the risk of transmitting hereditary disease from parent to offspring, has some unique features with wide social implications.

Patients' Awareness of a Potential Problem

The initiative in seeking medical advice is usually taken by patients, once they recognize that they may have a medical problem. The stimulus may range from the first signs of chronic disease to the onset of acute appendicitis or a normal life event such as a pregnancy. In preventive medicine, this initial phase is very problematical because the people concerned are healthy and most have a natural mental barrier against the realization that they are, in fact, vulnerable while feeling perfectly well. Before they can present themselves for further advice, they have to be informed both that a problem exists and that it could affect them personally. The message must be powerful enough to cross the "invulnerability barrier." This has always been a major problem in preventive genetics and is becoming even more important now that more acceptable preventive approaches are becoming available.

Consultation and Diagnosis

Once an individual is aware of an actual or potential problem, he presents himself to the doctor for diagnosis. Accuracy in genetic diagnosis is exceptionally important because the action taken as a result can have radical and life long consequences for both the presenting individuals and their offspring.

Information

Information is the principal tool of the clinical geneticist. It is absolutely essential to communicate the meaning of the diagnosis and the implied risks effectively because the "patient" must be placed in a position to take autonomous and independent action, and this obviously requires full understanding. Since genetic disease is so varied (and in some instances so variable), full communication can represent a major challenge. The doctor must be prepared to share professional knowledge fully and on an equal footing with the patient. Counseling takes time and requires reinforcement by educational aids such as leaflets and video tapes. Parents' associations are also very valuable because contact with other individuals with similar problems is often very helpful.

Negotiation

The communication of the diagnosis is followed by discussion of options and agreement on a course of action. In general, the balance of initiative and decision-making between doctor and patient varies with the nature of the problem. In acute situations, the initiative lies almost entirely with the doctor. For instance, few patients with acute appendicitis will disagree with the recommendation for immediate operation or with the choice of instruments. However, more chronic conditions blend progressively into the patient's daily life, and their successful management requires that the patients have increasing autonomy in integrating them into a normal existence. For instance, asthma, diabetes, or thalassemia can be managed only as joint cooperative enterprises. The geneticist works at the extreme end of this spectrum. He is often dealing with healthy adults at their most autonomous (i.e., taking responsible decisions for the well being of their family), rather than with sick people with all the elements of dependency and regression which that implies. This gives genetic counseling its unique tone. It is generally agreed that ultimately decisions are taken by the couple at risk, the doctor's responsibility being to give enough information and support for them to make the decisions they feel are right. One consequence of accepting the patient's autonomy is that genetic counselors are prepared to support the patient in almost any (legal) decision, as long as it is made responsibly even if it is contrary to the counselor's own instincts. The acceptance of the patient's autonomy also proves to have important implications for more general decision making, for instance, when new technologies for the prevention of genetic disease become available.

Action

Information on the risk of transmitting genetic disease may lead to various actions. Some may be taken by the patient alone, e.g., whether or not to use the information, or to alter marriage or reproductive behavior. Others require the assistance of the medical service, e.g., choices involving contraception, fetal diagnosis, or termination of pregnancy. Since reproduction is involved, all possible choices involve other people: the spouse, affected offspring, further offspring, the extended family, and society as a whole. Consequently, in making decisions, the patients are concerned with these responsibilities to others, as well as with the risk of transmitting genetic disease or genetic risk to their children. It is artificial to consider the interests of the fetus, the parents, and society separately from the couple at risk, because all of these interests are present and competing within the microcosm of the couple themselves, and the outcome is expressed in their choice of actions.

In summary, it is the central role of information that characterizes the practice of clinical genetics. The first step in the clinical transaction is to provide information to stimulate healthy individuals to seek advice. Once a genetic diagnosis is made, the geneticist's main tool is further information, which frequently enables the patient to take independent action. This shifts the balance of the medical transaction away from the clinical sphere of the doctor and toward the personal sphere of the patient, so that initiative, autonomy, and responsibility reside more with the patient than in most other branches of medicine. The linear arrangement of the clinical consultation summarized in Figure 1 is

Personal Sphere | *Clinical Sphere*

Patient's awareness of potential problem → Consultation → diagnosis → information → negotiation → *Action*

Figure 1 Patient–doctor interaction.

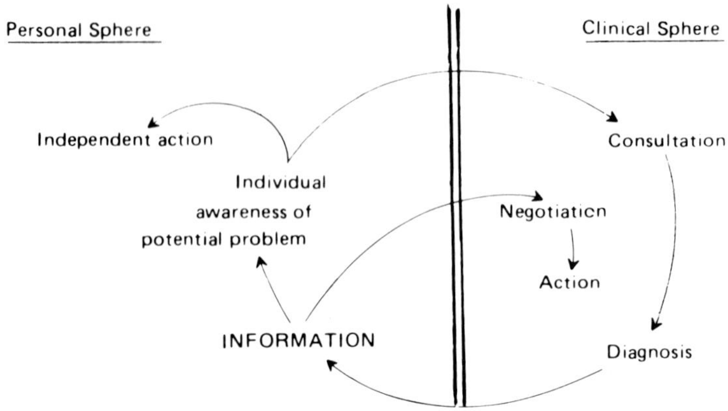

Figure 2 The general structure of medical consultations.

converted to the circular interaction summarized in Figure 2, and it seems that many of our problems in learning to deliver an effective service to the community arise from the unfamiliarity of this pattern and the associated shift in the balance of responsibility.

OPTIONS FOR ACTION ON THE KNOWLEDGE OF GENETIC RISK

In theory, people at genetic risk may discover the fact and seek to be more fully informed before marriage, after conception, or after the birth of the first affected child. The timing of the discovery of risk fundamentally affects the options available to the individual at risk. The ideal would be to discover the risk before marriage, so that all subsequent decisions concerning marriage and reproduction could be taken in an informed and responsible way. In Table 1, an effort has been made to summarize categories of hereditary diseases. It shows that even if all present available knowledge were fully applied, only a small minority of mothers at special genetic risk could discover the fact before marriage. More might discover it before conception. However, for the foreseeable future, most mothers carrying fetuses with severe abnormalities can discover that they are at special risk only during pregnancy or after the delivery of the first affected child. At present, most couples at risk for having children with serious hereditary disease discover the fact only after marriage, and usually only after the birth of their first affected child. Even then, unless the child is correctly diagnosed, many couples remain ignorant of a genetic risk until a sequence of reproductive disasters has demonstrated it

Table 1 Earliest Possible Time of Discovering a Special Risk of Transmitting Congenital Disease

	Time of acquiring risk				Earliest time and method of discovering risk						
					Preconception			In pregnancy		After birth	
Type of disease	Own conception	Marriage	Offspring's conception	Embryonic development	Special risk group	Family history	Prospective het. screening	Teratogenesis	Fetal diagnosis	Neonatal screening	Diagnosis of affected child
Chromosomal											
Nondisjunction	–	–	+	–	+ Few	–	–	–	+ Some	–	+
Translocation	+	–	+	–	–	+ Some	–	–	+ Some	–	+
Mendelian											
Dominant	+	–	+	–	–	+ Some	–	–	+ Some	–	+
X-linked	+	–	+	–	–	+ Some	–	–	+ Some	Some	+
Recessive	–	+	+	–	–	–	+ Some	–	+ Some	Some	+
New mutation											
Dominant	–	–	+	–	–	–	–	–	+ Rare[c]	–	+
X-linked	–	–	+	–	–	–	–	–	+ Rare[c]	–	+
Recessive	–	–	Remote effects only	–	–	–	–	–	–	–	–
Congenital malformation (nonmendelian)	–	–	–	+	+[a]	–	–	+[b]	+	Some	+

[a]Diabetic mother, for example.
[b]Rubella infection on drugs, for example.
[c]Would apply only to new mutations causing congenital malformation.

Table 2 Options Available to Individuals Who Know They May Transmit Hereditary Diseases to Their Offspring

Time	Possible course of action
Before marriage	1. Refrain from marriage (dominant and sex-linked)
	2. Avoid marrying another carrier (recessive)
After marriage (usually after birth of first affected)	3. Refrain from reproduction
	4. "Take the chance"
	5. Reproduce with fetal diagnosis and selective abortion
	6. Reproduce with a substitute genetic partner
	7. Divorce and reproduce with another partner
After the birth of an affected child	8. Accept affected infant and treat it
	9. Accept affected infant and not treat it
	10. Reject affected infant

unambiguously. This timing limits the number of possibilities available for subsequent evading action. The maximum range of options available to couples at risk is listed in Table 2.

Altered Marriage Behavior

Remarkably little detailed work has been done on the effect of genetic counseling on marriage. In particular, most studies having focused on the more comprehensive issue of fertility. One decision that could be taken prior to marriage is to refrain from marrying altogether—a choice most likely to be made by individuals at risk for carrying severe dominant or sex-linked conditions. There are no published figures on the effect of knowledge of this type of risk on subsequent marriage patterns. A second option, open to known heterozygotes for recessive conditions, is to choose only a "normal" marriage partner. However, there is good evidence that knowledge of thalassemia status obtained immediately prior to marriage does not affect marriage patterns, whether fetal diagnosis is or is not available (WHO, 1982; Stamatoyannopoulos, 1974). In summary, one of the two possible ways to avoid genetic disease by altering marriage behavior is highly unsatisfactory, and there is no evidence that the other has yet been seriously used. However, social patterns differ so much that it is perfectly possible that marriage behavior might be altered in certain communities and in certain situations. Earlier heterozygote screening, for instance in the high schools, has not yet been carried out on a large enough scale for any information to be available about its long-term effects on marriage behavior. If genetic information were available early enough, communities with a tradition of cousin marriage might use it in arranging marriages, while where the condition concerned affects ethnic minorities in a large unaffected "host" community, one effect could be to increase the rate of marriage "out." As the practice of genetic counseling spreads, more information will become available on all these aspects.

Voluntary Childlessness

There is, by contrast, plenty of evidence of decreased reproductive activity among couples knowing themselves at risk for the most severe genetic diseases, e.g., Huntington's chorea (Harper et al., 1982; Carter et al., 1983), Duchenne muscular dystrophy (Carter, 1973), cystic fibrosis (Kaback et al., 1984), and thalassemia (Modell et al., 1980). However, executing the decision not to reproduce further is not simple. It is usually achieved in the first instance by contraception. However, since everyone is not equally adept, and many are ambivalent, accidental pregnancies continue to occur. The couples may then have to fall back on first-trimester abortion, i.e., the decision not to reproduce is at least partly implemented through the indiscriminate abortion of all fetuses, only one-quarter of which would actually be affected. There are two implications. The first is that unless these means of implementing the decision not to reproduce further are available, genetic couseling for such conditions may be practically useless: indeed may be worse than useless. For instance, counseling for couples of prospectively detected heterozygotes was introduced in Ferrara in North Italy in the 1960s, but there was no consequent fall in the thalassemia major birth rate. Indeed there was some evidence of "reproductive compensation" (Aguzzi et al., 1978). This does not mean that people took no notice, but only that the means of acting on the information were not at hand. When contraception became more generally available in Italy, the thalassemia major birth rate fell by 30% in Ferrara, even before the introduction of fetal diagnosis (WHO 1983). Thus genetic counseling for reproductive risk is really an aspect of family planning. The second implication is that though the painful decision not to reproduce appears simple on paper, it has moral implications because it can be fulfilled only through efficient contraception and back-up early termination of pregnancy. It simply is not an available option where family planning is not yet accepted.

"Taking the Chance"

This is the only possible approach to obtaining further healthy children when family planning and fetal diagnosis are not available. It may also be chosen even when fetal diagnosis is available by groups who traditionally have high fertility and particular objections to mid-trimester abortion. For instance, in the United Kingdom most Muslim Pakistanis at risk for thalassemia will "take the chance," but most Cypriot at-risk couples would not dream of reproducing without fetal diagnosis. Counseled couples who do not consider that the condition they are at risk for is serious enough to justify mid-trimester abortion will usually also "take the chance." For instance, in the United Kingdom few British couples of West Indian origin at risk for having children with sickle cell disease request mid-trimester diagnosis, but African couples are more interested, Thus, the decision whether or not to accept fetal diagnosis is a very finely balanced one, the main consideration determining the point of balance being the grief and guilt associated with mid-trimester termination of pregnancy. Whatever the reason for the decision to "take the chance," it is usually associated with much anguish, and neonatal diagnosis, where possible, is usually sought.

Fetal Diagnosis

The option of reproducing using mid-trimester fetal diagnosis and selective abortion is naturally preferable for most families than not reproducing at all. Therefore, it is not surprising that those groups that have been shown to limit reproduction as a result of genetic counseling display great interest in fetal diagnosis. Although few studies have been done, most indicate that in Europe about 85% of mothers in the risk groups for important hereditary diseases are in favor of fetal diagnosis and selective abortion, and when they are aware of the risk, they adopt this approach to obtaining a healthy family.

Other Possibilities

The remaining options, to reproduce with a substitute genetic partner (sperm or egg donation) or to divorce and find another partner are not commonly resorted to at present as a solution for genetic problems, although precise figures are lacking. It is often stated that there is a high incidence of family breakdown where children have a severe congenital disease, but the many threads involved have not been adequately disentangled. For instance, the stresses involved in caring for a chronically damaged child need to be carefully distinguished from the reproductive risk inhibiting normal sexual relationships and the genetic risk limiting compensation by having normal children.

In conclusion, even when risk can be identified before marriage, what evidence is available indicates that the fetal diagnosis approach is the most popular one for couples at high genetic risk because it allows them to attain their biological objectives while discharging their responsibilities to their offspring and to society.

MEDICAL RESPONSIBILITY

The issue of fetal diagnosis also implies a set of special responsibilities for the medical staff concerned: (a) research; (b) protecting their patients and explaining their needs to the wider community; (c) educating the rest of the medical service and the community in general about genetic diseases; and (d) developing the service in order to bring the benefits of new developments to those most in need of them.

Research

Research is obviously a high priority because, although fetal diagnosis is the most acceptable option for many couples at high genetic risk, it is nevertheless extremely distressing. The area of research covered in this treatise, the movement of fetal diagnosis from the second to the first trimester, is probably the biggest single step possible in this direction, since for the majority of hereditary conditions there is not, and probably never will be, any alternative to intrauterine diagnosis.

Speaking for Our Patients

The fact that avoidance of hereditary disease often requires and will continue to require selective abortion makes at-risk couples particularly vulnerable to outside anti-abortion pressures. These pressures usually come from individuals who have no direct experience of hereditary disease and do not particularly wish to threaten those who do. However, their activities may add considerably to our patients' burdens. There is a general assumption that if one pressure group attempts to influence social policy, those who feel threatened will respond, both sides of the argument will be heard, and a reasonable final balance will be achieved. However, this does not happen for hereditary disease because our patients are particularly vulnerable. They are mostly pregnant women (or families busy with the care of chronically sick children) who also know that they can transmit genetic abnormalities and feel the consequent shame because of public ignorance about inheritence. In addition, many may belong to ethnic minorities. They have to make extremely difficult moral choices and are afraid of criticism of their feelings and actions. It would be hard to find a group less likely to stand up and speak out in their own defense and for the community in general. Nevertheless, a good genetics service is in the interest of the whole community because the entire population is at risk (even though only a small proportion know they are, either by having had an abnormal child or through heterozygote diagnosis).

We, therefore, have a special responsibility (to society as well as to our patients) to protect our patients' interests, to speak for them, and to create a forum in which their voices may be heard. This can best be done by objective description of their problems together with description of their choices among the various available options discussed above. However, we are not performing this function particularly well, probably because we share our patients' anxieties and are afraid to call attention to the importance of termination of pregnancy in genetic practice. This may account for the fact that there is a striking scarcity of clear statistical information of this kind, even though some of it would be fairly easy to acquire. For instance, what proportion of couples who produce a child with a severe metabolic disease actually obtain a clear diagnosis and genetic counseling? How many known or potential carriers of severe X-linked or dominant conditions never marry? How many pregnancies are actually terminated simply from fear of a genetic risk that cannot be diagnosed in the fetus (e.g., cystic fibrosis)? How many at-risk couples divorce? How many artificial inseminations by donor are done for genetic reasons?.

Community Education

It is extremely important for the community in general to realize that new mutation or chromosomal nondisjunction can happen to anyone and that almost everyone carries one or more recessive genes. Therefore, although genetic disease is uncommon, everyone is at risk for transmitting it to their children. It is our responsibility to bring about this wider understanding, which would reduce stigmatization and greatly relieve some of the burdens felt by our patients.

Provision of an Adequate Service

We also cannot avoid the obligation to follow through on the consequences of the new developments that we help to bring about. For instance, from the time that fetal diagnosis becomes possible for a condition, that condition becomes avoidable in principle, and from that time on a new element of responsibility is attached to all new births of affected children to identifiable mothers at risk. Subsequent births can occur only (a) by mistake (ignorance or diagnostic error) (b) by choice not to accept fetal diagnosis or termination of pregnancy on the part of the patient or the community; or (c) by an administrative decision limiting the necessary resources. When such developments occur, this unavoidable responsibility, although real, is rather shapeless, and part of the problem is to define it and attach it to specific individuals. Ultimately, of course, responsibiltiy for avoidable conditions should be transferred to the parents, to whom it properly belongs. However, particularly, when prospective identification of individuals at risk is concerned, there may be difficulties in identifying and constructing the appropriate medical channels.

Probably the most important ethical issue in the whole area of fetal diagnosis is the fact that, even in developed countries and even though we are aware of their high acceptability, preventive genetic services are delivered very inefficiently to the community. For instance, although in general over 80% of older women are interested in amniocentesis when it is offered, it is only in Denmark that this proportion actually get it. In the United Kingdom and the Netherlands from 30 to 50% may have amniocentesis, while in France probably less than 20% do. The discrepancy between the high potential demand and the number of fetal diagnoses actually performed leads to the continuing births of affected children to parents who would have had fetal diagnosis if they had been more fully informed. The fact that these births are now avoidable makes them more difficult for the parents to accept. Therefore, it is clearly a priority for us to work to increase the general awareness of risk and the possibility of prevention. However, this requires someone to be responsible, and this is part of the problem. For instance, who is responsible for the fact that mothers of advanced age are still so poorly advised of their genetic risk or that more than half the couples at risk for producing thalassemic children in the United Kingdom still go undetected? A really adequate service will not be provided until these responsibilities have been allocated and the appropriate groups have incorporated them into their professional training (i.e., until these new developments have made us bring about the appropriate social structures to deal with them). We are clearly making very slow progress with this at present.

THE ADVANTAGES OF, AND NEW PROBLEMS ASSOCIATED WITH, FIRST TRIMESTER FETAL DIAGNOSIS

The unsatisfactory nature of mid-trimester abortion as a solution for genetic problems is probably responsible for much of our hesitancy in promoting preventive genetics services. It also ensures that parents have emotional conflicts even when they are at risk for severe diseases, and decision-making is very finely balanced. Both individual decisions and public policy are likely to be critically influenced by the availability of an earlier approach to diagnosis, which is likely to increase the scope of prevention of genetic disease in every way.

In Developed Countries

For severe conditions where mid-trimester diagnosis is already available, most couples would prefer an earlier approach that gives more rapid results with less psychological conflict and greater privacy. It is also highly likely that when the less uniformly severe conditions are diagnosed before 12 weeks of gestations, parents will have less difficulty in deciding to abort, and more will choose to abort rather than to continue an affected pregnancy. Thus, earlier intervention will reduce many difficulties by increasing the ease and acceptability of fetal diagnosis as a means of avoiding hereditary disease. It is bound to raise new problems by increasing the demand for diagnosis, so there is a steadily increasing need for discussion of social and ethical issues and for keeping the community properly informed.

Nevertheless, the widest new implications arise from the increased acceptability of earlier fetal diagnosis as a solution for genetic problems. The new DNA technology may ultimately permit the identification of almost any inherited characteristic in the fetus as well as in adults, so that it will become possible to identify nonpathological genes and many genes associated with relatively mild clinical consequences. Geneticists are already asking themselves when they should and when they should not offer fetal diagnosis. The discussion earlier in this chapter indicates that such decisions can best be made in conjunction with the patients. For instance, when a new diagnostic test becomes available, the best approach may be to inform the affected families of the new development and document their reactions, i.e., whether they themselves would consider using the new test and whether they would recommend others at risk to do so. Their subsequent reproductive behavior and use of fetal diagnosis can be monitored, and if they find it useful, it should be offered more widely.

Fetal sexing is probably the most complicated example of nonpathological genetic diagnosis. Termination of pregnancy in the mid-trimester on grounds of fetal sex is generally unacceptable, but the possibility of sex selection in the first trimester, at a time when termination of pregnancy on social grounds is widely available, is a new issue. However, it is clear that sex selection as a primary indication for fetal diagnosis is generally offensive in industrialized societies, and there can be little doubt that its practice would endanger the entire genetics services by producing negative social reactions. However, it is important to be aware that the conclusion that it should not be offered is a pragmatic one, and does not absolutely exclude fetal sexing as a primary indication in exceptional cases. By contrast, there seems to be no contraindication to providing information on fetal sex when it becomes available within the context of genetic diagnosis. It may be requested by the parents, and can sometimes be integral to their decisions concerning the outcome of the pregnancy. The issue has been more fully discussed by Fletcher (1983a,b).

In this context, it is important to point out that first-trimester diagnosis, although a great advance on mid-trimester diagnosis, is by no means free of emotional stresses. From the psychological point of view, the evolution of the pregnancy is more rapid in the first than in the second trimester. The attention focused on the fetus by the ultrasound and diagnostic examinations and the extra emphasis arising from the parents' hopes and fears speeds up the perceptual evolution of the pregnancy. Thus, delays in diagnosis associated, for example, with tissue culture or DNA analysis are more significant than previously, and the need for rapid diagnosis is even greater.

In Developing Countries

The appropriateness of a preventive approach for genetic disease is influenced by numerous social constraints that can only be touched upon here. They differ between societies and tend particularly to favor fetal diagnosis as a solution for the problem of genetic disease in developing countries, because of the dominance of financial considerations.

In developed countries, the costs of medical care are usually distributed throughout society by different forms of insurance, so most couples at risk for producing affected offspring are free to choose their course of action mainly on emotional, social, and ethical grounds. However, where these arrangments do not exist, the burden of caring for an affected child falls directly on the family, and almost any form of treatment for chronic disease, whether it be for hemophilia, thalassemia, or an amino acid disorder or even early prophylactic antibiotics for sickle cell disease, may be prohibitively expensive. Therefore, most families must choose in the end to leave an affected child to live or die untreated. Selective abortion would be far preferable if it were available and ethically approved, and might more often be chosen even for less disabling conditions. The development of chorionic villus sampling combined with direct karyotyping, DNA analysis, and biochemical diagnosis together with early, simple abortion is an important step toward appropriate technology for developing countries, where problems such as unstable electricity supply and high levels of contamination often rule out reliable tissue culture. This may be the only realistic way to start a fetal diagnosis service in many countries, and there is also some evidence that first-trimester fetal diagnosis may make a very big difference in some societies where mid-trimester abortion is not acceptable.

Religion is at present one of the most important factors limiting the extension of fetal diagnosis services through its influence on abortion legislation. Although no religion favors abortion,many permit it under special circumstances, and an earlier approach may make a critical difference to whether fetal diagnosis can be accepted or not in some societies. For instance, there is already some evidence that first-trimester fetal diagnosis is acceptable to Muslim families who cannot accept mid-trimester diagnosis.

Many other factors affect the level of interest in fetal diagnosis in a community. Where family size is large because of reproductive compensation for high infant mortality, as in most of Africa, simply having further children may seem the simplest solution. However, as family size decreases with improved primary health care and population policies (e.g., in China), the preventive approach to congenital disease becomes progressively more important. Finally, the long-standing tradition of cousin marriage in many (mainly Muslim) societies is an additional indicator for genetic counseling and potentially for fetal diagnosis.

WHAT IS THE ULTIMATE REASONABLE OBJECTIVE IN FETAL DIAGNOSIS?

First-trimester fetal diagnosis is a major advance, but it is still not an ideal procedure. How could it be improved? Is diagnosis before or at conception a realistic idea? Ultimately it might prove possible to genotype, for example, the ovum before fertilization, and if it were cheap and easy it would prove a good approach. However, the appropriate technology is far inthe future, and there is reason to doubt the efficiency of the approach, even if it ever became feasible. The subject may be illuminated somewhat by looking at the issue of chromosomal nondisjunction, which is by far the major intrauterine cause of human hereditary disease. It occurs in women of all age groups and accounts for up to half of all spontaneous abortions. At least 15% of all recognized pregnancies end in spontaneous abortion. About 15–30% of women in developed countries will conceive a fetus with a chromosomal nondisjunction in the course of their reproductive lives, while in developing countries where family sizes are large, nearly all women must conceive such a fetus at least once. Fortunately, only those nondisjunctions that cause minimal disturbances of embryonic development allow the fetus to survive to birth, the majority miscarrying in early pregnancy. Although there is still room for diagnosis earlier than the present 9 to 10 weeks, it may not prove practical to operate earlier than 6 to 7 weeks of gestation because the number of spontaneous abortions and chromosomal anomalies would be too high for an efficient service. Conception and early winnowing in the usual way may ultimately remain the most practical approach. However, the importance of rapid diagnosis (e.g., within 48 hrs of sampling) should not be underestimated, since, from the psychological point of view, termination of pregnancy should be available as soon as possible. In short, it may not prove realistic to try to achieve diagnostic termination of pregnancy earlier than the majority of spontaneous abortions. This may not prove to be a bad thing, since it is the ultimate safeguard against a frivolous approach to the problems of human inheritance.

CONCLUSIONS

Possibly the most important ethical implication of th earlier approach is for public health education, because if mothers are to take advantage of early fetal diagnosis they need to have some idea of their potential risks before conception. Fortunately, another important effect of the earlier approach should be to increase our confidence in the preventive approach. It should enable us to break through our inhibitions about promoting fetal diagnosis more widely and encourage us to put together a suitable package of information about heathy reproduction for schools, couples getting married, and family planning clinics. We should seize the need to explain the risk of diagnosable hereditary diseases, such as thalassemia, sickle cell anemia, and Tay-Sachs disease, because it provides a valuable opportunity to convey clear information on recessive inheritance that can be used as a foundation when diagnosis of other common conditions such as cystic fibrosis becomes possible. Effective strategies for delivering this type of information and providing screening still need to be worked out.

REFERENCES

1. Aguzzi, S., Vullo, C., and Barrai, I. (1978). Reproductive compensation in families segregating for Cooley's anaemia in Ferrara. *Ann. Human Genet. London 42*:153.
2. Carter, C. O. (1973). *Current Status of Genetic Counselling and its Assessment*. In *Birth Defects* (A. G. Motulsky and W. Lenz eds.) Excerpta Medica, Amsterdam.
3. Fletcher, J. C. (1983a). *Ethics and Public Policy: Should Sex Choice Be Discouraged in Sex Selection of Children?* (N. G. Bennet, ed.). Academic Press, New York.
4. Fletcher, J. C. (1983b). *Is Sex Selection Ethical?* pp. 333–348. Alan R. Liss, New York.
5. Kaback, M., Zippen, D., Boyd, P., and Cantor, R. (1984). Reproductive behavior of families with CF children. Abstracts of International Cystic Fibrosis Meeting, Brighton.
6. Modell, B., Ward, R. H. T., and Fairweather D. V. I. (1980). Effect of introducing antenatal diagnosis on reproductive behaviour of families at risk for thalassemia major. *Br. Med. J. 1*:1347.
7. Stamatoyannopoulos, G. (1974). *Problems of Screening and Counselling for the Haemoglobinopathies*. In *Birth Defects* (A. G. Motulsky and W. Lenz, eds).
8. WHO (1983). Memorandum: Community control of hereditary anaemias. *Bull. WHO 61*:63–80.

16

Ethical Issues in Clinical Trials of First Trimester Prenatal Diagnosis

JOHN C. FLETCHER
Warren G. Magnuson Clinical Center, National Institutes of Health, Bethesda, Maryland

INTRODUCTION

Clinical trials comparing the safety and accuracy of first-trimester chorion villus sampling (CVS) as a method of prenatal diagnosis and mid-trimester amniocentesis (AM) are being mounted in several countries. The discussion below is about a proposed trial in the United States, but the issues involved are of concern to physician–researchers in other nations.

Clinical trials raise ethical issues of risks of harm, magnitude of benefits, and fairness in selection of subjects. A randomized clinical trial (RCT) requires careful consideration because a proven approach will be withheld (by chance) from some to compare the advantages and disadvantages of a new approach. Clinical research in prenatal or perinatal care also presents ethical complexities since the fetus, in addition to the mother, is a subject of research.

Three ethical issues will be discussed in this chapter: (a) ethical arguments against and for a trial, (b) questions of benefit and risk to pregnant women and fetuses, and (c) considerations of selection of subjects and their informed consent.

ETHICAL CHALLENGES TO A TRIAL

Some physicians may intuitively be opposed to a trial because they believe it would not be best for their patients to be in a position to lose perceived benefits of CVS. They may agree with criticisms of RCTs (Fried, 1974; Waldenstrom, 1983) as too compromising of the physician's fidelity to the best interests of the patient. From an egalitarian perspective, Veatch (1983) objected to strict randomization on grounds of fairness. He argued that economically disadvantaged subjects due the highest standard of justice were unduly restricted by randomization in their range of choices.

Is a Trial Unfair and Unnecessary?

If the physician's loyalty is only to the welfare of the individual patient or that some special patients' interest should not be unfairly limited by those of science, one could object to a trial of CVS. Aware of the obvious advantage of CVS for early diagnosis, some physicians may refuse to permit patients to enroll in a trial and possibly lose such benefits.

On a review of the risks of prenatal diagnosis, i.e., maternal morbidity and mortality, fetal loss, psychological risks of stress from the waiting period before and after AM, and depression following abortion for genetic indications, experience with CVS to date appears favorable.

An early report of CVS (Kazy et al., 1982) was remarkable for lack of complications such as bleeding or infection. Subsequent reports (Ward et al., 1983; Gustavii, 1984) include infrequent cases of vaginal bleeding that appear to clear up easily. Many reports stress the lack of discomfort to the research subject or patient. Although not systematically studied, infection appears rare (Brambati et al. 1984; Jackson, 1984a). Jackson et al. (1984) noted "small abnormalities resembling fluid collection or blood clots" on ultrasound scans 1 week after CVS that had resolved by 16 weeks.

No maternal death as a result of CVS has been reported. Simpson (1980) reviewed a series of 20,000 AM cases in which only one death due to amnionitis had occurred. The report stated further that "maternal deaths are known to have occurred from complications of therapeutic abortion." No study of maternal death specifically associated with abortion for genetic reasons has been done. However, the risks of mortality after abortion are well known. The risks of death from mid-trimester abortion are seven times higher than in first-trimester abortions, as shown in Table 1. Differences between risks of complications are also dramatic. Mid-trimester abortion by prostaglandin has a complication rate of 24 per 100 abortions. First-trimester abortion by dilatation and evacuation results in complications in less than 6 per 1000 abortions (Cates et al., 1977; Grimes and Cates, 1980). These differences

Table 1 Death-to-Case Rate for Legal Abortion by Weeks of Gestation United States, 1976–1980

Weeks of gestation	Deaths[a]	Abortions[a]	Rate[b]	Readjusted rate[c]
8	11	2,944,587	0.4	1.0
9–10	13	1,559,089	0.8	2.0
11–12	7	739,727	0.9	2.2
13–15	8	247,471	3.2	8.0
16–20	18	232,006	7.8	19.5
21	4	52,120	7.7	19.5

[a]Based on distribution of 3,998,152 abortions (69.23%) with weeks of gestation known.
[b]Deaths per 100,000 abortions.
[c]Based on an index rate for 8 menstrual weeks' gestation of 0.4 deaths/100,000 abortion.
Source: Lang, P. (1979/1980). Legal Abortion Deaths: 1976–1980: Table 19. Abortion Survey Report. Centers for Disease Control, Atlanta, Georgia.

are important to physicians concerned primarily for the safety of their patients.

Earlier (8–11 weeks) diagnosis and direct analysis of chromosomes reduces the stress of waiting for AM (16–18 weeks) and for its results, in some cases past 20 weeks. In a wanted pregnancy when the couple is also willing to use abortion to prevent an affected child, they face a real moral and emotional problem. The longer the conflict persists, the more serious and stressful will be their choices and the consequences. Perhaps the greatest difference between CVS and AM will be the psychological and ethical acceptability of the former by patients and families. Another positive feature of the timing of CVS noted by Jackson et al., (1984) and Ward (1983) is that patients and spouses enjoy more "privacy" since the pregnancy is not yet obvious to others.

Three studies (Blumberg et al., 1975; Donnai et al., 1981; Leschot et al., 1982) describe psychological risks of depression and/or family and marital conflict in patients after mid-trimester abortion for genetic indications. Some features of parents' problems after abortion of a wanted pregnancy are similar to mourning the loss of a newborn with serious handicaps (Kennell, 1970). Feelings of guilt are common in addition to feeling judged by others. The most detailed follow-up study concluded (Leschot, 1982, p. 107):

> The decision to terminate a second trimester pregnancy because of a malformed fetus is an event wth long term negative side-effects for the patient and her family.

Table 2 Fetal Loss, 25 June 1984

Centers	Total biop-sies	Success	Thera-peutic abor-tion	Con-tinued	Loss max.	Loss max.(%)	Loss adj.	Loss adj. (%)	Delivered
6	1007	969	23	917	29	3.2	20	2.2	156
25	1467	1405	170	1297	62	4.8	48	3.7	191

Source: Jackson (1984a). Division of Medical Genetics, Thomas Jefferson University, Philadelphia, Pa. 19107.

In my experience, counselors seldom, if ever, mention the increased emotional risks of genetic abortion after AM. However, some centers (Donnai et al., 1981) wisely provide special help and support to mothers during the abortion episode. Many investigators have commented on the appearance of reduced feelings of guilt or remorse after first-trimester genetic abortion following CVS. This question can be studied more carefully in the context of clinical trials.

Table 2, drawn from results of a voluntary registry of fetal loss (Jackson, 1984a), summarizes available results on CVS from six centers with the largest experience and for 25 other centers. Among the latter are 16 having fewer than 50 cases. The maximum loss columns represent all fetuses lost subsequent to a procedure on a confirmed viable fetus where there was no termination for diagnosis. The next two adjusted loss columns represent the editor's interpretation of reported losses. He removed any loss after a definite diagnosis of choromosome abnormality made from fetal tissue but unknown before the loss. He also removed any loss 8 weeks or more after CVS where there was no apparent connection between the procedure and the loss.

This information, while useful, provides no scientific basis on which to give risk estimates to patients prior to CVS. These figures should not be used to predict that rate of loss will be higher or lower than the risks of AM. Many things can go wrong in an uncontrolled case series, in a voluntary reporting system, and when zeal for a new procedure abounds. The registrar's decisions are open to question. For example, might some fetal losses in the adjusted column be due to spontaneous abortion rather than CVS? No conclusions should be drawn from these data; however, these are the best facts available until data from trials are compiled.

Counterarguments

In my view, two counterarguments can be used to refute claims of unfairness of an RCT of CVS and AM. The first argument is scientific but has ethical implications. Genuine questions exist about the key risks and accuracy of CVS. Rational considerations support a comparison with AM, if sound ethical reasons also support a trial. Some patients previously disposed to CVS will be more willing to be randomized, if they understood the unknowns of CVS.

Despite patient acceptability and psychological advantages, no sound scientific reasons yet exist for physicians to adopt a policy to recommend CVS for first-trimester fetal diagnosis. In the early days of a new procedure, physicians do their best to advise patients while stressing the uncertainties. Such a situation begs the question of the comparative significance of CVS. Suspension of judgment about which approach is better for most patients, while dealing with patients who look for expert advice, goes to the heart of the practice of medicine today.

Rather than rush to judgment about the advantages of CVS on largely psychological grounds, physicians can now adopt "the uncertainty that will lead us to discover better grounds for planning and acting" (Chalmers, 1983). The priority questions for study to gain "better grounds" are (NICHD, 1984):

> Is CVS associated with spontaneous abortions and other complications of pregnancy, with low birth weight, congenital malformations or other problems identified at later follow-up? And, is the accuracy of CVS comparable to that of AM, especially in the identification of chromosomally abnormal fetuses?

Very little is known with certainty about these key questions of safety and accuracy compared to what is known about AM. Table 3 shows

Table 3 Incidence of Spontaneous Abortion in Amniocentesis Cases and Controls in Three Studies

	Canadian Medical Research Council (1977)	National Institute of Child Health and Human Development Amniocentesis Registry (1978)	Medical Research Council, UK (1978)
Amniocentesis subjects	0.9%	2.8%	2.7%
Control subjects	1.6–1.9%	2.4%	1.3%

Source: Turnbull and MacKenzie (1983).

results of three studies of spontaneous abortion in AM cases and controls. However, authorities (Turnbull and MacKenzie, 1983) advise caution in use and interpretation of these AM studies. The studies used different categories, had difficulties in selection of controls, and did not randomize for ethical reasons. Compared to AM at a period early in its development, the risks of fetal loss in Table 2 appear roughly similar. Operator experience may have much to do with the highs and lows of this risk. However, one cannot be sure unless and until more understanding is gained about the relationship between the relative risks of CVS and the complex high background risk of natural fetal loss. Spontaneous abortion is higher in early pregnancy. How much higher is it due to advanced maternal age and chromosomal abnormalities in the fetus? This vexing, potentially answerable question has never been studied in relation to CVS and AM in a controlled trial.

Some basic biological and methodological questions have been raised about the accuracy and limits of diagnosis in the CVS approach (Simoni et al., Chapter 6, this treatise). Perhaps the chorion and villi do not truly represent the genetic condition of the fetus. Chromosomal mosaicism continues to be implicated in some CVS analyses (Jackson, 1984a). In present practice, such findings must be reconfirmed by a new CVS or an AM. Jackson et al. (1984) also notes problems in laboratory methods that yield a less than optimal number of mitotic metaphases in chromosomes or result in poor quality of chromosome morphology. The chromosomes do not band as well as those prepared after AM. Less confidence exists in the accuracy of cytogenetic studies after CVS than after AM.

Two conditions are required in most cases, before a sound scientific (and ethical) basis exists for a RCT (Levine 1981). First, some evidence must exist on which to anticipate some benefit. (Phase I cancer trials are possibly the most difficult setting for these judgments.) What is now known about CVS surely meets this criterion. Accurate diagnoses are being made, and healthy babies are born after the procedure. Second, researchers must be able to state with confidence that no scientifically valid reason exists to predict that CVS will be superior to AM. If physicians already knew that CVS was better, they would be ethically obliged to give it to patients and change policy about prenatal diagnosis (Shaw and Chalmers, 1970). What is unknown about CVS's risks and diagnostic accuracy meets the second criterion of uncertainty.

The second counterargument is based on an ethical principle, but scientific implications follow from it. If societies widely respect the principle of justice (or fairness) and also desire the benefits of medical research, an obligation arises to distribute the burdens (as well as the benefits) of research as fairly as possible (Commission for the Protection of Human Subjects of Biomedical and Behavioral Research, 1979). To offer potentially beneficial research only to those "in favor" with physicians is unfair. Likewise, to restrict the most risky research to social outcasts, a practice in the past, is also unjust. However, no obligation to distribute benefits arises until strong evidence is available that the treatment or device in question is a benefit. In medicine, the RCT is a fair way to test the question, if deeper considerations permit. Also, if the question is to be tested, a further duty exists to protect the most vulnerable subjects and not to overburden the already burdened with an unfair share of the risks. A later section will take up the issue of fairness in selection of subjects whose pregnancies are at higher risk. The previous section has hopefully persuaded the reader that the benefits of CVS have yet to be proved.

Before making a decision to begin research for the sake of potential benefits, the investigator's selection of subjects must pass reasonable tests based on principles of beneficence, nonmaleficence, and fairness. How beneficial, risky, and fair is the trial itself for the subjects who will participate? If these prior questions are satisfactorily answered, it follows that randomization may be the best and fairest strategy by which to study the question. This ethical aspect coincides well with scientific interests. As a research strategy, randomization has three advantages (Byar et al., 1976; Chalmers, 1983): (a) It eliminates bias from the assignment of patients to arms of the trial. (b) It yields comparison groups comparable in both known and unknown variables. (c) It guarantees the validity of the statistical tests of significance used to compare approaches. If genuine doubt exists about the better approach, chance assignment is also the fairest way to distribute risks and benefits to persons in the trial, if they are willing to consider their interests as equal to those of others in the trial. Each subject is in the same ethical position of advantage and disadvantage before entry. Also, unknown and unpredictable risks are more likely to come to light in a RCT than with other research strategies. Society and research subjects are thereby provided with more accountability. A good example is a finding about the risk of noncompliance in a placebo-controlled study of a cholesterol-lowering drug (Coronary Drug Project Research Group, 1980). This unforeseen risk was not appreciated until well after the trial. Ideally, consent to RCT means that subjects, too, adopt the same uncertainty about the "better" approach. Perhaps difficult to achieve psychologically, this attitude does succeed in establishing fairness in the trial. All are as equal as possible.

Does Abortion Make a Trial of Chorionic Villus Sampling Unethical?

Moral arguments against abortion that make fetal interests equal in all or most cases to interests of parents and others would also oppose a trial of CVS. The reasoning is that if one ought not to be doing abortions, then one ought not to do a trial that will both cause and lead to more abortions. Physicians (Lejeune, 1970) and ethicists (Ramsey, 1973) who have objected to prenatal diagnosis do not attack the technology. They argue that those who use it cannot escape the moral harm done by abortion. Two dominant themes appear in their arguments: (a) A basic purpose of medicine—to save life—is violated by the practice of abortion linked to prenatal diagnosis. (b) While some abortions may be justified, the practice itself tends to set aside certain fetuses as deserving of abortion and thus treat fetuses unequally and unjustly.

The strengths and weaknesses of this argument have been evaluated elsewhere (Callahan, 1970; Fletcher, 1978, 1982). Briefly, the strengths are (i) the protection afforded to every disabled life by the equality principle, (ii) the compassion toward the individual fetus regardless of handicap, and (iii) the consistency in moral judgments in cases ranging from minor to severe handicaps. Weaknesses lie in (a) increase of suffering to parents and families, (b) allowing great harm in some cases to the future child, (c) encouragement of passivity and resignation toward inherited disorders, and (d) potentially obstructing fetal therapy. One general and two specific responses can be made to an argument that categorically applies equality of every fetal life with every other life.

First, this view unnecessarily restricts the diversity of ethical principles required to resolve many types of moral conflicts in abortion cases and in research with human fetuses. Ethical views that rely only on one principle usually fail to meet the complexities and varieties of moral problems in diverse human communities (Walzer, 1983). Not all moral conflicts involving fetal interests are reducible to one type. For example, a set of special ethical considerations in fetal research has evolved (Commission for the Protection of Human Subjects of Biomedical and Behavioral Research, 1975; Code of Federal Regulations, 1983) that uses some features of the equality argument for one special problem—research with the fetus prior to abortion—but also uses tests of other principles, e.g., the maximization of benefit (beneficence) and the minimization of harm (nonmaleficence). These new ethical considerations of fetal research, however, are only a small set of an older and richer tradition of ethical guidance about choices in abortion. Guidance has gradually evolved for the many different problems and settings in which choices must be made. Abortion decisions have contexts as variable as incest, rape, unplanned pregnancy in the single or married state, and pregnancies following artificial insemination. The consent of the woman to the pregnancy is also a key element in ethical reasoning. Ethical reflection on wanted pregnancies at higher risk for genetic disorders is only one current in the wider stream of this evolving body of guidance.

The view that the interests of the newly fertilized embryo are equal to those of every other human life did not appear until the nineteenth century (Council on Science and Society, 1984). This argument differs markedly from an older moral tradition based on views of "animation" or "ensoulment" of the fetus. The older tradition has more in common with a developmental view of the moral status of the fetus than with the categorical view of embryonic and fetal equality. A developmental view refers to, but is not determined by, biological milestones in embryonic and fetal development (Sumner, 1981; Callahan, 1970; Grobstein, 1981). Embryonic and fetal development is a crucial partner for moral reasoning about abortion and research choices. However, the basic ethical principles that structure and shape such reasoning should be selected to keep continuity with an older tradition that encourages respect for the life and potential personhood of the fetus at every point in development of an increasingly recognizable human individual. In this view, the fertilizing egg already has some moral status demanding respect. The more the embryo and developing fetus grows and possesses some recognizable human features and crucial biological capacities, the more the moral status of the fetus approximates that of living persons. In many of the traditions of ancient and contemporary ethics, however, the fetus does not have the same moral status as a newborn or a fully developed human being (Birch and Cobb, 1981). Older and more pervasive moral traditions permit reasoning that balances fetal interests with those of mother, parents, and extended family. However, these traditions do not permit indifference toward embryonic or fetal life at any stage of development.

Second, in a trial of CVS, choices about abortion will be parental in origin and not a requirement of the research protocol. Abortion following a positive finding is not the only option. Statistically, most parents do choose abortion in this situation and are probably predisposed to do so. Genetic counselors and obstetricians should not, in my view, require a prior commitment to abortion as a condition of prenatal diagnosis. The choice should always be discussed, and the parents should be allowed to change their minds. In a trial, the approach to abortion choices will be the same as in current practice. Parents' decisions will not be experimentally manipulated to gain any other knowledge. Thus, the experiment will not exert any independent pressure for abortion.

The third point is that one of the long-range consequences of a trial may help to reduce overreliance on abortion after prenatal diagnosis. Perhaps fetal therapy will eventually be a result of safer, accurate, and earlier fetal diagnosis. Fetal therapy is now impossible for the choromosomal disorders found after CVS. However, long-range consideration of fetal interests should not dismiss the role of this trial as one of many steps toward such therapy. Fetal therapy is slowly growing as an integral speciality in medicine (Harrison et al., 1984). Anyone who wants to reduce the incidence of abortion for genetic disorders in the future would surely favor fetal therapy. However, the risks of learning must precede the benefits of treatment.

ISSUES OF BENEFIT AND RISK

From the standpoint of the interests of the women and fetuses in the trial, some tests can be applied from Federal (United States) regulations on research with pregnant women and fetuses. The key passages are the following (Code of Federal Regulations, 1983):

> §46.206 (a) No activity to which this subpart is applicable may be undertaken unless:
>
> (b) Except where the purpose of the activity is to meet the health needs of the mother or the particular fetus, the risk to the fetus is minimal and, in all cases, is the least possible risk for achieving the objectives of the activity.
>
> §46.207 (a) No fetus *in utero* may be involved as a subject in any activity covered by this subpart unless: (1) The purpose of the activity is to meet the health needs of the particular fetus and the fetus will be placed at risk only to the minimum extent necessary to meet such needs, or (2) the risk to the fetus imposed by the research is minimal and the purpose of the activity is the development of important biological knowledge which cannot be obtained by any other means.

The origins of these regulations lie in public and congressional concerns about fetal research strongly expressed in the early and mid-1970s. The Commission for the Protection of Human Subjects of Biomedical and Behavioral Research (1975) reported to Congress on the issue and also formulated a basic approach to federal regulations that embodied three concerns: (a) to protect fetuses in research, especially fetuses to be electively aborted; (b) to permit experiments that directly benefit fetuses, e.g., an experiment in fetal therapy; and (c) to permit experiments that do not directly benefit the fetus but increase biomedical knowledge that may result in benefits to fetuses and children in the future.

The first concern is not relevant to a proposed RCT of CVS. As noted above, when a trial begins, all fetuses are presumed wanted. Furthermore, no manipulation of abortion choices or procedures will be made in the context of a study. The second and third concerns are relevant tests.

A trial of CVS and AM "meets the health needs" of the mother much more directly than those of the fetus. The mother's risks of having an affected child are relevant to her health and participation in the family and society. Spontaneous abortion risks are also an important feature of obstetrical care. The mother's health needs will be directly met by diagnosis and expert care in case of spontaneous abortion. Table 4 shows the estimated risk of a chromosomal abnormality in women over 35 years of age, based on the European Collaborative Study (Ferguson-Smith, 1983). Beginning at age 35, the benefit of diagnosis for risk of a chromosomal abnormality (1.2%) is higher than the best collective estimate of the risk of fetal loss due to AM (0.5%). This benefit-to-risk relationship increases steadily with age. Prenatal diagnosis provides information vital to a mothers's well-being and choices about her pregnancy. Furthermore, answers to questions of safety in prenatal diagnosis will lead to fewer complications after the procedure and less loss of maternal life after abortion.

Table 4 Maternal Age-Specific Rates for Chromosome Abnormalities

Maternal age	Trisomy 21	All aberrations (%)
35	0.39	1.22
36	0.50	1.32
37	0.64	1.50
38	0.81	1.73
39	1.04	2.06

Source: Ferguson-Smith (1983).

By comparison, after finding of abnormality in the fetus, the health needs of the fetus are brought to light, but these needs are not "met" in any usual sense of the term, especially when compared to the health needs of the mother. Some fetuses will survive, and babies subsequently will be delivered who might have been otherwise aborted by anxious parents without benefit of prenatal diagnosis. If the findings are negative, the "health" of the fetus is clarified, but the only way it is "improved" is by avoidance of abortion. This consequence of diagnosis is probably not what the Commission for the Protection of Human Subjects of Biomedical and Behavioral Research, (1975, p. 6) intended by "meeting health needs," e.g.,

> Therapeutic research refers to research designed to improve the health condition of the research subject by prophylactic, diagnostic or treatment methods that depart from standard medical practice but hold out a reasonable expectation of success.

From the standpoint of fetal interests, the clearest way to view the trial is as a nontherapeutic or investigative experiment to gain biomedical knowledge with a very high probability of benefit to fetuses and children in the near and distant future. Future unwanted losses of fetal life will be prevented more effectively when the safest method of prenatal diagnosis is established. Amniocentesis, the current method of choice, has never been studied in a randomized trial. Much will be learned about spontaneous abortion, maternal age factors, and the optimal time to do prenatal diagnosis. These findings will lead to more accurate standards of safety. Finally, the potential benefit to fetal therapy has been noted.

Minimal Risk

In the context of maternal and fetal interests, the key question is whether the trial passes a test of minimal risk, defined in the regulations as follows (Code of Federal Regulations 1983):

> §46.102 (g) "Minimal risk" means that the risks of harm anticipated in the proposed research are not greater, considering probability and magnitude, than those ordinarily encountered in daily life or during the performance of routine physical or psychological examinations or tests.

In the following discussion of the ethical significance of "minimal risk" in a proposed trial, these assumptions are made:

1. Pregnant women (2500) between 35 and 39 years of age will be randomized to CVS (done no later than 10.5 weeks) and an AM (done no earlier than 16 weeks).
2. "Risks of daily life" include the following:
   (a) An average risk of chromosomal abnormalities in this age group of 1.56% (between 1 and 2 in each 100)
   (b) A natural risk of spontaneous abortion entering week 10 of 13.6%
   (c) A natural risk of spontaneous abortion entering week 16 of 2%
3. Amniocentesis is a "routine" test for pregnant women over 35 years of age.
4. The risks of added fetal loss due to the procedures are the following:
   (a) For AM, no greater than 0.5%
   (b) For CVS, no less than 2% and no greater than 5%.

Discussion

The NICHD (1984) request for proposals for a RCT of CVS uses the figure of 2500 patients. The 35 to 39-year-old age group will be the only participants in the model for a trial now being considered in several countries.

The risk of chromosomal abnormality was derived by taking the average (in Table 4) of the risks for 35 to 39-year olds in the column "all aberrations." The risks of spontaneous abortion by week of pregnancy are shown in Table 5. Figure 1, based on epidemiological research in three New York City hospitals (Stein et al., 1980), shows the high incidence of spontaneous abortion associated with maternal age. The selection of 13.6% as the specific risk of natural fetal loss entering week 10 is based on data reported by Gustavii (1984) (Table 6), who used Swedish records of all women treated for spontaneous abortion in 1980 and 1981. The risk of spontaneous abortion entering week 16 was placed at 2% based on an extension of the Swedish data and comparison to the AM control patients' experience reported in Table 3. In proper perspective, these risks of background spontaneous abortion begin and extend over a period in pregnancy to 28 weeks, i.e., 10–28 weeks and 16–28 weeks, respectively.

Although the Commission did not discuss the issue of whether AM is a routine "physical" test, a good case can be made that, considering the "ordinary" risks of pregnancy in this age group, AM is a routine test for

Table 5 Life Table of Spontaneous Abortions by Week of Pregnancy

Week	Probability of spontaneous abortion < 28 weeks[a]
6	10,105
8	8,122
10	6,733
12	4,856
14	3,202
16	2,385
18	1,841
20	1,380
22	981
24	604
26	329

[a]Per 100,000 pregnancies.
Source: Harlap et al. (1980).

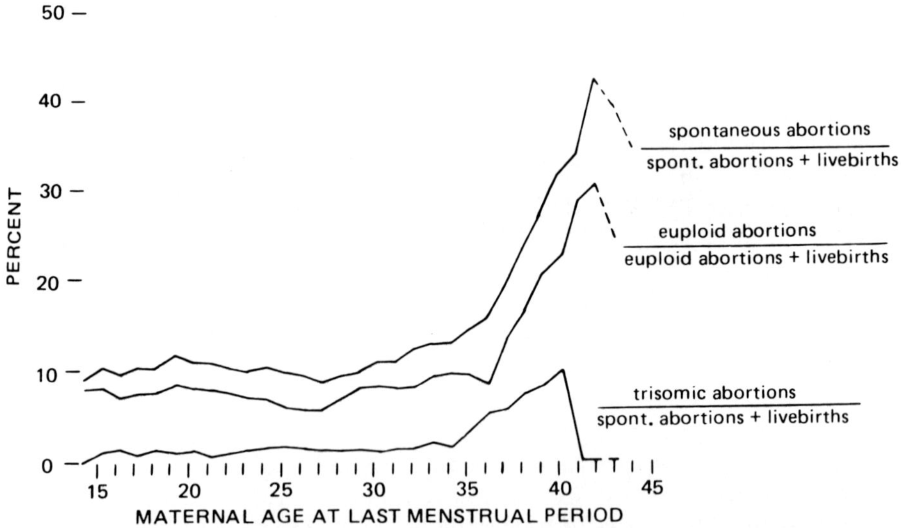

Figure 1 Estimated rates (%) of spontaneous abortion, euploid abortion, and trisomic abortion by maternal age for private and public patients combined. Curves were smoothed by estimating rates at each maternal age using the number of events observed at each age and the two adjacent ages. ———, Denominator less than 25. From Stein et al. (1980).

Table 6 Fetal Losses at Given Gestational Periods, Related to Age of Mother

Maternal age (years)	No. of pregnancies (week 7)	Fetal loss rate (%) in gestational period (nth week & later):[a]			
		8th	10th	12th	14th
Under 30	3787	7.4	6.1	4.1	2.1
30–34	1829	8.6	6.7	4.3	2.2
35–39	616	16.0	13.6	8.7	4.1
40 and over	105	33.3	22.2	10.3	2.8
All ages	6337	9.1	7.2	4.7	2.3

[a]These loss rates are cumulative: for example, of 3787 fetuses at the 7th week in women under 30 a total of 294 (7.8%) were lost, 14 between weeks 7 and 8 leaving 3773 fetuses at the 8th week of which a total of 280 (7.1%) were lost, and so on.
Source: Gustavii (1984).

pregnant women over 35 who want it. Little argument is needed to show that pregnancy is a risk-laden area of daily life. Perhaps as much as 50% of implanted embryos fail to develop and are discharged from the mother's body after dying. Between 1 and 2 women in every 100 over 35 will give birth to a baby with a chromosome abnormality. The risks of spontaneous abortion are imminently treatable, and death is rare in developed nations, but the risks are real. Two other precedents support a view that AM is a routine test. The NICHD (1978) supported a trial in the United States of AM's safety and accuracy. On the basis of this trial, physicians in the United States adopted a policy to recommend AM for mid-trimester diagnosis. Furthermore, the Ethics Advisory Board of the (then) Department of Health, Education, and Welfare approved waivers of the regulations (Levine, 1979) for a nontherapeutic study of fetoscopy as a technique to diagnose the hemoglobinopathies. The risk of miscarriage in fetoscopy was recently reported as 7.5% (Golbus, 1984). This risk is several times higher than the best estimate of the risk of AM for fetal loss.

What burden of fetal loss can be estimated from the research itself? Table 7, which builds on the assumptions above, describes expected fetal loss in an RCT of 2500 women ages 35–39 years of age. Amniocentesis adds 6 losses to a background of 25 (+ 24%). On the lowest estimate of 2%, CVS adds 19 losses to a background of spontaneous abortion of 170 (+ 11%).

Table 7 Projected Added Abortion Risks (Spontaneous Rate vs. Chorionic Villus Sampling[a]

	Weeks	%	Cases (No.)	AM (No.)	Total
Spontaneous abortion	10-28	13.6	170	6	176
	16-28	2.0	25	6	31
Chorionic villus sampling		2 (1.5)[b]	19	6	25
		3 (2.5)	31	6	36
		4 (3.5)	44	6	50
		5 (4.5)	56	6	62

[a]Projected RCT of 2500 subjects, in two groups if 1250 each; 2500 total. The women are 35–39 years old.
[b]Figures in brackets are after subtracting abortion risk for AM, thus reflecting the added burden of CVS in a randomized trial.

The worst outcome, in this way of anticipating fetal loss, assumes that the risk of added loss could be as high as 5%. Then the research adds 6 losses after AM (+25%) and 56 after CVS (+33%) against the respective backgrounds of spontaneous abortion.

In research with CVS when the risks are predictably low (2–3%), the risk of fetal loss can be acceptably termed as minimal, because considering the "probability and magnitude" of the natural risk of spontaneous abortion, fetal loss will be less than that expected after AM as a routine procedure. On the other hand, if a higher risk level (4–5%) were probable, the expected fetal loss would not be within the scope of minimal risk. Even considering the background spontaneous abortion risks, the added fetal losses would be higher than in routine practice of prenatal diagnosis. On these terms, it may be ethically acceptable for physicians to offer it to some very high-risk patients, but unacceptable to do research in an RCT of CVS.

However, considering the probabilities of fetal loss, two reasons support the view that the lower risks (2–3%) will most likely result. First, only centers with proven experience and a required number of cases of CVS will do the trial. One can expect results similar to the six most experienced centers cited in Table 2. Second, if one controls for all cases and has a reliable method to predict fetal loss [ultrasound examinations (Jackson, 1984b)], the comparability of the two groups for fetal loss will be more assured.

To recapitulate, the argument that the added risk of fetal loss due to research in a RCT of CVS is minimal requires these steps: (a) considering the daily risks of pregnancy in this age group, (b) assuming that AM is a routine test with a minimal risk of fetal loss, and (c) weighing the most probable fetal loss due to CVS compared to AM against the magnitude of the natural risk of fetal loss in each stage of pregnancy, then (d) the probable risks of fetal loss from CVS are also minimal.

The regulation also stipulates that the research must in all cases be the least possible risk to achieve the objectives of the activity. The strategy of randomization meets this requirement since all fetuses, like their mothers, will enter from the same position of advantage and disadvantage. In a multicenter trial, some differences will appear between centers themselves. If one grants some unavoidable differences between centers, then the rule can be satisfied on the assumption that in all cases in each center, the least possible risk will be distributed as fairly as possible. Otherwise, all fetal research would have to be done in only one center, a conclusion surely not intended by the Commission.

If one would study AM at 16 weeks in unrandomized diagnostic cases, is it not ethically acceptable to do a RCT with CVS as one alternative if the risks of fetal loss are no greater, considering probability and magnitude, than the risks of AM as a routine diagnostic procedure? The only objection to this reasoning could arise from a view of strict equality of each fetus at 10 weeks of gestation with each fetus at 16 weeks. If one counts each loss independently of background losses, the added abortions would not pass a test of minimal risk. However, the regulation's language about probability and magnitude invites reasoning that balances interests in a trial. Also, in the consideration of fetal interests, as noted above, the most pervasive moral traditions allow for morally relevant differences between the earliest stages of pregnancy and later stages. The following passage from Grobstein's account of fetal development considers the question of the moral status of the fetus from the standpoint of the criterion of "recognition" of human likeness (Grobstein, 1981, p. 102):

> Examination of human embryos shows that structural characteristics recognizably human to a lay person are present at least by twelve to thirteen weeks of development. This is at the end of the first trimester, the time at which it has been traditional to change the term embryo to fetus as the designation for the developing human. Although the fetus at this stage has a lot of developing to do and is by no means a miniature

> person needing simply to be scaled up by growth, a number of critical features for recognition are present. The head is disproportionately large and the legs are tiny, but the general body configuration is recognizably human. In contrast to earlier stages, a definite face is present, a critical characteristic for human recognition. Also, hands and feet, including fingers and toes, are well defined and unquestionably human. It is important to note that responsive movements at this stage are quite stong and that spontaneous movement is beginning. Although the fetus is very small, almost any observer is likely to regard it as human and at least a person-to-be.

Any research with CVS will be done well before the stage described by Grobstein. The "recognition factor" should be seen as the least objective element in a series of considerations of fetal moral status. More objective standards, such as responsiveness, capacity to experience pain, brain development, and viability, have been introduced in the search for norms that provide milestones in fetal development. By these more objective standards, research with CVS on the first-trimester fetus, developmentally viewed as a late human embryo, falls well within the intent of a rule of minimal risk. The point of quoting Grobstein at some length is that, by the standard likely to be most widely respected by nonscientists and parents, the research involves only minimal moral risks.

Assuming that a case has been made that the risks of a trial to the fetus are minimal, the considerations may move to fairness in selection of subjects and informed consent.

SELECTION OF SUBJECTS FOR RESEARCH

In several places, the discussion assumes that the only source of research subjects for a RCT of CVS will be pregnant women age 35 or older. What are the arguments aginst extending the scope further? Should not other pregnancies at risk for genetic disorders be included? Is it unfair to the older mothers, as a group, to bear the burdens of the research alone? Conversely, if dramatic benefits come to one randomized group rather than another, would it be unfair to exclude others at risk to trasmit genetic diseases from these benefits?

The main point of ethical significance is that so many more candidates with low risks of disorders are in the 35 to 39-year-old group than in groups with higher risks for recessive and X-linked disorders. Pregnancies in advanced maternal age are the vast majority of cases of prenatal diagnosis in most countries. Maternal age cases may vary depending on resources, personnel, research interests, and policy about indications for prenatal diagnosis. Switzerland's medical geneticists reported that in 1981–1983, of a total of 12,038 cases, 7816 (64.9%) were for indications of maternal age of + 35 years (Swiss Society for Medical Genetics, 1984). However, diagnosis was given for 3175 cases (26.4%) of women under 35 years of age who expressed anxiety about a chromosomal abnormality and requested service. Other indications, such as, previous neural tube defects, recessive disorders, and X-linked diseases, were only 1% of total cases. Norway, a country whose Parliament has limited the number of AM procedures to about 500 annually, performed 555 total cases, 370 (66%) of which were for maternal age, but the age limit is 38 years (K. Berg, personal communication, 1984). The incidence of prenatal diagnosis for maternal age must be at least between 65 and 75% of total cases in countries that provide genetic services.

The more quickly and effectively a trial can be done, the sooner the knowledge about benefits and risks can be applied to high-risk groups. The sheer size of the advanced maternal age group prevents any ethical problem of overburdening them. Their genetic risks are low, and, in the design of the trial that will be most widely followed, they have a choice not to be randomized and select either AM or CVS for themselves.

Inclusion of higher-risk pregnancies with low frequency of genetic disorders and a different history of spontaneous abortion would lead to some serious adverse consequences:

The trial would take much longer to accumulate significant numbers of cases to compare.

Women at high risk would be much less willing to be randomized.

The women who previously had had AM, as many in higher risk groups have, would strongly favor CVS.

The spontaneous abortion history of younger women is different and the "reproductive histories" (Vogel, 1984) of heterozygote mothers are controverted.

Some recessive disorders are found more frequently in cultural groups with strong objections to mid-trimester abortion.

These consequences would clearly threaten the scientific merit and the ethical acceptability of a trial.

Other groups of at-risk pregnancies for chromosomal disorders might be considered in the interest of fairness, unless sound scientific reasons prevented this goal. Examples are pregnancies of (a) carriers of balanced translocations, (b) first degree family history of chromosomal abnormality, (c) previous birth of trisomy 21, and (d) previous spontaneous abortion of trisomy 21.

CONSIDERATIONS OF INFORMED CONSENT

After proposed research has met tests of benefit, risk, and fairness, the issues of informing patients and seeking consent must be examined. Research in pregnancy is difficult from the perspective of consent because the most partial person toward the fetus is asked to consider a choice impartially. Parents anxious about a pregnancy may be willing to "try anything" that holds out hope of knowledge. They will hear information in a strongly biased way. In the light of these emotional factors, the chance that information will not be well understood is high. Despite these problems, investigators who conduct meetings to inform parents and prepare consent documents should set adequate goals for the quality of their spoken and written communications to seek consent. The integrity of the written or signed consent document presupposes the deeper ethical integrity of the understanding between investigator and research subject. To achieve this understanding is hard work well worth the time invested, because misunderstandings, such as information about risks, are avoided that can trouble subjects deeply.

Quality of verbal and written communications in consent negotiations can be evaluated in terms of (1) helpfulness in making choices, (2) clarity of explanation of risks and benefits, (3) clarity in explaining differences between research and practice, and (4) aids to retention of the most important information.

Figure 2 shows the design of a RCT of CVS that is likely to be widely followed. Since much depends on identification and referral from general practitioners and obstetricians, these doctors should have an explanation of the trial well in advance. Additionally, they should have the opportunity in a meeting with the investigators to ask questions and express any ethical reservations, such as those described in the first part of this chapter. The consent process really begins from the referral souce to the researcher, and misimpressions can easily begin there as well. Clear written explanations in the trial in the hands of the referring physician can also lead to more clarity in his or her preparation of the patient.

The third step in the trial's design is counseling about CVS and AM. Ideally, the spouse should be present. Flexibility and extra effort for this step will benefit the couple and lead to more achievement of qualitative

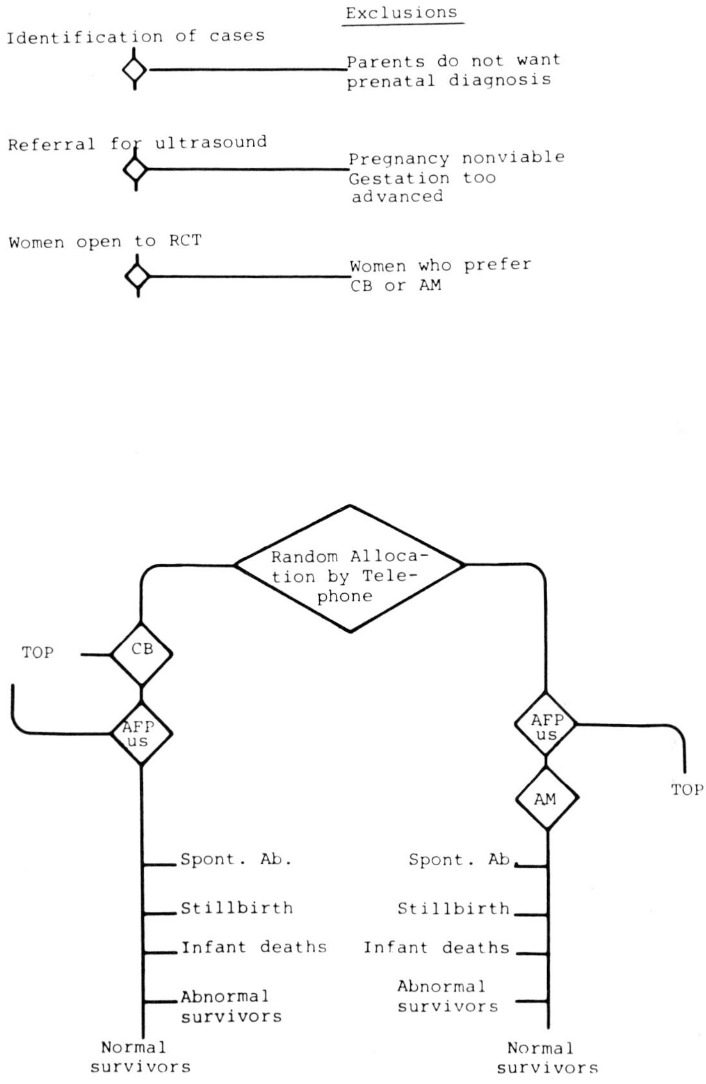

Figure 2 Proposed flow diagram for randomized clinical trial (RCT) of chorion biopsy (CB) and amniocentesis (AM) for prenatal diagnosis. From Chalmers (1984).

outcomes in the consent process (Fletcher and Boverman, 1980; Boverman, 1983). The content of the verbal and written explanations should include the following elements in language clear to the couple:

1. An explanation of the purpose of the study, namely, to compare two approaches to prenatal diagnosis. The background risks of chromosomal abnormalities should be given, with risks for the pregnancy and risks for the general population. What will be expected of the patient in examinations and follow-up studies and in each procedure, including the timing, should be described. Visual aids will help with the less familiar CVS procedure. Chorionic villus sampling should be described as a "research procedure," or an approach in a "research" stage of development too early to tell about its benefits and risks in comparison to AM.
2. A description of the risks should include the following:
   a. Background risk of spontaneous abortion
   b. Estimated added risk of fetal loss due to procedures
   c. Risk of complications from procedures
   d. Differential risk of maternal complications and death after abortion
   e. Emotional risks of post-AM abortion
   f. Risks of inclusive and inaccurate diagnosis for AM and CVS
3. A description of the benefits to be reasonably expected are the following:
   a. Reassurance, if no chromosome abnormality, and statistical likelihood of this finding
   b. Knowledge of the abnormality, if any, and statistical likelihood of this finding
   c. Support and proper referral for option chosen by parents if abnormality found: termination of pregnancy, preparation for birth of affected child, etc.
   d. In the event of the abortion option, explain where it will be done, by whom, and that expert help will be offered during hospitalization
   e. Explain benefit of earlier timing of CVS balanced by unknowns of fetal loss and accuracy of diagnosis
   f. Knowledge of sex of fetus, if desired.
4. An explanation should be given of randomization, the concept defined simply, and that the doctors will not make the choice. The purpose of using randomization should be explained. The subject

should know that she has a clear choice to say "no" to the study and still receive the method of her choice, by referral from her physician. If she declines the trial, no penalty or loss of benefits to which she is otherwise entitled will be involved. Furthermore, she may change her mind after deciding to participate. (In studies that actually follow self-selected groups, this option should be accompanied by an explanation of examinations and other follow-up involved.)

5. A statement about confidentiality and privacy, including no personal identifiers in reports, protection of choices about abortion, and protection of preference not to know sex of fetus.
6. A statement that prenatal diagnosis may involve remote risks to future child (risks of CVS are unknown and part of study), but harms of AM are not evident on follow-up studies that have been done.
7. The number of research subjects in the study.

A final consideration is that sufficient time should be given for questions and discussion, as well as an interval provided for the couple to decide without appearance of pressure. An offer of referral for consultation may be made for any ethical or special religious concerns they may show.

CONCLUSIONS

This chapter presented an ethical argument for a randomized trial of chorion villus sampling and amniocentesis. Some objections to a trial, based on physician loyalty to patients and moral criticism of abortion, were discussed and counter arguments made. The major ethical challenge to a trial is from the standpoint of fetal interests because of the lack of clear health benefits to each particular fetus in the trial. The argument used above favors a RCT of CVS because of the benefits it would bring to fetuses in the very near and distant future. By analysis of the components of minimal risk, as defined in U.S. federal regulations for fetal research, a case was made that the most probable risks of added fetal loss by CVS in a trial will be less than the current risks of AM, when one considers the background risks of spontaneous abortion in each period of pregnancy and the experience of the investigators to be involved in a trial. The chapter then discussed considerations of fairness in selection of subjects and elements in the process of informed consent.

The approach taken in this chapter is based on a two-step approach to analysis of ethical questions in technology (Fletcher, 1983). The first step is to assemble the best evidence on the question at hand and the consequences of alternatives. Since empirical data or the best estimates or science cannot dictate ethical directives, the second step must call on ethical principles and traditions of guidance that have the widest support in the society, lest the approach that is recommended fail for lack of historical continuity and precedents. The argument drew on three ethical principles (beneficence, nonmaleficence, and fairness) and a moral tradition of balanced consideration of fetal interests that has ancient roots, historical precedents, and a pervasive contemporary respect in the society. These ethical principles are widely respected and used for the resolution of contemporary problems in fetal and other research. The argument concludes that when the available evidence is evaluated by the criteria that flow from these ethical principles, such a trial is ethically acceptable.

ACKNOWLEDGMENTS

The research for this chapter was supported by a grant from the Norwegian Marshall Fund and by support from the Clinical Center, National Institutes of Health, for a 6-month work study project in 1984. The author greatly appreciates help of those investigators of CVS who made field visits possible in 1984 to observe and discuss the procedure: B. Modell and H. Ward (London), B. Brambati (Milan), B. Gustavii (Lund), and J. Philip and J. Bang (Copenhagen). Helpful comments and technical assistance were given by K. Berg and A. Heiberg (Oslo), L. Jackson (Philadelphia), and S. Fabro (Washington, D.C.). Betty O. Perry prepared and typed the manuscript.

REFERENCES

1. Birch, C. and Cobb J. (1984). *The Liberation of Life*, p. 167. Cambridge University Press, Cambridge.
2. Blumberg, B. D., et al., (1975). The psychological sequelae of abortion performed for a genetic indication. *Am. J. Obstet. Gynec. 122*:799–808.
3. Boverman, M. (1983). Mental health aspects of the informed consent process. In *Research Ethics* (K. Berg and K. E. Tranøy) p. 229 New York, Alan R. Liss.
4. Brambati, B., Simoni, G., Danesino, C., et al. (1985). First trimester fetal diagnosis of genetical disorders. Clinical evaluation of 250 cases. *J. Med. Gen. 22*:92–99.
5. Byar. D. P. et al. (1976). Randomized clinical trials. *N. Engl. J. Med. 295*:74–80.

6. Callahan, D. (1970). *Abortion: Law, Choice, and Morality*, p 377. Macmillan, New York.
7. Cates, W. et al. (1977). The effect of delay and method choice on the risk of abortion morbidity. *Famil. Plann. Perspect. 9*:266.
8. Chalmers. I. (1983). Scientific inquiry and authoritarianism in perinatal care and education. *Birth 10*:151.
9. Chalmers, I. (1984). Randomized trial to compare first trimester chorion villus sampling with second trimester amniocentesis for prenatal diagnosis. (Unpublished).
10. Code of Federal Regulations (1983). Protection of human subjects. Activities directed towards fetuses in utero as subjects. 45 CFR 46.208.
11. Commission for the Protection of Human Subjects of Biomedical and Behavioral Research (1975). *Research on the Fetus*, Report and Recommendations. DHEW Publication No. (OS) 76–127, Washington, D.C.
12. Commission for Protection of Human Subjects of Biomedical and Behavioral Research (1979). *The Belmont Report* p. 7. FR Document 79–12065. U.S. Government Printing Office, Washington, D.C.
13. Coronary Drug Project Research Group (1980). Influence of adherence to treatment and response of cholesterol on mortality in the coronary drug project. *N. Engl. J. Med 303*:1308.
14. Council on Science and Society (1984). Report of a Working Party. *Human Procreation* p 3. Oxford University Press, Oxford.
15. Donnai, P. et al., (1981). Attitudes of patients after "genetic" termination of pregnancy. *Brit. Med. J. 282*:621–3.
16. *Ferguson-Smith, M. A. (1983). Prenatal chromosome analysis and its impact. Brit. Med. Bull. 39*:356.
17. Fletcher, J. C., and Boverman, M. (1980). Involving the patient's family in informed consent. Presentation: American Psychological Association, Montreal.
18. Fletcher, J. C. (1978). Prenatal diagnosis. Ethnical issues. In *Encyclopedia of Bioethics* (W. T. Reich, ed.), p. 1336–1346. Free Press, New York.
19. Fletcher, J. C. (1982). *Coping with Genetic Disorders* p 127. Harper and Row, San Francisco.
20. Fletcher, J. C. (1983). *Is sex selection ethical?* In *Research Ethics,* K. Berg, K. E. Tranoy (eds) p. 334. Alan R. Liss, New York.
21. Fried, C. (1974). *Medical Experimentation.* American Elsevier, New York.
22. Golbus, M. S. (1984). Fetoscopy and fetal sampling. In '*Unborn Patient, Diagnoses and treatment* (M. R. Harrison, M. S. Golbus, and R. A. Filly, eds.), p. 137. Grune & Stratton, Orlando, Florida.
23. Grobstein, C. (1981). *From Chance to Purpose*, p 102. Addison-Wesley Publishing Company, Reading, Massachusetts.
24. Grimes, D. A., and Cates, W. (1979). Complications from legally induced abortion. *Obstet. Gynecol. Surv. 34*:177.
25. Gustavii, B. (1974). Chorionic biopsy and miscarriage in first trimester. *Lancet 1*:562.
26. Harlap, S. Shiono P. H., Ramcharan, s. (1980). A life table of spontaneous abortions and the effects of age, parity, and other variables. In *Human*

abortions and the effects of age, parity, and other variables. In *Human Embryonic and Fetal Death,* (I. H. Porter and E. B. Hook, eds.), p. 148. Academic Press, New York.

27. Harrison, M. R., Golbus, M. S. and Filly, R. A. (1984). *Unborn Patient. Prenatal Diagnosis and Treatment.* Grune and Stratton, Orlando, Florida.
28. Jackson, L. (1984a). Fetal loss. *CVS Newsletter,* June 25, 1984.
29. Jackson, L. (1984b). Data collection for monitoring obstetric risk of early fetal diagnosis. Geneva: World Health Organization, p 2.
30. Jackson, L., Wapner, R., Grebner, E., and Barr, M. (1984). Fetal diagnosis by chorionic villus sampling. In *Human Prenatal Diagnosis* (K. Filkins and J. F. Russo, eds.), pp. 285–310. Dekker, New York.
31. Kazy, Z., Rozovsky, I. S., and Bakharev, V. (1982). Chorion biopsy in early pregnancy. A method of early prenatal diagnosis for inherited disorders. *Prenat. Diag. 2*:39–45.
32. Kennell, J. H. (1970). The mourning response of parents to the death of a newborn infant. *N. Engl. J. Med. 283*:344–349.
33. Lejeune, J. (1970). On the nature of man. *Am. J. Human Genet. 22*:121–128.
34. Leschot, N. J. et al. (1982). Therapeutic abortion on genetic indications. A detailed followup study of 20 patients. In *On Prenatal Diagnosis* (M. Verjaal and J. H. Leschot, eds.). p. 85 Rodopi, University of Amsterdam.
35. Levine, C. (1979). Ethics advisory board approves waivers for fetoscopy research. IRB 1:8.
36. Levine, R. J. (1981). *Ethics and Regulation of Clinical Research*, p 126. Urban & Schwarzenberg, Baltimore.
37. NICHD (1978). Amniocentesis Register. *The Safety and Accuracy of Midtrimester Amniocentesis.* U.S. Department of Health, Education, and Welfare, Washington, D.C.
38. NICHD (1984). *Cooperative Clinical Comparison of Chorion Villus Sampling and Amniocentesis.* RFA 84-10, p 3. U.S. Department of Health Education and Welfare, Washington, D.C.
39. Ramsey, P. (1973). Screening. An ethicist's view. In *Ethical Issues in Human Genetics: Genetic Counseling and the Use of Genetic Knowledge*, (B. Hilton et al., eds.) p. 147. Plenum, New York.
40. Shaw L. W. and Chalmers T. C. (1970) Ethics in cooperative trials *Ann. NY Acad. Sci. 169*:487–495.
41. Simpson, N. E. (1980). Genetic amniocentesis, In Prenatal Diagnosis, Past, Present, and Future, Report of an International Workshop. Sp. Iss. *Prenat. Diag.* p 5.
42. Stein, Z., et al. (1980). Maternal age and spontaneous abortion, in *Human Embryonic and Fetal Death* (I. H. Porter and E. B. Hook eds.), p. 122. Academic Press, New York.
43. Sumner, L. W. (1981). *Abortion and Moral Theology.* Princeton University Press, Princeton, New Jersey.
44. Swiss Society for Medical Genetics (1984). Summary of the results of prenatal diagnosis in Switzerland 1981–1983. *Mediz. Genet. (No. 12).*:11.
45. Turnbull, A. C. and MacKenzie, I. Z. (1983). Second trimester amniocentesis and termination of pregnancy. *Br. Med. Bull. 39*:315–321.
46. Veatch, R. (1983). Justice and research design: The case for a semi-randomization clinical trial. *Clin. Res. 31*:12–22.

47. Vogel, F. (1984). Clinical consequences of heterozygosity for autosomal-recessive diseases. *Clin. Genet.* *25*:392–401.
48. Waldenstrom, J. (1983). The ethics of randomization. In *Research Ethics* (K. Berg and K. E. Tranøy eds), p 245. Alan R. Liss, New York.
49. Walzer, M. (1983). *Spheres of Justice* p 5. Basic Books, New York.
50. Ward, R. H. T. (1983). First trimester chorionic villus sampling Table 1. (unpublished) University College Hospital, London.
51 Ward, R. H. T., Modell, B, Petrou, M., Karagözlu, F., and Dobratsos, E. (1983). Method of sampling chorionic villi in first trimester of pregnancy under guidance of real time ultrasound. *Br. Med. J.* *286*:1542–1543.
52. WHO, Working group on Fetal Diagnosis of Hereditary Disease. (1983). Report HMG/WG83.2 World Health Organization, Geneva.

Index

C

G

H